D1244276

The Cardiology Intensive Board Review

Third Edition

The Cardiology Intensive Board Review

Third Edition

Editors

Leslie Cho, MD, FACC
Director, Women's Cardiovascular Center
Section Head, Preventive Cardiology and Rehabilitation
Robert and Suzanne Tomsich Department of Cardiovascular Medicine
Cleveland Clinic
Cleveland, Ohio

Brian P. Griffin, MD, FACC
John and Rosemary Brown Chair in Cardiovascular Medicine
Section Head, Cardiovascular Imaging
Department of Cardiovascular Medicine
Heart and Vascular Institute
Cleveland Clinic
Cleveland, Ohio

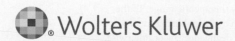

Philadelphia • Baltimore • New York • London
Buenos Aires • Hong Kong • Sydney • Tokyo

Acquisitions Editor: Julie Goolsby
Product Development Editor: Andrea Vosburgh
Production Project Manager: David Saltzberg
Design Coordinator: Joan Wendt
Manufacturing Coordinator: Beth Welsh
Marketing Manager: Stephanie Manzo
Prepress Vendor: Integra Software Services Pvt.Ltd.

Third edition

Copyright © 2015 Wolters Kluwer Health

Copyright © 2009 Lippincott Williams & Wilkins, a Wolters Kluwer business. Copyright © 2003 Lippincott Williams & Wilkins. All rights reserved. This book is protected by copyright. No part of this book may be reproduced or transmitted in any form or by any means, including as photocopies or scanned-in or other electronic copies, or utilized by any information storage and retrieval system without written permission from the copyright owner, except for brief quotations embodied in critical articles and reviews. Materials appearing in this book prepared by individuals as part of their official duties as U.S. government employees are not covered by the above-mentioned copyright. To request permission, please contact Wolters Kluwer Health at Two Commerce Square, 2001 Market Street, Philadelphia, PA 19103, via email at permissions@lww.com, or via our website at lww.com (products and services).

9 8 7 6 5 4 3 2 1

Printed in China

Library of Congress Cataloging-in-Publication Data

Cardiology intensive board review question book.
The cardiology intensive board review / editors, Leslie Cho, Brian P. Griffin.--3rd edition.
    p. ; cm.
Preceded by: Cardiology intensive board review question book / edited by Leslie Cho, Brian P. Griffin, Eric J. Topol. 2nd ed. c2009.
    Includes bibliographical references and index.
    ISBN 978-1-4511-7671-1
    I. Cho, Leslie, editor.   II. Griffin, Brian P., 1956- , editor.   III. Title.
    [DNLM: 1. Cardiovascular Diseases--Examination Questions.   2. Cardiovascular Diseases--drug therapy--Examination Questions.   3. Heart--physiology--Examination Questions.   WG 18.2]
    RC669.2
    616.1'20076--dc23

                                    2014031891

This work is provided "as is," and the publisher disclaims any and all warranties, express or implied, including any warranties as to accuracy, comprehensiveness, or currency of the content of this work.

This work is no substitute for individual patient assessment based upon healthcare professionals' examination of each patient and consideration of, among other things, age, weight, gender, current or prior medical conditions, medication history, laboratory data and other factors unique to the patient. The publisher does not provide medical advice or guidance and this work is merely a reference tool. Healthcare professionals, and not the publisher, are solely responsible for the use of this work including all medical judgments and for any resulting diagnosis and treatments.

Given continuous, rapid advances in medical science and health information, independent professional verification of medical diagnoses, indications, appropriate pharmaceutical selections and dosages, and treatment options should be made and healthcare professionals should consult a variety of sources. When prescribing medication, healthcare professionals are advised to consult the product information sheet (the manufacturer's package insert) accompanying each drug to verify, among other things, conditions of use, warnings and side effects and identify any changes in dosage schedule or contradictions, particularly if the medication to be administered is new, infrequently used or has a narrow therapeutic range. To the maximum extent permitted under applicable law, no responsibility is assumed by the publisher for any injury and/or damage to persons or property, as a matter of products liability, negligence law or otherwise, or from any reference to or use by any person of this work.

RRS1409

To our families and to the cardiovascular disease fellows past, present, and future

Contributors

Bhuvnesh Aggarwal, MD
Cardiovascular Medicine Fellow
Cleveland Clinic
Cleveland, Ohio

Craig R. Asher, MD, FACC
Cardiology Fellowship Director
Department of Cardiology
Cleveland Clinic Florida
Weston, Florida

Bryan J. Baranowski, MD
Staff Electrophysiologist Department of Cardiovascular
Medicine
Cleveland Clinic
Cleveland, Ohio

Luke J. Burchill, MBBS, PhD
Advanced Cardiac Imaging Fellow
Department of Cardiovascular Medicine
Cleveland Clinic
Cleveland, Ohio

Leslie Cho, MD, FACC
Director, Women's Cardiovascular Center
Section Head, Preventive Cardiology and Rehabilitation
Robert and Suzanne Tomsich Department of
    Cardiovascular Medicine
Cleveland Clinic
Cleveland, Ohio

Jodie M. Fink, PharmD
Pharmacotherapy Residency Program Director
Department of Pharmacy
Cleveland Clinic
Cleveland, Ohio

Gary S. Francis, MD
Professor of Medicine
Department of Cardiovascular Medicine
University of Minnesota Medical Center
Minneapolis, MN

Baris Gencer
Research Cardiologist
Interventional Cardiology Unit
Division of Cardiology
University Hospital
University of Geneva
Geneva, Switzerland

Brian P. Griffin, MD, FACC
John and Rosemary Brown Chair in Cardiovascular
    Medicine
Section Head, Cardiovascular Imaging
Department of Cardiovascular Medicine
Heart and Vascular Institute
Cleveland Clinic
Cleveland, Ohio

Wael A. Jaber, MD
Staff Cardiologist
Department of Cardiovascular Medicine
Cleveland Clinic
Cleveland, Ohio

Miriam S. Jacob, MD
Staff Physician
Section of Heart Failure and Cardiac Transplantation
Heart and Vascular Institute
Cleveland Clinic Foundation
Cleveland, Ohio

Douglas E. Joseph, DO
Staff Physician
Section of Vascular Medicine
Department of Cardiovascular Medicine
Cleveland Clinic
Cleveland, Ohio

Alexander Kantorovich, PharmD
Clinical Assistant Professor of Pharmacy Practice
Chicago State University
College of Pharmacology
Chicago, Illinois

Hemantha K. Koduri, MD, FACP, FHM
Clinical Fellow in Vascular Medicine
Cleveland Clinic Heart and Vascular Institute
Cleveland Clinic
Cleveland, Ohio

Amar Krishnaswamy, MD, FACC
Associate Program Director
Interventional Cardiology Fellowship Program
Department of Cardiovascular Medicine
Cleveland Clinic
Cleveland, Ohio

Venu Menon, MD
Director, Cardiovascular Medicine Training Program
Department of Cardiovascular Medicine
Cleveland Clinic
Cleveland, Ohio

Michael A. Militello, PharmD
Clinical Specialist in Cardiovascular Disease
Department of Pharmacy
Cleveland Clinic
Cleveland, Ohio

Debabrata Mukherjee, MD, MS, FACC
Chairman, Department of Internal Medicine
Chief, Cardiovascular Medicine
Professor of Internal Medicine
Texas Tech University
El Paso, Texas

Gian M. Novaro, MD, MS, FACC, FASE
Director, Echocardiography
Department of Cardiology
Cleveland Clinic Florida
Weston, Florida

Parag R. Patel, MD
Advanced Cardiac Imaging Fellow
Cleveland Clinic
Cleveland, Ohio

Dermot Phelan, MD, PhD
Section of Cardiovascular Imaging
Department of Cardiovascular Medicine
Cleveland Clinic
Cleveland, Ohio

Michael B. Rocco, MD, FACC
Staff Cardiologist
Department of Cardiovascular Medicine
Cleveland Clinic
Cleveland, Ohio

Marco Roffi, MD
Staff Interventional Cardiologist
Interventional Cardiology Unit
Division of Cardiology
University Hospital
University of Geneva
Geneva, Switzerland

Ellen Mayer Sabik, MD, FACC, FASE
Staff Cardiologist
Department of Cardiology
Cleveland Clinic
Cleveland, Ohio

Maran Thamilarasan, MD
Staff Cardiologist
Section of Cardiovascular Imaging
Department of Cardiovascular Medicine
Cleveland Clinic
Cleveland, Ohio

Donald A. Underwood, MD
Head, Electrocardiography
Section of Clinical Cardiology
Department of Cardiovascular Medicine
Heart and Vascular Institute
Cleveland Clinic
Cleveland, Ohio

Amanda R. Vest, MD
Advanced Heart Failure and Cardiac Transplantation Fellow
Department of Cardiovascular Medicine
Cleveland Clinic
Cleveland, Ohio

Preface

The third edition of this book has been updated to reflect changes in guidelines and practice since the last edition. The aim of the book remains the same: to help those certifying or recertifying prepare for the cardiovascular board examination. As in prior editions, we have included subjects, images, and tracings that are important not only for examinations but also relevant to clinical practice. The questions are presented in formats that are commonly used on the boards.

We would like to thank all of the contributors to this and prior editions, our colleagues and fellows from whom we learn on a daily basis, and especially our families who support and encourage our academic activity in addition to our busy clinical practices. We hope you enjoy the book and find it helpful.

Leslie Cho, MD
Brian P. Griffin, MD

Abbreviations

AAA	abdominal aortic aneurysm		CHD	coronary heart disease
ABI	ankle brachial index		CHF	congestive heart failure
ACC	American College of Cardiology		CI	confidence interval
ACE	angiotensin-converting enzyme		CK-MB	MB fraction of creatine kinase
ACEI	angiotensin-converting enzyme inhibitor		CPK	creatine phosphokinase
ACS	acute coronary syndrome		CRP	C-reactive protein
ACTH	adrenocorticotropic hormone		CS	coronary stenting
AED	automated external defibrillator		CT	computed tomography
AFib	atrial fibrillation		CTA	computed tomographic angiography
AHA	American Heart Association		CTEPH	chronic thromboembolic pulmonary hypertension
AI	aortic insufficiency		CXR	chest X-ray
AMI	acute myocardial infarction		DC	direct current
AP	action potential		DTI	direct thrombin inhibitor
aPTT	activated partial thromboplastin time		DVT	deep venous thrombosis
AR	aortic regurgitation		ECG	electrocardiogram
ARB	angiotensin receptor blocker		EF	ejection fraction
AS	aortic stenosis		EGD	esophagogastroduodenoscopy
ASA	atrial septal aneurysm		EMD	electromechanical dissociation
ASD	atrial septal defect		EMS	emergency medical service
AV	atrioventricular		EP	electrophysiology
AVNRT	atrioventricular nodal reentrant tachycardia		ESR	erythrocyte sedimentation rate
AVR	aortic valve replacement		ET	exercise training
AVRT	orthodromic atrioventricular reentrant tachycardia		FDA	Food and Drug Administration
β-AR	beta-adrenoreceptor		FEV_1	forced expiratory volume in the first second of expiration
bFGF	basic fibroblast growth factor			
BMI	body mass index		GI	gastrointestinal
BNP	brain natriuretic peptide		GP	glycoprotein
BP	blood pressure		GU	genitourinary
bpm	beats per minute		HBE	His bundle electrogram
BUN	blood urea nitrogen		HF	heart failure
CABG	coronary artery bypass grafting		HIT	heparin-induced thrombocytopenia
CAD	coronary artery disease		HR	heart rate
cAMP	cyclic adenosine monophosphate		HRA	high right atrium
CBC	complete blood count		HRR	hazard rate ratio
cDNA	complementary DNA		HTN	hypertension
CHB	complete heart block		IABP	intraaortic balloon pump

ICD	implantable cardioverter–defibrillator		PJRT	permanent junctional reciprocating tachycardia
IgE	immunoglobulin E		PMI	point of maximum impulse
IgG	immunoglobulin G		PO	oral(-ly)
INR	international normalized ratio		PT	prothrombin time
IQR	interquartile range		PTCA	percutaneous transluminal coronary angioplasty
IRBBB	incomplete right bundle branch block		PVARP	post-ventricular atrial refractory period
ISA	intrinsic sympathomimetic activity		PVC	premature ventricular contraction
ISR	in-stent restenosis		QOL	quality of life
IV	intravenous(-ly)		RA	right atrium(-al)
IVC	inferior vena cava		RAO	right anterior oblique
JNC	Joint National Committee		RAS	renal artery stenosis
JVP	jugular venous pulse		RBBB	right bundle branch block
LA	left atrium(-al)		RCA	right coronary artery
LAD	left anterior descending artery		RCC	right coronary cusp
LBBB	left bundle branch block		RR	risk ratio
LCC	left coronary cusp		RT-PCR	reverse transcriptase-polymerase chain reaction
LCx	left circumflex artery		RUSB	right upper sternal border
LDL	low-density lipoprotein		RV	right ventricle(-ular)
LDH	lactate dehydrogenase		RVH	right ventricular hypertrophy
LMWH	low-molecular-weight heparin		RVSP	right ventricular systolic pressure
LV	left ventricle(-ular)		SAM	systolic anterior motion
LVEF	left ventricular ejection fraction		SBE	subacute bacterial endocarditis
LVH	left ventricular hypertrophy		SC	subcutaneous(-ly)
LVOT	left ventricular outflow tract		SERCA2	sarcoplasmic-endoplasmic reticulum calcium ATPase type 2
MAT	multifocal atrial tachycardia		SL	sublingual(-ly)
MET	metabolic equivalents		SSS	sick sinus syndrome
MI	myocardial infarction		STEMI	ST-segment elevation myocardial infarction
MR	mitral regurgitation		SVR	systemic vascular resistance
MRA	magnetic resonance angiography		SVT	supraventricular tachycardia
MRI	magnetic resonance image(-ing)		TAO	thromboangiitis obliterans
MS	mitral stenosis		TdP	torsades de pointes
MTHFR	methylenetetrahydrofolate reductase		TEE	transesophageal echocardiography
MV	mitral valve		TIA	transient ischemic attack
MVP	mitral valve prolapse		TID	transient ischemic dilation
NCC	noncoronary cusp		TIMI	thrombolysis in myocardial infarction
NSAID	nonsteroidal anti-inflammatory drug		tPA	tissue plasminogen activator
NSR	normal sinus rhythm		TR	tricuspid regurgitation
NTG	nitroglycerin		TTE	transthoracic echocardiogram
OR	odds ratio		TVR	target vessel revascularization
P	pulse		UA	unstable angina
PA	pulmonary artery		UA/ NSTEMI	unstable angina and non–ST-segment elevation myocardial infarction
PAD	peripheral arterial disease		UFH	unfractionated heparin
PCI	percutaneous coronary intervention		VF	ventricular fibrillation
PCWP	pulmonary capillary wedge pressure		VSD	ventricular septal defect
PDA	patent ductus arteriosus		VT	ventricular tachycardia
PE	pulmonary embolus		VTE	venous thromboembolism
PEA	pulseless electrical activity		VTI	velocity time integral
PET	positron emission tomography			
PFO	patent foramen ovale			

Contents

chapter 1

Arrhythmia

Bryan J. Baranowski

QUESTIONS

1. Which of the following antiarrhythmic medications would be the best choice for treatment of a patient with atrial fibrillation (AFib) and significant renal insufficiency?

   a. Propafenone
   b. Sotalol
   c. Dofetilide
   d. Flecainide

2. Which of the following antiarrhythmic medications has active metabolites?

   a. Amiodarone
   b. Sotalol
   c. Dofetilide
   d. Flecainide

3. A patient arrives at the emergency department with symptomatic narrow complex tachycardia. The patient is hemodynamically stable. The decision is made to administer intravenous (IV) adenosine. Under which of the following circumstances should the dosage of adenosine be reduced?

   a. The patient is taking theophylline.
   b. The patient is taking dipyridamole.
   c. The patient has significant valvular regurgitation.
   d. The patient has a significant left-to-right shunt.

4. Which of the following medications is contraindicated for use with dofetilide?

   a. Digoxin
   b. Diltiazem
   c. Verapamil
   d. Propranolol

5. Which of the following antiarrhythmic drugs may be more likely to have proarrhythmia at increased heart rates?

   a. Sotalol
   b. Flecainide
   c. Quinidine
   d. Dofetilide

6. Which of the following statements is *true* regarding antiarrhythmic drugs with reverse-use dependence?

   a. Antiarrhythmic drugs with reverse-use dependence have greater efficacy for arrhythmia prevention than termination and have less risk for ventricular proarrhythmia at slower heart rates.

   b. Antiarrhythmic drugs with reverse-use dependence have less efficacy for arrhythmia prevention than termination and have greater risk for ventricular proarrhythmia at slower heart rates.

   c. Antiarrhythmic drugs with reverse-use dependence have greater efficacy for arrhythmia prevention than termination and have greater risk for ventricular proarrhythmia at slower heart rates.

   d. Antiarrhythmic drugs with reverse-use dependence have less efficacy for arrhythmia prevention than termination and have less risk for ventricular proarrhythmia at slower heart rates.

7. Which of the following is *true* regarding the Cardiac Arrhythmia Suppression Trials (CAST I and II)?

   a. The treatment drugs increased mortality for patients without heart disease.

   b. All class IC antiarrhythmic drugs were found to decrease mortality.

   c. The treatment drugs effectively suppressed premature ventricular complexes (PVCs).

   d. The antiarrhythmic drugs studied were flecainide, propafenone, and moricizine.

8. Which of the following antiarrhythmic drugs is the most potent sodium channel blocker?

   a. Flecainide

   b. Lidocaine

   c. Disopyramide

   d. Procainamide

9. Which of the following effects is expected when administering adenosine to a patient with recent cardiac transplantation (denervated heart)?

   a. No effect

   b. Diminished effect

   c. Enhanced effect

   d. Delayed effect

10. A patient presents with regular narrow QRS tachycardia. A 12-lead electrocardiogram (ECG) demonstrates an r′ in lead V_1 that was not seen on ECG when the patient was in sinus rhythm. An esophageal electrode shows a 1:1 atrial-to-ventricular relationship during tachycardia. The ventriculoatrial (VA) interval is measured as 55 milliseconds. Which of the following is the most likely diagnosis?

    a. Orthodromic atrioventricular reentrant tachycardia (AVRT)

    b. Atrial tachycardia

    c. AV nodal reentrant tachycardia (AVNRT)

    d. Permanent junctional reciprocating tachycardia (PJRT)

11. A 17-year-old patient who is known to have Wolff-Parkinson-White syndrome presents with a regular narrow complex tachycardia with a cycle length of 375 milliseconds (160 bpm) that occurred with a sudden onset. You note

that there is a 1:1 atrial-to-ventricular relationship and that the RP interval is 100 milliseconds. The best initial treatment is

a. IV procainamide.

b. atropine.

c. vagal maneuvers.

d. catheter ablation.

12. A 25-year-old patient presents with the sudden onset of tachycardia and is found to have a regular narrow QRS tachycardia with a cycle length of 340 milliseconds (176 bpm). An ECG appears to show P waves visible just after each QRS complex. You place an esophageal electrode and confirm a 1:1 atrial-to-ventricular relationship with a VA interval of 110 milliseconds. During the tachycardia, there is spontaneous development of left bundle branch block (LBBB), and a slower tachycardia with a VA interval of 150 milliseconds is now seen. What is the most likely diagnosis for the second tachycardia?

a. AVNRT

b. Orthodromic AVRT using a right-sided accessory pathway

c. Orthodromic AVRT using a left-sided accessory pathway

d. Ventricular tachycardia (VT) with 1:1 VA conduction

13. A 65-year-old man presents after an arrest while eating at a local restaurant. On arrival, paramedics documented ventricular fibrillation (VF), and he was successfully resuscitated. He has a history of myocardial infarction (MI) and congestive heart failure (CHF). Serum electrolytes are remarkable only for mild hypokalemia. MI is ruled out by ECG and serial blood tests of myocardial enzymes. Subsequent evaluation includes cardiac catheterization, which shows severe three-vessel coronary artery disease (CAD) and severe left ventricular (LV) systolic dysfunction. A nuclear myocardial perfusion scan shows a large area of myocardial scar without significant viability in the territory of the left anterior descending coronary artery. The decision is made to treat the CAD medically. Which of the following is the best management strategy for his arrhythmia?

a. PO amiodarone

b. Implantable cardioverter defibrillator (ICD) implantation if an electrophysiologic (EP) study shows inducible VT or VF

c. ICD implantation

d. β-Blocker medication

14. A 55-year-old woman has CAD and moderately severe LV systolic dysfunction (LV ejection fraction, 34%). Routine ambulatory Holter monitoring shows asymptomatic frequent ventricular ectopy with PVCs and occasional runs of nonsustained VT. Which of the following statements about the management of this patient is *true*?

a. Implantation of an ICD is indicated.

b. Implantation of an ICD is indicated if an EP study shows inducible VT.

c. Treatment with amiodarone is indicated, and if the arrhythmia recurs, then an EP study is indicated.

d. No treatment is indicated unless the arrhythmia becomes symptomatic.

15. A patient arrives at the emergency department after experiencing multiple shocks from his ICD. The shocks were not preceded by any symptoms. He is noted to be in sinus rhythm on presentation, and, while on the monitor, he receives several more shocks from the ICD without any arrhythmias noted. Which of

the following is the most appropriate initial step in the management of this patient?

    a. Immediately arrange for a programmer for interrogation and reprogramming of the ICD.

    b. Arrange for urgent surgery in the EP laboratory.

    c. Initiate antiarrhythmic drug therapy.

    d. Place a "donut" magnet over the ICD site.

16. Which of the following is most important for successful resuscitation of an adult patient with out-of-hospital cardiac arrest?

    a. IV epinephrine

    b. Early direct current (DC) shock defibrillation

    c. IV antiarrhythmic drugs

    d. Early intubation

17. Which of the following rhythms documented at the time of resuscitation from cardiac arrest carries the poorest prognosis for long-term survival?

    a. Asystole

    b. Electromechanical dissociation (EMD) or pulseless electrical activity (PEA)

    c. VF

    d. VT

18. Which of the following rhythm disturbances is most commonly documented for an adult with out-of-hospital sudden cardiac death resuscitated within the first 4 minutes after arrest?

    a. Asystole

    b. EMD or PEA

    c. Monomorphic VT

    d. VF

19. Which of the following treatment options has been most consistently shown to be effective for the primary prevention of sudden cardiac death in patients with CAD and recent MI?

    a. D-Sotalol

    b. β-Blocker medications

    c. Amiodarone

    d. Dofetilide

20. Which of the following is the most common condition associated with sudden cardiac death in the United States?

    a. Hypertrophic cardiomyopathy

    b. CAD

    c. Valvular heart disease

    d. Dilated cardiomyopathy

21. A 55-year-old man is referred for recurrent syncope. The episodes consist of a prodrome of weakness and nausea followed by loss of consciousness. Physical examination is unremarkable. ECG and exercise treadmill stress test were normal. Which of the following is the most appropriate next step?

    a. EP study

    b. Signal-averaged ECG

    c. Head-upright tilt-table testing

    d. Ambulatory Holter monitoring

22. A 40-year-old woman presents to the emergency department with tachycardia. An ECG shows regular narrow complex tachycardia at 160 bpm. Atrial activity is difficult to discern in the tracing, but during tachycardia, there appears to be an "r'" in lead V_1 that is not present on an ECG during sinus rhythm recorded a few months earlier. Which of the following is the most likely diagnosis?

    a. AVNRT

    b. AVRT

    c. Atrial tachycardia

    d. Atrial flutter

23. An 80-year-old man with chronic AFib of 15 years' duration is admitted with recurrent episodes of dizziness and a recent episode of syncope. He has normal LV function and no evidence of CAD. In-hospital telemetry confirms the presence of slow ventricular rate and frequent pauses (4 seconds) that correlate with his lightheadedness. His medications consist of warfarin sodium (Coumadin). The most appropriate course of action includes which of the following?

    a. Reassuring the patient and instructing him to come back if he has recurrence of syncope

    b. Prolonged monitoring with a loop recorder

    c. EP testing to evaluate for ventricular arrhythmia

    d. Permanent pacemaker implant

    e. ICD implant

24. A decision was made in the previous case to proceed with a permanent pacemaker. Which would be the most suitable pacing modality?

    a. Dual-chamber system programmed to DDDR

    b. Dual-chamber system programmed to DDDR with mode switching

    c. Dual-chamber system programmed to DDIR

    d. Single-chamber system in the ventricle programmed to VVIR

    e. Single-chamber system in the atrium programmed to AAIR

25. Which one of the following is *true* about "pacemaker syndrome"?

    a. Symptoms usually include fatigue, dizziness, and hypotension.

    b. It occurs equally in atrial-based and ventricular-based pacing systems.

    c. It does not occur in patients who have 1:1 VA conduction.

    d. It can be treated with fludrocortisone.

    e. It is treated by increasing the VVI baseline pacing rate.

26. Of the following patients, who is the most likely to carry the diagnosis of sick sinus syndrome (SSS)?

    a. A 65-year-old woman with a resting sinus arrhythmia varying from 70 to 85 bpm

    b. A 30-year-old with sinus pauses 1.5 seconds in duration

    c. A 20-year-old athletic man with sinus bradycardia at 25 bpm while sleeping

    d. A 73-year-old man with persistent AFib and a ventricular rate of 40 bpm during peak treadmill test

    e. A 70-year-old with sinus bradycardia and AV block secondary to a β-blocker overdose

27. A 76-year-old patient with dilated cardiomyopathy and LBBB on baseline ECG is undergoing evaluation for syncope. Placement of a catheter near his bundle during EP testing is most likely to

   a. induce AFib.

   b. induce VT.

   c. perforate the atrium.

   d. perforate the ventricle.

   e. induce complete heart block (CHB).

28. A 25-year-old patient with a history of depression is brought to the emergency room after ingesting some of her mother's prescription medications, including diltiazem and metoprolol. Her pulse rate is 25 bpm, and her BP is 90/50 mmHg. Her ECG shows sinus bradycardia and high-grade AV block. In preparation for temporary pacemaker placement, which of the following is most likely to be effective?

   a. IV calcium gluconate

   b. Isoproterenol infusion

   c. IV atropine

   d. IV magnesium sulfate

   e. IV glucagon

29. A young patient is admitted to the intensive care unit with amitriptyline overdose. Three hours after gastric lavage, he develops hypotension and wide complex tachycardia that is recurrent despite cardioversion. Appropriate management includes which of the following?

   a. IV bretylium

   b. Temporary pacemaker with overdrive pacing

   c. IV calcium gluconate

   d. IV hypertonic sodium bicarbonate

   e. IV magnesium sulfate

30. An 80-year-old undergoes dual-chamber pacemaker placement for CHB. Excellent ventricular and atrial capture thresholds were obtained at the time of the implant. The pacemaker programmed parameters are as follows: mode, DDD; lower rate, 70 bpm; upper rate, 130 bpm; atrial sensitivity, 0.25 mV (most sensitive setting); ventricular sensitivity, 1.00 mV; AV delay, 175 milliseconds; pace/sense configuration, bipolar. The next day, the following rhythm strip was recorded (Fig. 1.1): This rhythm strip shows

   a. normal pacemaker function for the programmed parameters.

   b. atrial noncapture.

   c. ventricular noncapture.

   d. atrial undersensing.

   e. ventricular undersensing.

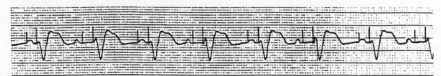

Figure 1.1

31. A 50-year-old man with chronic obstructive pulmonary disease related to chronic smoking presents to the emergency room with palpitations. ECG shows narrow

QRS tachycardia at 165 bpm. His BP is 125/60 mmHg. Expiratory wheezes are heard on lung examination. His medications include albuterol inhaler and theophylline. The most appropriate initial treatment includes which of the following?

   a. Adenosine IV bolus
   b. Digoxin loading over 6 hours
   c. Verapamil IV bolus
   d. Propafenone IV bolus
   e. Immediate cardioversion

32. A 55-year-old woman returns to the clinic after a recent dual-chamber pacemaker placement. She reports frequent palpitations and fatigue. These episodes last for several minutes before stopping. A Holter monitor recorded the following rhythm (Fig. 1.2): The pacemaker is programmed to mode DDD; lower rate, 80 bpm; upper rate, 150 bpm; AV delay, 200 milliseconds; postventricular atrial RP, 150 milliseconds. The latter part of this rhythm strip shows

   a. VT induced by the pacemaker.
   b. initiation of atrial tachycardia with atrial tracking.
   c. pacemaker-mediated tachycardia.
   d. pacemaker function failure with inappropriate rapid ventricular pacing.
   e. artifact.

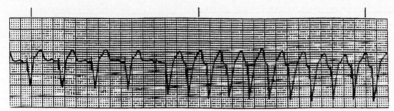

Figure 1.2

33. An 82-year-old man receives a dual-chamber pacemaker for SSS. Routine trans-telephonic check (without and with magnet) shows the following strips (Fig. 1.3). Which of the following is *true*?

   a. The pacing mode is VVI secondary to automatic mode switch.
   b. There is consistent atrial capture on the magnet strip.
   c. There is consistent ventricular capture.
   d. Ventricular sensing cannot be determined by the available strips.
   e. Atrial sensing cannot be determined by the available strips.

Free Running

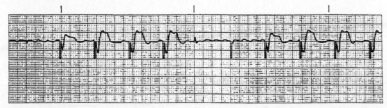

Magnet

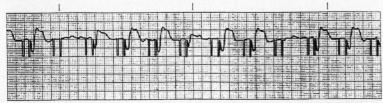

Figure 1.3

Questions 34–37

The following tracings (Figs. 1.4, 1.5, 1.6, and 1.7) are obtained during EP evaluation of AV conduction in different patients. HRA (*high right atrium*) and HBE (*His bundle electrogram*) are the intracardiac electrograms, recording from the high right atrium and the His bundle regions, respectively. Which of the following is *true* for these tracings?

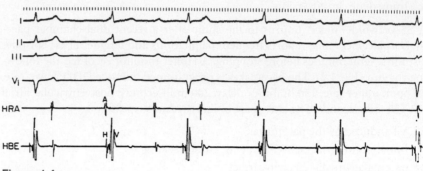

Figure 1.4

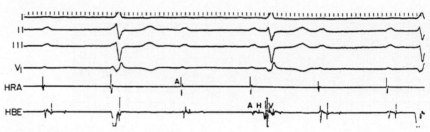

Figure 1.5

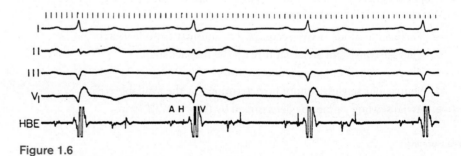

Figure 1.6

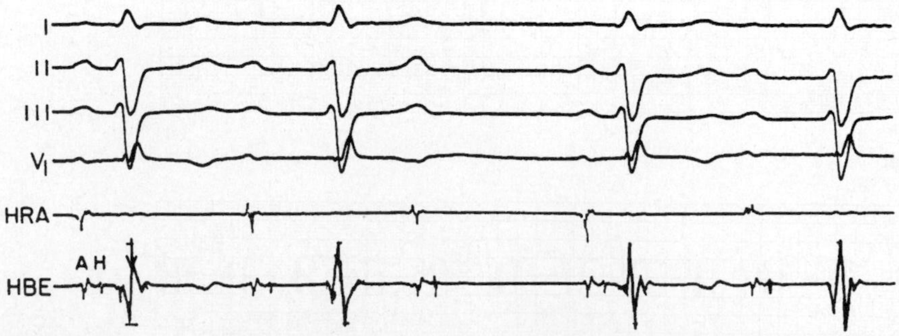

Figure 1.7

a. CHB at the level of the AV node

b. CHB at the infra-Hisian (below the His bundle) level

c. Second-degree AV block at the AV node level

d. Second-degree AV block at an infra-Hisian level

e. First-degree AV block

38. A 38-year-old woman with congenital CHB undergoes a dual-chamber permanent pacemaker. A 12-lead ECG obtained after the procedure shows normal sinus rhythm (NSR) with atrial tracking (a sense–V pace behavior). The ventricular-paced complex has a right bundle branch block (RBBB) morphology. Further evaluation should include

a. obtaining a portable anteroposterior chest X-ray (CXR) to evaluate lead position.

b. obtaining a two-view (anteroposterior and lateral) CXR to evaluate lead position.

c. repeating the 12-lead ECG.

d. requesting a pacemaker interrogation.

e. reassuring the patient without ordering further tests.

39. Which of the following is *true* regarding EP testing of the conduction system?

a. It is indicated in patients with symptomatic third-degree heart block to identify the level of block.

b. An abnormal sinus node recovery time is an indication for pacemaker placement.

c. A normal sinus node recovery time rules out the diagnosis of SSS.

d. Patients with evidence of infra-Hisian block during EP testing should be considered for permanent pacing.

e. Ambulatory ECG is less reliable than EP testing in evaluating SSS.

40. Which of the following statements is *true* regarding Brugada syndrome?

a. It is characterized by ST elevation and a pseudo-RBBB pattern in the right precordial leads with persistent ST elevation.

b. The ECG manifestations can be exacerbated by sotalol.

c. It is the leading cause of death in young men in the Middle East.

d. AFib is the most frequently reported arrhythmia.

e. It is effectively treated with β-blockers.

41. In patients with long-QT syndrome

a. EP testing is indicated to evaluate for inducible ventricular arrhythmias.

b. the mechanism of torsades de pointes (TdP) is believed to be related to early afterdepolarization.

c. sotalol is effective for the treatment of the associated ventricular tachyarrhythmias.

d. hyperkalemia increases the risk of TdP.

e. cardiac arrest typically occurs at rest in LQT1 syndrome.

42. A 75-year-old man is admitted with upper gastrointestinal (GI) bleeding. His ECG shows sinus rhythm at 90 bpm, with a PR of 220 milliseconds, RBBB, and left anterior fascicular block. He had one episode of near syncope 2 days before this admission. His current hematocrit is 20. You are consulted regarding the need for a pacemaker. Which of the following is *true*?

   a. You should proceed with permanent pacemaker placement in the setting of bifascicular block.

   b. You should proceed with ICD placement.

   c. You should perform EP testing to evaluate the AV conduction system.

   d. You should reassure the patient and suggest no further testing.

   e. You should prescribe β-blockers to slow down the sinus rate.

43. Which of the following criteria is most helpful in differentiating supraventricular tachycardia (SVT) from VT in a patient presenting with wide complex tachycardia?

   a. The patient is older than 65 years.

   b. The tachycardia rate is >160 bpm.

   c. The patient is awake with a BP of 110/65 mmHg.

   d. There is an RS pattern in V_2.

   e. There is AV dissociation.

44. A 76-year-old man walks into the emergency room reporting palpitations and dizziness. A 12-lead ECG shows wide complex tachycardia at a rate of 160 bpm. His BP is 110/50 mmHg. He reports that he recently sustained an MI. He has not had any similar symptoms before. Which of the following should be included in further evaluation and treatment of his arrhythmia?

   a. Verapamil, 10-mg IV bolus, to treat SVT with aberrancy, as the patient is hemodynamically stable

   b. Immediate DC cardioversion

   c. Procainamide, 15 mg/kg IV over 30 to 60 minutes

   d. Immediate cardiac catheterization and angioplasty, as needed

   e. Digoxin, 1 mg IV over 6 hours in four divided doses

45. A 55-year-old man had a pacemaker initially implanted 8 years ago over the left prepectoral area. Two months earlier, his old pacemaker reached end-of-life, and he underwent replacement of the pacemaker using the existing leads. He is presenting now with dull pain, swelling, and mild erythema over the pacemaker pocket site that started 1 week earlier, together with low-grade fever. He reports some purulent drainage from the incision site. Blood cultures were drawn. The best course of action is

   a. to prescribe PO antibiotics for 2 weeks.

   b. to admit the patient for IV antibiotics and pacemaker-system extraction.

   c. to prescribe long-term suppressive PO antibiotics, as the pacemaker and leads system are too old to be extracted.

   d. to remove the recently implanted pulse generator on the left, leaving the old leads in place, and implant a new pacemaker system on the right prepectoral area.

   e. to incise and drain the pacemaker pocket and allow it to heal with secondary intention with daily change of dressing.

46. Which of the following is a *correct* statement concerning external cardioversion of AFib?

   a. Acute MI is a contraindication to cardioversion, as it results in further myocardial damage.

   b. A nonsynchronized shock should be delivered because the rhythm is irregular.

c. Inadequate synchronization may occur with peaked T waves, low-amplitude signal, and malfunctioning pacemakers.

d. Digoxin therapy should be discontinued for 48 hours before elective cardioversion.

e. Patients with pacemakers should not undergo cardioversion because of the risk of pacemaker damage.

47. In patients with Wolff-Parkinson-White syndrome, with which of the following is acute pharmacologic treatment of AFib best achieved?

a. Diltiazem

b. Lidocaine

c. Verapamil

d. Procainamide

e. Adenosine

48. A 75-year-old patient with a history of ischemic cardiomyopathy develops worsening heart failure symptoms during episodes of AFib despite a controlled ventricular rate. Which of the following is included in a reasonable trial of pharmacologic therapy?

a. Flecainide

b. Sotalol

c. Verapamil

d. Disopyramide

e. Amiodarone

49. Which of the following is *true* regarding the use of digoxin in AFib?

a. It is superior to placebo for the acute conversion of AFib.

b. It controls ventricular rate during exercise in most patients.

c. It can control ventricular rate at rest in many patients.

d. It effectively maintains sinus rhythm after cardioversion.

e. Because of its hepatic clearance, it is safe to use in patients with renal insufficiency.

50. Which of the following statements regarding flecainide as a treatment of AFib is *true*?

a. It may contribute to an increase in the digoxin level.

b. It may be used without an AV nodal blocking agent because of its potent effect on the AV conduction system.

c. It has been shown to be effective and safe for use in patients with hypertrophic cardiomyopathy.

d. It has no effect on the acute conversion of AFib but only on maintenance of sinus rhythm postcardioversion.

e. It is used for the treatment of AFib but not atrial flutter.

51. Which of the following mechanisms is responsible for AFib occurring in the immediate postoperative period after a maze procedure?

a. Change in the atrial refractory period as a result of the surgical manipulation

b. Autonomic imbalance as a result of the surgical intervention

c. Misplacement of a suture line

d. An incomplete or omitted suture line

e. Inhibition of atrial natriuretic peptide secretion as a result of the surgical manipulation

52. The following tachycardia was induced during EP testing of a 36-year-old woman with recurrent palpitations (Fig. 1.8). Which of the following is the most likely diagnosis?

a. AVNRT

b. Orthodromic reentrant tachycardia

c. Antidromic reentrant tachycardia

d. VT

e. Idiopathic left VT

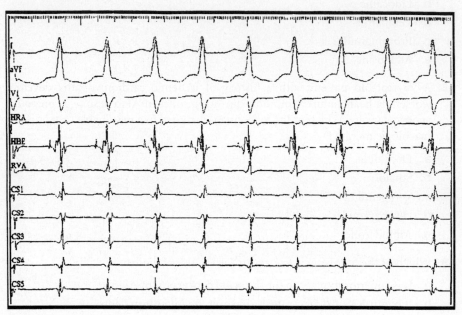

Figure 1.8

ANSWERS

1. **a.** Propafenone. Sotalol and dofetilide are primarily excreted by the renal route and should be used cautiously, if at all, in patients with significant renal insufficiency. Flecainide primarily undergoes hepatic elimination (approximately 70%) but has 25% renal elimination. The route of elimination for propafenone is 99% hepatic.

2. **a.** Amiodarone. Sotalol, dofetilide, and flecainide do not have significant active metabolites. Amiodarone is metabolized to the active metabolite desethylamiodarone.

3. **b.** The patient is taking dipyridamole. Dipyridamole potentiates the effect of adenosine by interfering with metabolism; therefore, a reduced dose of adenosine is recommended. Although not a part of this question, it is important to remember that adenosine also needs to be used with extreme caution in heart transplant patients as a markedly exaggerated response to adenosine can be seen in the denervated heart. An increased dose of adenosine is recommended in the presence of methylxanthines such as theophylline, which antagonizes the effect of adenosine (blocks receptors), and other factors such as slow circulation time, valvular regurgitation, and left-to-right shunts that reduce the effectiveness of adenosine.

4. **c.** Verapamil. Verapamil may increase serum levels of dofetilide because of interference with renal excretion and hepatic metabolism.

5. **b.** Flecainide. Flecainide is a class IC antiarrhythmic drug, and these agents exhibit "use dependence." This refers to the property of increased drug effect at increased heart rates. Sotalol and dofetilide are class III antiarrhythmic drugs that exhibit "reverse-use dependence"—that is, greater drug effect at slower heart rates. Quinidine has effects on both sodium and potassium channels. While the effects on the sodium channels are use dependent, it is far less pronounced compared with the Ic agents such as flecainide. The potassium-blocking properties and resulting QT prolongation are more pronounced at slower heart rates— reverse-use dependent.

6. **c.** Antiarrhythmic drugs with reverse-use dependence have greater efficacy for arrhythmia prevention than termination and have greater risk for ventricular proarrhythmia after AFib termination (at slower sinus rates) than during AFib. Antiarrhythmic drugs with use dependence, such as sotalol and dofetilide, have greater antiarrhythmic effect at slower heart rates. Consequently, drug efficacy is enhanced at the relatively slower rates in sinus rhythm, making these drugs more effective for prevention of AFib than those drugs with use dependence. Likewise, for proarrhythmia, the antiarrhythmic drugs with reverse-use dependence are more likely to produce ventricular proarrhythmia after conversion to sinus rhythm at the relatively slower sinus rate or with a postconversion pause.

7. **c.** The treatment drugs effectively suppressed premature ventricular complexes (PVCs). CAST studied the concept that PVC suppression in the postinfarction period would reduce the incidence of sudden cardiac death. Patients without heart disease were, therefore, excluded from these studies. CAST I studied flecainide, encainide, and moricizine versus placebo. Demonstration of effective suppression of PVCs by one of the drugs was necessary before a patient could be randomized to drug or placebo treatment. Propafenone, another class IC antiarrhythmic drug, was not studied. CAST I was prematurely terminated by the safety committee after only a 10-month average follow-up because of significantly increased incidence of arrhythmic death and nonfatal cardiac arrests in the flecainide and encainide treatment groups. CAST II was a continuation of

the study with only moricizine versus placebo, but this study was also terminated early because of an increased incidence of cardiac arrest in the moricizine treatment group.

8. **a.** Flecainide. All of these drugs are class I antiarrhythmic medications and have sodium channel–blocking properties to various degrees. Class IC agents, such as flecainide, have the most potent sodium channel–blocking effects, and class IB agents, such as lidocaine, have the least potent sodium channel–blocking effects.

9. **c.** Enhanced effect. Patients with denervated hearts are supersensitive to the effects of adenosine.

10. **c.** AV nodal reentrant tachycardia (AVNRT). Atrial tachycardia and PJRT are long RP tachycardias and, therefore, would not have such a short VA interval. PJRT is a special type of orthodromic AVRT that involves a posteroseptal accessory pathway with decremental (AV nodal-like) conduction properties and, hence, has a long RP (long VA) interval. Because of the time required to reach the accessory pathway for the retrograde portion of the arrhythmia circuit, orthodromic AVRT generally has a VA interval longer than 70 milliseconds. Therefore, a VA interval shorter than 70 milliseconds excludes orthodromic AVRT and makes AVNRT the most likely diagnosis. A small r′ wave (pseudo r′ wave) can sometimes be seen at the terminal portion of the QRS (usually best in lead V_1). This deflection represents retrograde activation of the atrial (a retrograde P wave) occurring shortly after the QRS complex.

11. **c.** Vagal maneuvers. A sudden onset of a regular narrow complex tachycardia with a cycle length of 375 milliseconds and an RP interval of 100 milliseconds is a short RP tachycardia (the PR interval would be 375 milliseconds – 100 milliseconds = 275 milliseconds, so the RP is shorter than the PR). This patient most likely presents with orthodromic AVRT, a reciprocating tachycardia circuit that involves antegrade conduction through the AV node and retrograde conduction through the accessory pathway (however, AVNRT is also possible). As the AV node is a necessary component of the arrhythmia circuit, AV nodal blockade effectively terminates this type of tachycardia. Vagal maneuvers, such as Valsalva, coughing, or carotid sinus massage, may be quite effective and avoid the potential risks associated with administration of medications. Verapamil and other drugs that block AV conduction, such as β-blockers and adenosine, may be quite useful for termination of AVRT. This should not be confused with the management of AFib in the setting of Wolff-Parkinson-White syndrome, in which administration of AV nodal blocking drugs, such as verapamil, is contraindicated due to a concern for uninhibited and thus rapid AV conduction of the AP, which if rapid enough can induce ventricular fibrillation. When AV conduction is occurring through both the AV node and AP, retrograde, concealed conduction into the AP can limit its antegrade conduction properties. If preexcited, AFib with IV procainamide or DC cardioversion is the correct management. A precautionary note regarding the use of adenosine for regular narrow QRS tachycardia in patients with Wolff-Parkinson-White syndrome: Adenosine may precipitate AFib and result in a very rapid ventricular response (preexcited tachycardia). Atropine has no role in the treatment of these types of arrhythmia. Catheter ablation is not generally an acute treatment option for this arrhythmia, although this approach may be an excellent option for chronic treatment (cure).

12. **c.** Orthodromic AVRT using a left-sided accessory pathway. A regular narrow QRS tachycardia that has VA interval prolongation with the development of bundle branch block is most consistent with an orthodromic AVRT using an accessory pathway ipsilateral to the bundle branch. During AVRT, the antegrade limb of the circuit is the AV node and His-Purkinje/bundle branch system, and the retrograde limb is the accessory pathway. Block in a bundle branch ipsilateral

to an accessory pathway creates a larger circuit, as the antegrade limb must now use the contralateral bundle branch, and therefore, the VA interval increases. This results in an increase in the tachycardia cycle length (a slower tachycardia). Of note, a slower tachycardia with bundle branch block itself does not necessarily have the same significance. Other types of tachycardia may slow because of a change in conduction of other components of the tachycardia circuit, such as the conduction through the AV node (A–H interval). Thus, it is important to demonstrate VA interval prolongation during bundle branch block to implicate an ipsilateral accessory pathway participating in AVRT.

13. **c.** ICD implantation. Cardiac arrest with VT or VF in the absence of reversible causes (e.g., MI, severe electrolyte or metabolic disorders) is a class I indication for ICD implantation. ICD implantation for such patients is superior to amiodarone drug therapy, as demonstrated in the Antiarrhythmics Versus Implantable Defibrillator (AVID) trial. The Canadian Implantable Defibrillator Study examined a similar population of patients and, although not statistically significant, showed a strong trend for the superiority of ICDs. Demonstration of inducible VT or VF in these types of patients is not necessary.

14. **b.** Implantation of an ICD is indicated if an EP study shows inducible VT. The Multicenter Automatic Defibrillator Implantation Trial (MADIT) evaluated patients with CAD, ischemic cardiomyopathy with an LV ejection fraction of <35%, and nonsustained VT. This study showed that for patients with inducible VT at baseline EP study and after administration of IV procainamide, treatment with an ICD was superior to treatment with antiarrhythmic drugs. A follow-up study, MADIT II, assessed the role of ICD implantation in patients with an ischemic cardiomyopathy and an ejection fraction ≤30%. Nonsustained VT was not required to undergo ICD implant, nor was an EP study. The study was terminated early after an average follow-up of 20 months because the ICD significantly reduced all-cause mortality (14.2% versus 19.8% for conventional therapy). This study helped expand ICD implant indications. This is a class I indication for ICD implantation.

15. **d.** Place a "donut" magnet over the ICD site. The patient is having inappropriate or spurious shocks from the ICD, most likely caused by detection of electrical noise from a malfunction of the ICD lead. It is imperative that further shocks be prevented immediately, not only for patient comfort but also to prevent induction of life-threatening ventricular arrhythmias (including ventricular arrhythmia storm) caused by the ICD shocks. The most effective action at this point is placement of a magnet over the ICD site. This prevents the ICD from delivering any therapies. It would not be optimal to delay the prevention of further shocks while waiting for an ICD programmer. Of note, unlike pacemakers, ICDs do not have an asynchronous pacing response to application of a magnet.

16. **b.** Early direct current (DC) shock defibrillation. The two most crucial factors that determine the value of out-of-hospital resuscitation for patients who experience sudden cardiac death are citizen-bystander cardiopulmonary resuscitation and early DC shock defibrillation.

17. **a.** Asystole. EMD or PEA and, in particular, asystole tend to be found in increasing proportions as the time since arrest increases. This is likely caused by degeneration of prolonged VF. When VF is the documented rhythm at the time of resuscitation, the long-term survival is approximately 25%. When EMD or PEA is the documented rhythm, the long-term survival rate drops to approximately 6%, and it drops even further, to approximately 1%, when asystole is documented.

18. **d.** VF. The initial rhythm documented in a patient who undergoes sudden cardiac death is dependent on the time elapsed since the arrest. Most episodes of sudden cardiac death (approximately 65% to 85%) that are documented electrocardiographically are caused by malignant ventricular arrhythmias such as VF. Monomorphic VT is uncommonly documented as a cause of out-of-hospital sudden cardiac death, perhaps caused by degeneration of unstable VT to VF. Asystole and EMD or PEA are found in greater proportions as the time since arrest increases, as these rhythms are likely the result of prolonged VF.

19. **b.** β-Blocker medications. Several randomized trials of the use of β-blocker medications for patients after MI have shown efficacy for the prevention of sudden cardiac death (including propranolol, timolol, metoprolol, and acebutolol). Trials of amiodarone in this setting have provided mixed results. Two large randomized trials, the European Myocardial Infarct Amiodarone Trial (EMIAT) and the Canadian Amiodarone Myocardial Infarction Arrhythmia Trial (CAMIAT), examined the use of amiodarone in patients after MI and did not show a reduction in overall mortality with the use of amiodarone. The Polish Amiodarone Trial showed that amiodarone improved survival only in patients with preserved LV function after MI. The Survival with Oral D-sotalol (SWORD) trial studied the use of the D-isomer of sotalol (D-sotalol) in patients with recent MI and LV dysfunction. This study found worse survival in the group treated with D-sotalol than in the group treated with placebo. The Danish Investigations of Arrhythmias and Mortality on Dofetilide (DIAMOND) studies showed that dofetilide had a neutral effect on total mortality compared with placebo in the treatment of post-MI patients with LV dysfunction.

20. **b.** CAD. CAD is the predominant disease process associated with sudden cardiac death in the United States, accounting for 64% to 90% of cases. The other cardiomyopathies, such as dilated and hypertrophic cardiomyopathies, together account for approximately 10% to 15% of cases of sudden cardiac death.

21. **c.** Head-upright tilt-table testing. Syncope in the absence of structural heart disease is most likely neurally mediated (vasovagal). The head-upright tilt-table test is the most appropriate test to evaluate for this condition. This test initiates the vasovagal episode by maximizing venous pooling, sympathetic activation, and circulating catecholamines. In general, the test involves at least 30 minutes of 70-degree head-up tilt angle without a saddle support. An addition of a catecholamine challenge with isoproterenol is sometimes used. Among symptomatic patients, the sensitivity of the head-upright tilt-table test is approximately 85%. The specificity of the head-upright tilt-table test is good, with the frequency of an abnormal tilt-table test in control subjects being 0% to 15%. In the absence of structural heart disease, EP study, ambulatory Holter monitoring, and the signal-averaged ECG are low yield.

22. **a.** AVNRT. An "r'" in lead V_1 during regular narrow complex tachycardia that is not present during sinus rhythm indicates the inscription of the P wave in the terminal QRS, is consistent with a very short VA interval, and is very specific for AVNRT.

23. **d.** Permanent pacemaker implant. This patient has evidence of symptomatic bradycardia on Holter monitoring, which constitutes a class I indication for permanent pacemaker placement. He has AV conduction system disease with no obvious reversible causes, which is most probably caused by idiopathic fibrosis (Lev disease). Prolonged monitoring will probably show more episodes of bradycardia, which was already seen during telemetry, and which places this elderly patient at risk for syncope and injury. EP testing for ventricular arrhythmia is not indicated in view of the absence of structural heart disease. Likewise, ICD is not indicated.

24. **d.** Single-chamber system in the ventricle programmed to VVIR. This patient is in chronic AFib, and, therefore, physiologic pacing in the atrium cannot be achieved. Furthermore, conversion and long-term maintenance of sinus rhythm in this situation are very unlikely. Therefore, there is no indication for placement of an atrial lead. DDDR with mode switching and DDIR will behave like a VVIR system in this patient, at the expense, however, of an additional lead (atrial) and a more expensive dual-chamber pacemaker.

25. **a.** Symptoms usually include fatigue, dizziness, and hypotension. Pacemaker syndrome is caused by pacing the ventricle asynchronously, which results in AV dissociation or VA conduction. Symptoms consist of fatigue, dizziness, dyspnea, and weakness, with or without hypotension. The mechanism is believed to be related in part to atrial contraction against a closed AV valve and release of atrial natriuretic peptide. It occurs with ventricular pacing and therefore is worsened by increasing pacing rate and relieved by allowing intrinsic conduction (if present) by lowering the pacing rate, programming rate hysteresis, or upgrading to a dual-chamber system. Therapy with fludrocortisone and other volume-expansion modalities is not helpful.

26. **d.** A 73-year-old man with persistent AFib and a ventricular rate of 40 bpm during peak treadmill test. The 73-year-old man with AFib and slow ventricular rate during exercise is the classic example of SSS. This usually indicates degenerative disease of the cardiac conduction system involving the AV node as well as the sinus node. Function of the sinus node can only be assessed after AFib has been terminated, usually by DC cardioversion. In this patient's case, it would not be uncommon to manifest a long postconversion pause, followed by either marked sinus bradycardia or complete sinus node arrest with a resulting junctional or ventricular escape rhythm (hopefully) following cardioversion. The finding of sinus arrhythmia varying by 15 bpm in an older patient, the profound nocturnal bradycardia in young athletes, and the sinus pauses in young patients are related mostly to a high vagal tone and do not indicate sinus node disease.

27. **e.** Induce complete heart block (CHB). Patients with true complete LBBB are at risk for developing transient CHB during catheter manipulation in the septal region of the tricuspid valve. This is caused by transient traumatic block of the right bundle branch. A similar scenario can result when placing a Swan-Ganz catheter in patients with LBBB.

28. **e.** IV glucagon. This patient has an overdose of diltiazem and metoprolol. These drugs slow sinoatrial and AV conduction. Calcium and magnesium have no effect in reversing these bradycardic effects. Isuprel and atropine are not likely to overcome the β-blockade of metoprolol. IV glucagon acts on a specific receptor. This results in an increase in intracellular cyclic adenosine monophosphate, which enhances both sinoatrial and AV node conduction despite the presence of β-blockade.

29. **d.** IV hypertonic sodium bicarbonate. Amitriptyline has sodium channel–blocking properties and induced QRS widening and VT. Increasing the extracellular sodium concentration by the administration of sodium bicarbonate decreases the association of this drug with the sodium channel.

30. **d.** Atrial undersensing. This rhythm shows evidence of atrial undersensing. The pacemaker is programmed to DDD. In this mode, an appropriately sensed P wave should cause inhibition of the atrial spike; a ventricular spike is then delivered after the programmed AV interval or inhibited by an intrinsic R wave. In this strip, the P wave is present in each complex. However, in complexes 2, 4, 6, and 8, an atrial spike follows the intrinsic P wave because the intrinsic P wave was not appropriately sensed by the pacemaker. The noncapture of the atrium following the atrial spike on complexes 2, 4, 6, and 8 is anticipated as the atrium would still have been refractory from the preceding P wave. Capture of the atrium on complexes 1, 3, 5, and 7 is suggested by the P wave that is different in morphology (wider) than the intrinsic P wave. Atrial undersensing occurring early after implantation may be the result of lead dislodgment. A CXR should be obtained to assess lead position. Other possibilities include inappropriate programmed sensitivity, which can be assessed on a device check. Finally, inflammation at the lead tip–endocardium interface can result in a decrease in sensing amplitude. This may improve over several weeks as the lead matures and inflammation resolves.

31. c. Verapamil IV bolus. Adenosine is commonly used to terminate SVT. However, this patient is on theophylline, which is an effective blocker of the adenosine receptor. Propafenone might be poorly tolerated by this patient because of its associated β-blocking activity, which might increase airway resistance. Digoxin shortens the refractory period of the atrium and might potentially accelerate an atrial tachycardia. Immediate cardioversion is not needed, as the patient appears hemodynamically stable, and it would be reasonable to attempt pharmacologic therapy initially with verapamil.

32. c. Pacemaker-mediated tachycardia. In this strip, there is evidence of atrial undersensing (fifth complex). As a result, the fifth ventricular-paced beat comes "late" relative to atrial activation. This allows enough time to go by for the AV node to recover its conduction properties. This allows retrograde P-wave conduction following ventricular pacing, which is sensed by the pacer (because of short programmed postventricular atrial refractory period [PVARP]), and results in ventricular triggered pacing, causing a pacemaker-mediated tachycardia or endless-loop tachycardia. Acute treatment of this condition includes the application of a magnet to inhibit atrial sensing, thereby breaking the tachycardia loop. The spontaneous termination of these episodes in this patient is most probably related to intermittent atrial undersensing, which interrupts the tachycardia loop. Further prevention of these episodes includes reprogramming the PVARP, AV delay, or atrial sensitivity. Pacemaker-mediated tachycardia is an abnormal consequence of normal pacemaker function.

33. a. The pacing mode is VVI secondary to automatic mode switch. The initial rhythm strip shows background AFib with VVI pacing, most probably related to automatic mode switch. The absence of atrial pacing suggests adequate atrial sensing (of the fibrillation), which resulted in the mode switch behavior. Atrial pacing cannot be determined in the presence of AFib. There is adequate ventricular sensing, as determined on the nonmagnet strip (fifth complex—the small intrinsic QRS is sensed by the pacemaker which results in inhibition of pacing); however, there is intermittent ventricular capture noted (ventricular pacing spike followed by a lack of ventricular depolarization).

34. a. CHB at the level of the AV node. In this tracing, there is NSR with CHB and a narrow escape rhythm that is junctional in origin. This is apparent in the HBE tracing, in which the atrial deflections are completely dissociated from the H–V deflections. Therefore, the atrial impulse entering the AV node is not conducting down to the His bundle (A is not followed by His potential), indicating that the level of block is at the level of the AV node.

35. b. CHB at the infra-Hisian (below the His bundle) level. In this tracing, there is NSR with CHB and a relatively wide escape rhythm. In the HBE tracing, each atrial deflection is followed by an initial His deflection and a third, smaller deflection, H′, indicating that there is conduction delay within the His bundle itself. This is suggestive of significant His-Purkinje conduction disease. Therefore, the atrial impulse enters the AV node, conducts down to the His bundle (normal AH interval), where it encounters conduction delay (a "split" His made up of both an H and an H′), and then fails to propagate to the ventricle, indicating that the level of block is at or below the level of the bundle of His. There is obvious AV dissociation with a ventricular escape rhythm.

36. **d.** Second-degree AV block at an infra-Hisian level. In this tracing, the surface ECG shows NSR with 2:1 AV block. The HBE tracing shows constant AH with 2:1 block below the level of the His bundle.

37. **d.** Second-degree AV block at an infra-Hisian level. In this tracing, the surface ECG shows NSR with second-degree type I AV block (Wenckebach). This pattern of block is usually localized to the AV node. However, in rare circumstances the block can occur within or below the His bundle. The wide QRS seen on the surface leads are a clue in this case that the patient has conduction disease below the level of the AV node; however, the site of block can only be determined by reviewing the His bundle recordings. In this situation, the HBE tracing shows progressive prolongation in the HV interval before it blocks in a 3:2 conduction pattern. Therefore, the conduction delay is not at the level of the AV node but at or below the His bundle. As opposed to Wenckebach in the AV node, which is usually benign in nature, this type of infra-Hisian block indicates His-Purkinje conduction system disease and is an indication for pacemaker placement, as it may progress to CHB.

38. **b.** Obtaining a two-view (anteroposterior and lateral) CXR to evaluate lead position. The presence of an RBBB-paced QRS complex pattern suggests that the ventricular lead may be in the LV. The lead may enter the LV through an atrial septal defect or ventricular septal defect or via perforation of the interventricular septum. It may also be inadvertently introduced into an artery and passed retrogradely through the aortic valve. Another possibility is placement into one of the LV branches of the coronary sinus. Although sometimes an apical position in the RV in a rotated heart can potentially give an RBBB-paced pattern, a two-view CXR should be obtained to rule out LV positioning. A single-view portable AP will not distinguish an LV from an apical RV placement. If LV placement is confirmed on the lateral radiograph, repositioning of the lead is indicated.

39. **d.** Patients with evidence of infra-Hisian block during EP testing should be considered for permanent pacing. Patients with symptomatic CHB do not need EP testing because the decision for a permanent pacemaker is already made. The sensitivity and specificity of sinus node recovery time are approximately 70%, making this test less than ideal; in most cases, the decision as to whether to implant a pacemaker in cases of suspected sinus node dysfunction depends on symptoms and correlation with ambulatory monitoring rather than results of EP testing. Patients with infra-Hisian block tend to have an unpredictable course and should be considered for permanent pacing.

40. **a.** It is characterized by ST elevation and a pseudo-RBBB pattern in the right precordial leads with persistent ST elevation. Brugada syndrome has been described worldwide but is most common in Asian countries and is the leading cause of death in young men in part of Thailand. It is characterized by ST-segment elevation and a pseudo-RBBB pattern in the right precordial leads with persistent ST elevation. These features can be induced with sodium channel blockers such as flecainide and ajmaline. (Sotalol is a potassium channel blocker.) It is related to a mutation in the sodium channel gene. Mutations in SCN5A, which encodes the α-subunit of the cardiac sodium channel gene, have been found in up to 30% of families with Brugada syndrome. It is associated with a high incidence of sudden cardiac death resulting from VF. Risk assessment and therapy remain poorly defined at this time, but the implantation of an ICD has been advocated in patient with a Brugada pattern on their ECG and additional risk factors including a history of syncope or sudden cardiac death.

41. **b.** The mechanism of torsades de pointes (TdP) is believed to be related to early afterdepolarization. The pathognomonic arrhythmia associated with long-QT syndrome is TdP. The mechanism is believed to be related to early afterdepolarization and triggered activity. Sotalol causes QT prolongation and is contraindicated in patients with long QT. Hypokalemia, not hyperkalemia, is associated with an increase of TdP in this situation. EP testing is of no value and is not indicated for the risk stratification of patients with long-QT syndrome. Cardiac arrest occurs typically with vigorous activity and infrequently during sleep in LQT1 syndrome. Acute arousal events (emotion or noise) are much more likely to trigger events in LQT1 and LQT2 than LQT3. Events in LQT3 syndrome are common during sleep.

42. **c.** You should perform EP testing to evaluate the AV conduction system. The patient had an episode of near-syncope, which could be related to his GI bleeding, but the possibility of intermittent heart block in the setting of bifascicular block cannot be ruled out. This is a class I indication for EP testing to evaluate AV conduction. If there is evidence of abnormally prolonged HV interval, then a permanent pacemaker should be considered. If the syncopal episode was remote from the GI bleeding and based on the clinical history of the events there was a concern for intermittent high-degree AV block causing symptoms, then empiric placement of a PPM without an EP study prior would carry a class IIa indication. There is no indication for ICD placement in this setting. β-Blockers would blunt a reactive tachycardia resulting from the patient's anemia.

43. **e.** There is AV dissociation. In patients presenting with wide complex tachycardia, the presence of AV dissociation is highly specific for VT. All the other listed parameters suffer from significant overlap between SVT and VT.

44. **c.** Procainamide, 15 mg/kg IV over 30 to 60 minutes. Wide complex tachycardia occurring after MI is most likely to be VT. Verapamil is contraindicated in this setting, as it might lead to hypotension and VF. DC cardioversion can be used if the patient does not respond to antiarrhythmic therapy or if he becomes hemodynamically unstable. Procainamide is the drug of choice because it treats ventricular as well as supraventricular arrhythmia. There is no role for digoxin and no need for urgent cardiac catheterization in this situation.

45. **b.** To admit the patient for IV antibiotics and pacemaker-system extraction. This presentation is consistent with pacemaker-system infection, which occurred following the recent pulse generator replacement. Antibiotics PO or IV without extraction of the pacemaker system have limited efficacy in eradicating the infection. The patient should undergo pacemaker-system extraction, followed by IV antibiotics, until negative blood cultures are obtained. A new pacemaker system can then be implanted on the right side.

46. **c.** Inadequate synchronization may occur with peaked T waves, low-amplitude signal, and malfunctioning pacemakers. Cardioversion is the delivery of electric energy synchronized on the R wave. A synchronized shock should be used in AFib. A nonsynchronized shock may result in VF if they fall near the middle of the T wave when there is a marked dispersion of refractoriness within the ventricle. Improper synchronization may occur in a situation in which more than one peaked signal exists, such as with pacemakers and peaked T waves. On the other hand, a low QRS signal may not synchronize at all. In patients with pacemakers, the pads are positioned at least 3 inches away from the pulse generator to minimize damage. MI and digoxin intake are not contraindications for DC cardioversion as long as digoxin toxicity is not suspected.

47. **d.** Procainamide. Procainamide can slow down conduction across the accessory pathway and potentially converts AFib. Diltiazem (Cardizem) and verapamil

cause hypotension and a reflex increase in sympathetic activation and may result in increased ventricular response and in rare circumstances can lead to VF. Adenosine is of no use in this setting. Lidocaine has little effect on the refractory period of the accessory pathway.

48. **e.** Amiodarone. Amiodarone may allow maintenance of sinus rhythm in patients with AFib and cardiomyopathy. In low doses, the side effects are minimized. Flecainide and disopyramide are not used in patients with cardiomyopathy because of their potential for proarrhythmia and their negative inotropic effects. Verapamil is not effective for maintenance of sinus rhythm. Sotalol might not be tolerated in patients with heart failure and has the potential for proarrhythmia in patients on diuretics prone to hypokalemia.

49. **c.** Digoxin can control the ventricular rate at rest in patients with AFib, but not with exercise. It is as effective as placebo for the acute conversion of AFib and does not help in maintaining NSR.

50. **a.** It may contribute to an increase in the digoxin level. Flecainide (amiodarone, propafenone [Rythmol], and verapamil) can increase digoxin level. Flecainide can regularize and slow the atrial rhythm in patients with AFib and can, therefore, lead to increased ventricular response because of improved conduction of the atrial impulses through the AV node. It is, therefore, important to use an AV nodal blocking agent in patients with AFib treated with flecainide. It is used for AFib as well as flutter; however, it needs to be used with caution in atrial flutter patients, as it may slow the cycle length of the flutter circuit and result in more rapid conduction to the ventricle. There are no definite data on its safety in patients with hypertrophic cardiomyopathy. It is effective for acute conversion as well as maintenance of NSR postconversion.

51. **a.** Change in the atrial refractory period as a result of the surgical manipulation. The occurrence of AFib post-cardiac surgery is believed to be related to shortening of the refractory period of atrial tissue as it recovers from surgical manipulation, cardioplegia, and, potentially, ischemia. This nonuniformity of recovery results in reentry as the mechanism of AFib.

52. **a.** AVNRT. This tracing shows AVNRT. It is a narrow complex tachycardia using the slow pathway of the AV node in the antegrade direction (long AH) and the fast pathway of the AV node in the retrograde direction (short HA). It is unlikely to be orthodromic reentrant tachycardia in which the retrograde limb of the circuit is an accessory pathway, because the QRS-A time is very short (atrium and ventricle are activated almost spontaneously), not long enough to involve ventricular activation as part of the circuit. Because the QRS is narrow, VT is not a likely diagnosis. Idiopathic LV-VT can sometimes be narrow but has an RBBB morphology on the surface ECG.

SUGGESTED READINGS

The Antiarrhythmics Versus Implantable Defibrillators (AVID) Investigators. A comparison of antiarrhythmic-drug therapy with implantable defibrillators in patients resuscitated from near-fatal ventricular arrhythmias. *N Engl J Med.* 1997;337:1576–1583.

Budaj A, Kokowicz P, Smielak-Korombel W, et al. Lack of effect of amiodarone on survival after extensive infarction. Polish Amiodarone Trial. *Coron Artery Dis.* 1996;7:315–319.

Cairns JA, Connolly SJ, Roberts R, et al. Randomised trial of outcome after myocardial infarction in patients with frequent or repetitive ventricular premature depolarisations: CAMIAT. Canadian Amiodarone Myocardial Infarction Arrhythmia Trial Investigators [published erratum appears in *Lancet.* 1997;349(9067):1776]. *Lancet.* 1997;349:675–682.

The Cardiac Arrhythmia Suppression Trial (CAST) Investigators. Preliminary report: effect of encainide and flecainide on mortality in a randomized trial of arrhythmia suppression after myocardial infarction. *N Engl J Med.* 1989;321:406–412.

The Cardiac Arrhythmia Suppression Trial II Investigators. Effect of the antiarrhythmic agent moricizine on survival after myocardial infarction. *N Engl J Med.* 1992;327:227–233.

Connolly SJ, Gent M, Roberts RS, et al. Canadian Implantable Defibrillator Study (CIDS): study design and organization. CIDS Co-Investigators. *Am J Cardiol.* 1993;72:103F–108F.

Connolly SJ, Sheldon R, Roberts RS, et al. The North American Vasovagal Pacemaker Study (VPS). A randomized trial of permanent cardiac pacing for the prevention of vasovagal syncope. *J Am Coll Cardiol.* 1999;33:16–20.

Julian DG, Camm AJ, Frangin G, et al. Randomised trial of effect of amiodarone on mortality in patients with left-ventricular dysfunction after recent myocardial infarction: EMIAT. European Myocardial Infarct Amiodarone Trial Investigators [published erratum appears in *Lancet.* 1997;349(9059):1180 and 1997;349(9067):1776]. *Lancet.* 1997; 349:667–674.

Moller M. DIAMOND antiarrhythmic trials. Danish Investigations of Arrhythmia and Mortality on Dofetilide. *Lancet.* 1996;348: 1597–1598.

Moss AJ, Hall WJ, Cannom DS, et al. Improved survival with an implanted defibrillator in patients with coronary disease at high risk for ventricular arrhythmia. Multicenter Automatic Defibrillator Implantation Trial Investigators. *N Engl J Med.* 1996;335:1933–1940.

Waldo AL, Camm AJ, de Ruyter H, et al. Survival with oral D-sotalol in patients with left ventricular dysfunction after myocardial infarction: rationale, design, and methods (the SWORD trial). *Am J Cardiol.* 1995;75: 1023–1027.

chapter 2

Valvular Heart Disease

Dermot Phelan • Maran Thamilarasan

Case 1

A 60-year-old man presents to the emergency room with complaints of weakness, lethargy, and severe dyspnea. One week prior, his family notes that he complained of chest pressure that lasted for several hours. On physical examination, he appears to be in respiratory distress. Blood pressure (BP) is 80/50 mmHg. Heart rate is 130 bpm. His oxygen saturation is 87% on room air. Chest examination reveals diffuse crackles. Cardiac examination reveals a nondisplaced point of maximum impulse (PMI). Third and fourth heart sounds are heard, as is an apical systolic murmur. No thrill is present. Electrocardiogram reveals inferior Q waves without ST-segment elevation. He is urgently intubated and pressors are started. An intra-aortic balloon pump is placed. A surface echocardiogram reveals a normal-sized left atrium and a mild jet of mitral regurgitation (MR).

1. What test do you perform first?

   a. Cardiac catheterization

   b. Transesophageal echocardiography (TEE)

   c. Right heart catheterization with an oxygen saturation run

   d. Administration of thrombolytic therapy

2. A TEE is performed urgently (Fig. 2.1 shows a 3D view of the mitral valve from above). What is the most likely diagnosis?

   a. Endocarditis involving the mitral valve

   b. Posterior papillary muscle rupture as it has a single blood supply

   c. Anterior papillary muscle rupture as it has a single blood supply

   d. Severe mitral valve prolapse secondary to recent myocardial infarction

Case 2

A 65-year-old woman presents to your office for follow-up of a murmur she was told about several years prior. She denies any symptoms, but is not very active. Her past medical history is significant for hypertension and diabetes, both of which have been well controlled. On examination, she is in no acute distress. BP is 125/75 mmHg, with a resting heart rate of 70 bpm. Lungs are clear. Cardiac examination reveals a displaced PMI. S_1 is soft. S_2 reveals an increased P_2 component. There is a right ventricular (RV) lift. An S_3 is present. There is a grade III/VI holosystolic murmur heard at the apex radiating to the base. She has no peripheral

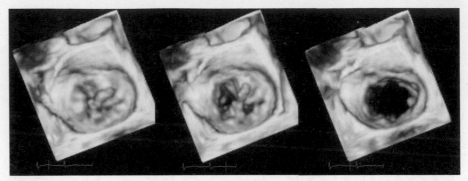

Figure 2.1

edema. Chest X-ray demonstrated cardiomegaly with prominence of the central pulmonary vasculature.

3. An echocardiogram is performed on this patient (Fig. 2.2). Left ventricular (LV) systolic dimension is 4.7 cm. Ejection fraction is 45%. There is posterior leaflet prolapse. There is a very eccentric jet of MR, which is read out as 2+. Which of the following is most likely?

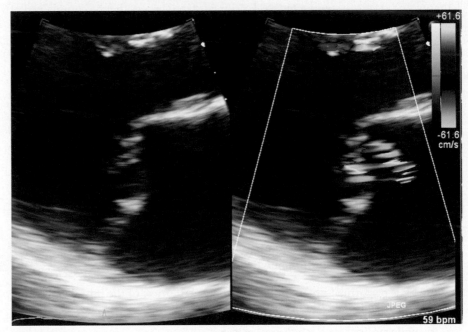

Figure 2.2

    a. MR is unlikely to account for her presentation.

    b. She likely has more severe MR than is evident on the echocardiogram.

    c. Her LV function is better than it appears on the echocardiogram.

    d. TEE is unlikely to be helpful here.

4. What do you recommend next?

    a. Stress echo, to assess LV and PA (pulmonary artery) pressures post stress

    b. Mitral valve surgery

    c. Start an angiotensin-converting enzyme inhibitor (ACEI) and reassess in 3 months

    d. Start a β-blocker

Case 3

A 40-year-old woman is referred to your office for evaluation of a murmur heard during a routine physical examination. She is asymptomatic. She used to jog 2 to 3 miles a day without problems but over the past few years has stopped exercising. She had frequent febrile illnesses as a child, but her past medical history is otherwise unremarkable.

Physical Examination

BP 120/70 mmHg, pulse 73 bpm.

She is in no acute distress.

Jugular venous pulse (JVP) is not elevated.

Chest is clear.

Cardiac—PMI not displaced. Regular rate and rhythm. S_1 is increased in intensity. S_2 is normal. A high-pitched diastolic sound is heard at rest and is heard best between the apex and left sternal border, 0.10 seconds after S_2. This is followed by a low-pitch decrescendo murmur with pre-systolic accentuation.

Abdomen—No organomegaly.

Extremities—No edema. Normal distal pulses. Good capillary refill.

An echocardiogram is performed (Fig. 2.3); proximal flow convergence radius (PFCR) using color 3D across the mitral valve indicates an orifice area of 1.2 cm². Resting PA pressures are 35 mmHg. Splittability score is 5. LV size and function are normal.

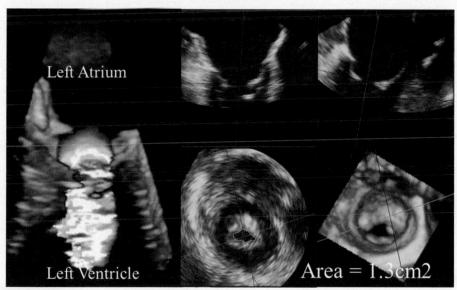

Figure 2.3

5. Which of the following would be the most reasonable next step in management?

    a. Immediate referral for surgery
    b. Immediate referral for percutaneous valvuloplasty
    c. Stress echocardiogram, to assess for mitral pressures post stress
    d. Follow-up in 2 years

6. A stress echocardiogram is performed. Patient exercises for 6 metabolic equivalents (METs). Right ventricular systolic pressure post stress is estimated at 70 mmHg. Which of the following would be an appropriate next step?

a. Consideration for percutaneous valvuloplasty
b. Mitral valve replacement
c. Start β-blocker and return for follow-up in another 2 years
d. Start digoxin

Case 4

A 50-year-old woman presents to you for evaluation. She complains of easy fatigability, as well as abdominal fullness and right upper quadrant pain. She also notes marked swelling in her legs. She has recently been diagnosed with asthma and is also undergoing evaluation for recurrent diarrhea. On examination, she has a BP of 100/60 mmHg. Heart rate is 96 bpm. There is elevation in jugular venous pressure, with a large a wave and a prominent v wave. Lungs are clear. Cardiac examination reveals a nondisplaced PMI. Rhythm is regular. S_1 and S_2 (including P_2) are normal. A diastolic murmur is heard along the sternal border, which increases with inspiration. A pansystolic murmur is also heard in this area. Hepatomegaly is present, along with ascites and peripheral edema.

7. What is the most likely cause of this patient's signs and symptoms?

   a. Rheumatic heart disease
   b. Carcinoid
   c. Primary pulmonary hypertension
   d. Cirrhosis of the liver secondary to chronic hepatitis

Case 5

A 28-year-old man is referred to your office for a second opinion regarding his hypertension. On physical examination, he is in no acute distress. BP is 160/90 mmHg, symmetric in both arms. Pulse rate is 75 bpm. Cardiac examination reveals a nondisplaced PMI. S_1 is normal. It is followed by a high-pitched sound widely transmitted throughout the precordium. A short II/VI systolic ejection murmur is heard. S_2 is normal.

8. What is the most important diagnostic test to perform next?

   a. Check plasma catecholamines.
   b. Check serum potassium level.
   c. Check lower extremity BP.
   d. Check plasma cortisol levels.

Case 6

A 59-year-old man presents for further evaluation of recurrent congestive heart failure. He appears to be in no acute distress on your evaluation. BP is 100/60 mmHg. Carotid upstrokes are weak, but not delayed. Chest examination shows minimal bibasilar rales. PMI is displaced and sustained. A summation gallop is present. There is an increased P_2. There is mild peripheral edema. An echocardiogram reveals a dilated LV with an ejection fraction of 25%. The aortic valve does have some calcification, with restricted leaflet excursion. Peak/mean gradients are 25/15 mmHg. By the continuity equation, the aortic valve area is calculated as 0.7 cm^2.

9. What is your next step?

   a. Immediate referral for aortic valve replacement (AVR)
   b. Referral for cardiac transplant
   c. Dobutamine echocardiogram
   d. Start an ACEI

10. With dobutamine echocardiography, the gradients across the valve increase to 60/40 mmHg, and the calculated valve area stays at 0.7 cm². What do you recommend?

   a. AVR
   b. Continued medical management
   c. Cardiac transplant evaluation
   d. Balloon aortic valvuloplasty

11. Alternatively, how would you interpret the following results: an increase in stroke volume by 5% and an increase in peak/mean gradients to 30/19 mmHg without a significant change in the aortic valve area?

   a. Patient has true severe aortic stenosis (AS) and should proceed to surgery.
   b. Patient has pseudo-AS and should be managed with medical therapy alone.
   c. Patient has a lack of contractile reserve and should be managed with medical therapy alone.
   d. Patient has a lack of contractile reserve but should still be considered for AVR.

Case 7

A 32-year-old man with known bicuspid aortic valve is referred to you for management of aortic insufficiency (AI). He is completely asymptomatic and jogs 3 miles a day as well as doing other aerobic exercise for 30 minutes daily. He has a grade III/VI systolic and diastolic murmur at his left sternal border, a collapsing pulse on examination, and his BP 170/70 mmHg. An echocardiogram reveals a mildly dilated LV (end-diastolic dimension of 6.0 cm) with an ejection fraction of 65%. There is prolapse of the conjoined aortic leaflet with 3 to 4+ insufficiency.

12. What is your recommendation?

   a. Referral for surgery
   b. Addition of vasodilator therapy
   c. Observation for now, return for follow-up in 3 years
   d. Cardiac catheterization

13. What do you tell him is his yearly risk of sudden death?

   a. <1%
   b. 2%
   c. 3% to 5%
   d. >5%

14. The above patient undergoes a gated computed tomography angiography of the thorax (Fig. 2.4), what would you recommend?

   a. Observation with echocardiography every 6 months
   b. Start a β-blocker and reassess in 6 months
   c. Refer to computed tomographic (CT) surgery for surgical replacement of his aortic valve
   d. Referral for surgical intervention to repair or replace his aortic valve and to replace his ascending aorta

Case 8

A 76-year-old woman has been accepted for AVR for severe symptomatic AS. Your opinion is sought by the cardiothoracic surgeon regarding best management of reported concomitant valvular lesions. On review of the echocardiogram you confirm severe AS. In addition, you note a morphologically normal mitral valve, mild

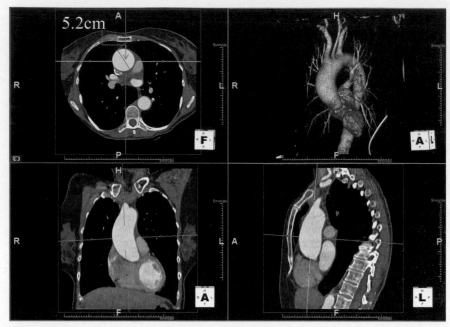

Figure 2.4

MR, and moderate tricuspid regurgitation (TR) associated with annular dilation (45 mm). There is also mild pulmonary hypertension.

15. What do you recommend?

    a. AVR alone

    b. AVR with mitral and tricuspid valve repair

    c. AVR with tricuspid valve replacement

    d. AVR with tricuspid valve repair if feasible

    e. AVR and mitral valve repair alone

Case 9

A 46-year-old woman with chronic obstructive pulmonary disease is referred by her pulmonologist for evaluation of a murmur and concern that her symptoms of shortness of breath with moderate exertion may be related to severe MR diagnosed on an outside echocardiogram. On examination, her body mass index is 19 kg/m^2, BP is 130/75 mmHg, and her heart rate is 75 bpm and regular. Her apex beat is nondisplaced. On auscultation, S$_1$ and S$_2$ are normal; there is a mid-systolic click with a grade IV/VI late systolic murmur heard best at the apex. An echocardiogram is performed (Fig. 2.5A).

16. Assuming an aliasing velocity of 40 cm/s and an MR V_{max} of 5 m/s, based on the PFCR seen here, what is the estimated effective regurgitant orifice area (EROA)?

    a. 0.4 cm^2

    b. 0.45 cm^2

    c. 0.18 cm^2

    d. Not enough information to calculate an EROA

17. A continuous-wave signal is provided through the mitral valve (Fig. 2.5B); based on the data provided how would you classify this MR?

    a. 1+, mild

    b. 2+, moderate

    c. 3+, moderately severe

    d. 4+, severe

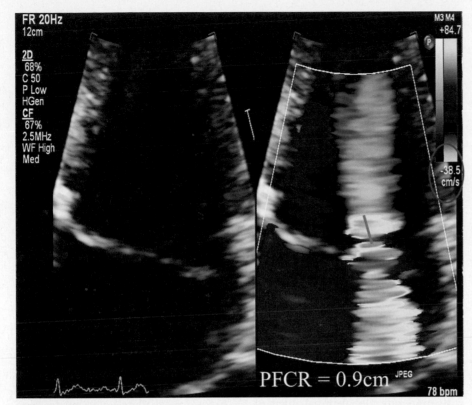

Figure 2.5A

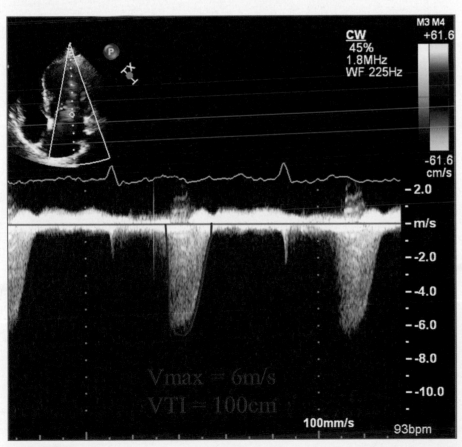

Figure 2.5B

Case 10

A 45-year-old man with rheumatic mitral stenosis presents for further evaluation. In the past 2 to 3 years, he has noted progressive dyspnea with less than moderate activity. He was started on a β-blocker 1 year ago, but remains symptomatic. Echocardiogram reveals a mean mitral gradient of 4 mmHg with a valve area of 1.6 cm². As there was a discrepancy between the degree of symptoms and resting hemodynamics you proceed to a stress echocardiogram that revealed a post stress PA pressure of 70 mmHg and a mean transmitral gradient of 17 mmHg. You decide to send this patient for percutaneous intervention.

18. What is the most appropriate test to order at the time of or prior to the valvuloplasty procedure?

    a. Transesophageal echocardiogram

    b. 24-Hour electrocardiographic monitoring to assess for paroxysmal atrial fibrillation

    c. Cardiac CT to assess for aortic calcification

    d. Stress nuclear perfusion study

Case 11

A 65-year-old man is referred to you for evaluation of a heart murmur. He denies any symptoms at this time. On physical examination, he is in no acute distress. BP is 135/75 mmHg; pulse is 82 bpm and regular. Carotid upstrokes are diminished. The PMI is sustained and displaced. A$_2$ is soft. A late-peaking systolic murmur is heard at the base. You order an echocardiogram. This reveals LV hypertrophy with moderate global impairment of LV function, calculated ejection fraction of 35%. There is severe calcific AS, with peak/mean gradients of 75/45 mmHg. Aortic valve area is 0.5 cm².

19. What is the role of AVR in this setting?

    a. It is absolutely indicated.

    b. It is absolutely not recommended.

    c. There is some evidence/opinion that would favor valve replacement.

    d. Dobutamine echocardiography is needed to determine whether this is truly severe AS.

Case 12

A 76-year-old woman is referred to your clinic with recent onset of exertional chest pain. She has a long-standing history of hypertension and atrial fibrillation. On examination, her body surface area is 2.0 m², BP is 150/100 mmHg, and heart rate is 80 to 90 bpm and irregular. The carotid upstroke is delayed and diminished. The apex beat is nondisplaced but sustained. S$_1$ is normal, and S$_2$ is soft and paradoxically split. There is a grade II/VI ejection systolic murmur heard best at the right upper sternal border that radiates to the carotids. An echocardiogram reports normal ejection fraction with a stroke volume of 55 mL. The peak and mean gradients across the aortic valve are 44/28 mmHg. The dimensionless index is 0.21 and the calculated aortic valve area is 0.83 cm². You review the echocardiogram (Fig. 2.6) and confirm the accuracy of the left ventricular outflow tract (LVOT) diameter and are satisfied that multiple windows were used to obtain the gradients.

20. Which of the following statements is *true*?

    a. The patient has moderate AS confirmed by gradients across the valve and should be followed up in 6 months with a repeat echocardiogram.

    b. The echocardiogram shows inconsistent data and should be repeated.

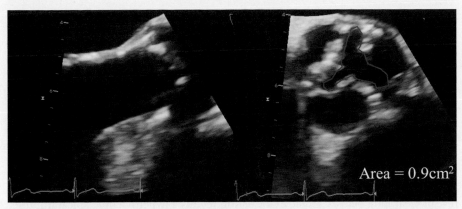

Area = 0.9cm²

Figure 2.6

c. This is a definite contraindication to AVR.

d. The rate of mortality, for a patient with these findings, is higher compared with patients with severe AS and high gradients across the aortic valve, but aortic valve surgery has resulted in better outcomes in these patients.

Case 13

A 75-year-old man is referred to you for evaluation of aortic regurgitation. He has no symptoms at this time. His past medical history is significant only for hypertension. On physical examination, he is in no acute distress. BP is 170/60 mmHg. Arterial pulses are brisk. A bisferiens pulse is noted in the brachial artery. The apical impulse is displaced and hyperdynamic. S_1 is not loud, and no opening snap is heard. A high-frequency holodiastolic murmur is heard, loudest along the right sternal border. A late diastolic apical rumble is heard as well.

21. You order an echocardiogram. Which of the following are you most concerned about?

a. Aortic valve commissural anatomy

b. Degree of AI

c. Aortic root dimension

d. Mitral valve

22. The above patient returns for follow-up 6 months later. He now reports symptoms of marked exertional dyspnea. An echocardiogram is read as 2+ central aortic regurgitation, with an LV end-diastolic dimension of 6.9 cm and an ejection fraction of 50%. What do you do next?

a. Cardiac catheterization with aortography

b. Start an ACEI, reassess in 6 months

c. Continue observation

d. Start a β-blocker, reassess in 6 months

Case 14

A 56-year-old man presents to the emergency room with the sudden onset of chest pain. He is tachypneic on presentation. O_2 saturation is 82% on room air. BP is 80/60 mmHg. Heart rate is 125 bpm. Lung examination reveals diffuse bilateral crackles. Cardiac examination reveals a nondisplaced PMI. S_1 is soft. P_2 is loud. An S_3 is present. A short decrescendo diastolic murmur is heard at the upper sternal border. Extremities are cool. Electrocardiogram reveals inferior ST-segment elevation. He is promptly intubated, and pressors are started. A brief echocardiogram is performed at the bedside. The study is difficult, but reveals premature closure of the mitral valve. There is hypokinesis of the inferoposterior walls.

23. Which of the following would be your next course of action?

a. Transesophageal echocardiogram, emergent cardiac surgical consultation

b. Intra-aortic balloon pump to stabilize hemodynamics, followed by emergent angiography

c. Administer thrombolytics

d. Send patient for magnetic resonance imaging (MRI)

Case 15

A 77-year-old patient is admitted to the hospital for urosepsis. His past medical history is significant only for having undergone AVR 5 years prior. On examination, he is febrile to 102°F. Heart rate is 106 bpm. Carotid upstrokes are full. Chest examination reveals clear lung fields. Cardiac examination reveals a hyperdynamic apical impulse, which is not displaced. S_1 and S_2 are normal. An early-peaking systolic murmur is heard at the sternal border. No diastolic murmur is heard. An echocardiogram is performed. Peak/mean gradients are 50/30 mmHg. LVOT VTI (velocity time integral) is 36 cm and aortic valve VTI is 78 cm. The aortic valve itself is not well seen. Flow in the descending thoracic aorta is normal. An echocardiogram 2 years prior had revealed peak/mean gradients of 24/12 mmHg. LVOT VTI was 19 cm and aortic valve VTI 41 cm.

24. What do you conclude about prosthetic aortic valve function?

a. He has prosthetic valve stenosis

b. No evidence for dysfunction

c. He has severe prosthetic valve regurgitation

d. He likely has endocarditis

25. The above patient remains febrile despite 1 week of antibiotic therapy. Electrocardiogram reveals a new long first-degree atrioventricular (AV) block. The patient becomes progressively dyspneic. A short, regurgitant murmur is heard. What do you recommend?

a. TEE with surgical consultation

b. TEE

c. Change antibiotic regimen

d. Monitor closely with daily electrocardiogram

Case 16

A 56-year-old man with mitral stenosis presents for evaluation. He has NYHA class II-III shortness of breath.

Physical Examination

He is in no acute distress.

JVP is mildly elevated.

Pulse is regular at 80 bpm.

Chest is clear.

Cardiac: Nondisplaced PMI. Opening snap heard 0.09 milliseconds after S_2. Long diastolic rumble. No peripheral edema.

Echocardiogram reveals a planimetered mitral valve area of 1.2 cm². Mean gradient 10 mmHg. Pressure half-time of 185 milliseconds.

He undergoes percutaneous valvuloplasty. The following morning, on examination, you note that he is comfortable. His oxygen saturation is 100% on room air. Opening snap is 0.12 milliseconds after S_2. A shorter decrescendo diastolic rumble is heard. You obtain a predischarge echocardiogram. The report indicates a pressure half-time of 180 milliseconds.

26. What do you do next based on the echocardiogram?

   a. There was a less-than-optimal result from the valvuloplasty. No significant change in mitral valve area was achieved. You plan to send him for another procedure or surgery.

   b. There was an error in half-time measurement. You order a repeat assessment of pressure half-time later that day.

   c. Repeat echocardiogram with planimetry of mitral valve area.

   d. Consider TEE to see the valve opening better.

27. The echocardiogram reveals a small left-to-right shunt at the atrial level by color. What do you recommend?

   a. Observation

   b. Referral for percutaneous closure

   c. Referral for surgical closure

   d. Indefinite anticoagulation

Case 17

An 80-year-old man underwent successful AVR with a bioprosthetic valve 4 months ago. He presents to your office for a routine follow-up visit. He is asymptomatic. He is in sinus rhythm. Echocardiogram reveals a normally functioning prosthetic valve. Chamber dimensions are normal with normal biventricular function. He has no clinical history of embolic events.

28. Which of the following should you recommend?

   a. Antibiotic prophylaxis, office visits if he feels unwell

   b. Antibiotic prophylaxis, with yearly office visits

   c. Warfarin therapy indefinitely

   d. Clopidogrel therapy indefinitely

Case 18

A 28-year-old 20-week pregnant woman is referred to your clinic after being diagnosed with mitral valve prolapse and severe MR on an echocardiogram ordered by her obstetrician. She reports no symptoms prior to pregnancy but since being told her diagnosis is extremely worried and has noticed some shortness of breath on exertion (New York Heart Association [NYHA] class II). She is clinically euvolemic.

29. What do you recommend?

   a. Antibiotics at the time of delivery

   b. Commence afterload reduction with an ACEI given her new onset symptoms

   c. Refer to an experienced surgeon for consideration for mitral valve repair as there is a high likelihood of successful durable repair

   d. Commence afterload reduction with diuretics and hydralazine

   e. No therapy at present but follow carefully with serial clinical and echo evaluation

Case 19

A 67-year-old woman is referred to your office for evaluation of a heart murmur. She describes symptoms of significant and limiting exertional dyspnea. On examination, she is normotensive. Pulse rate is 67 bpm and regular. Cardiac examination reveals a sustained but nondisplaced PMI. S_1 and S_2 are normal. An S_4 is present. A loud III/VI systolic ejection murmur is heard throughout the precordium. Carotid upstrokes are delayed and diminished. An echocardiogram is performed (Fig. 2.7); continuous-wave Doppler evaluation reveals a 4.5-m/s jet across the LVOT.

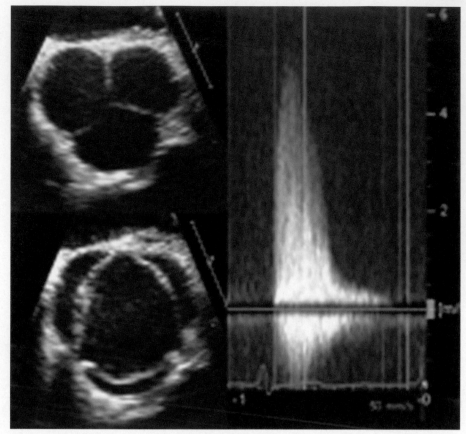

Figure 2.7

30. Which of the following would you do next to arrive at a diagnosis?

  a. TEE

  b. Repeat echocardiogram with amyl nitrate

  c. Stress echocardiogram

  d. Dobutamine echocardiogram

  e. The Pedoff probe has picked up an MR signal, the MR appears mild on all other views, no need for further investigation

Case 20

A 30-year-old woman presents to your office for a routine physical examination. She is asymptomatic. BP is 95/65 mmHg, with a resting heart rate of 65 bpm. Physical examination is remarkable for a mild pectus deformity. On cardiac auscultation, a mid-systolic click is heard. The click is heard earlier in systole with standing, and later in systole with squatting. No murmur is heard at rest, but a soft systolic murmur becomes audible with dynamic maneuvers.

31. Echocardiography demonstrates no high-risk features. What is the role of aspirin therapy in such patients who have had no evidence of embolic events?

  a. Should be prescribed to all patients

  b. May play a role, if a murmur is heard

  c. There is no clear role for aspirin therapy in such patients

Case 21

A 50-year-old man with severe AI is referred to you for a second opinion. He is asymptomatic. An echocardiogram reveals a mildly dilated LV (end-diastolic dimension of 6.2 cm and end-systolic dimension of 3.5 cm) with a normal ejection fraction.

He has already undergone a stress echocardiogram. He exercised for 14 METs. No symptoms or electrocardiographic changes were noted. Resting ejection fraction was calculated at 65%. Post stress, the ejection fraction is 60%. No segmental wall motion abnormalities were seen.

32. What do you recommend?

  a. Surgical intervention

  b. Continue with vasodilator therapy and reassess in 6 months

  c. Cardiac catheterization

  d. Stress nuclear ventriculogram

Case 22

A 70-year-old man presents to your office with complaints of exertional dyspnea. He is mildly hypertensive on examination. Carotid upstrokes are brisk, with a secondary upstroke. A loud III/VI systolic murmur is heard along the sternal border radiating to the neck. S_1 and S_2 are normal. An S_4 is heard. The murmur increases in intensity with Valsalva and decreases with handgrip.

33. An echocardiogram reveals a <2-m/s jet across the LVOT. What is your next step?

  a. Repeat the echocardiogram, but have Doppler interrogation performed in other views and with a nonimaging transducer. The degree of AS has been underestimated

  b. Repeat the echocardiogram with amyl nitrate

  c. Transesophageal echocardiogram to better assess the valves

  d. Coronary angiography

Case 23

A 26-year-old woman with a history of hypertrophic obstructive cardiomyopathy is referred for consideration for septal myectomy. She has NYHA class III dyspnea on exertion despite maximal medical therapy. On echocardiography, there is severe asymmetric septal hypertrophy with severe systolic anterior motion of the mitral valve. There is a late-peaking gradient across the LVOT of 60 mmHg, which increased to 105 mmHg with Valsalva. She has a structurally normal mitral valve on cardiac MRI with moderately severe posteriorly directed MR (Fig. 2.8).

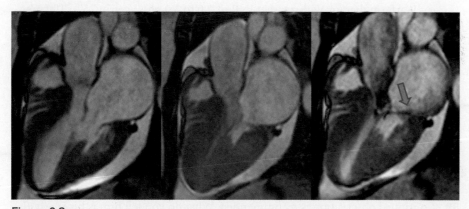

Figure 2.8

34. What would you advise her regarding surgery?

  a. She will probably require mitral valve replacement at the time of surgery.

  b. She will probably require mitral valve repair during surgery.

  c. She will probably not need surgery on her mitral valve.

  d. She may need plication of her papillary muscles.

Case 24

A 62-year-old man with a history of rheumatic heart disease presents to your office with complaints of exertional dyspnea. No constitutional complaints are present. He had undergone a mitral valve replacement with a bileaflet tilting disk mechanical valve 11 years prior. He is normotensive with a heart rate of 73 bpm. On examination, you note a grade II/VI holosystolic murmur at the apex. An echocardiogram is performed, which reveals normal LV and RV function. Peak mitral gradient is 30 mmHg. Mean transmitral gradient is 7 mmHg. Pressure half-time is 80 milliseconds.

35. What is your next diagnostic step?

    a. Fluoroscopy of the valve

    b. Transesophageal echocardiogram

    c. Invasive assessment of hemodynamics

    d. Draw blood cultures

36. Which of the following would be the expected physical findings in this patient if the valve were functioning normally?

    a. Prominent closing click, soft and brief diastolic rumble

    b. Prominent opening and closing clicks, soft and brief diastolic rumble

    c. Prominent opening click, long diastolic rumble

    d. Prominent closing click, systolic murmur

37. If the patient had a ball-and-cage valve instead, what would you expect to hear?

    a. Prominent closing click, soft and brief diastolic rumble

    b. Prominent opening and closing clicks, soft and brief diastolic rumble

    c. Prominent opening click, long diastolic rumble

    d. Prominent closing click, systolic murmur

38. Recommended antithrombotic therapy for a patient with a mechanical mitral valve replacement without a prior thromboembolic event or other high-risk features is

    a. Warfarin therapy with a target international normalized ratio (INR) of 3.0 to 4.0

    b. Warfarin therapy with a target INR of 2.5 to 3.5

    c. Warfarin therapy with a target INR of 2.0 to 3.0 plus aspirin 75 to 100 mg

    d. Warfarin therapy with a target INR of 2.5 to 3.5 plus aspirin 300 mg

    e. Warfarin therapy with a target INR of 2.5 to 3.5 plus aspirin 75 to 100 mg

Case 25

A 65-year-old man presents to your office for evaluation of valvular heart disease. He is asymptomatic. He walks 5 miles a day without difficulty. An echocardiogram reveals severe AS, with a maximum aortic jet velocity of 4.7 m/s by Doppler echocardiography. LV systolic function is preserved. There is mild LV hypertrophy (wall thickness 1.4 cm). He walks on a treadmill for 9 minutes, with a normal hemodynamic response.

39. Continued observation is recommended. What do you tell him is his yearly risk of sudden death, provided he remains asymptomatic?

    a. <2%

    b. 5%

    c. 5% to 10%

    d. >10%

40. What is the likelihood that he will become symptomatic, or come to surgery, within the next 3 years?

   a. 10%
   b. 10% to 25%
   c. 25% to 50%
   d. >50%

Case 26

A 52-year-old man who previously underwent AVR with a tilting disk valve presents to you several months following a documented transient ischemic attack (TIA). He has no symptoms at present. Workup at the time of his TIA included carotid Dopplers, and transthoracic and transesophageal echocardiogram. These were unremarkable. The valve was well seated and was functioning normally. No thrombus was seen. Only minimal aortic atheroma was seen. No intracardiac shunt was identified. He has been on warfarin throughout and has maintained an INR between 2 and 3. INR was 2.2 at the time of his TIA. On examination, he is in no acute distress. BP is 120/80 mmHg; pulse is 68 and regular. Carotid upstrokes are full and not delayed. Crisp valve closure sound is heard along with a short, early-peaking systolic ejection murmur at the base. No S_3 is heard. P_2 is normal. No peripheral edema is noted.

41. Which of the following would you recommend?

   a. Start ASA (acetylsalicylic acid), 325 mg/day.
   b. Increase warfarin, to achieve an INR of 3.5 to 4.5.
   c. Increase warfarin, to achieve an INR of 4.0 to 5.0.
   d. Start ASA, 81 mg/day, and increase warfarin, to achieve an INR of 2.5 to 3.5.

42. If his transesophageal study had revealed a small (1 to 2 mm) echodensity on the valve strut—suggestive of thrombus—but no obstruction to valve function, what should have been done?

   a. Intravenous heparin
   b. Bolus thrombolytic therapy
   c. Reoperation
   d. Intravenous IIb/IIIa inhibitors

Case 27

You are following a 50-year-old man with moderate mitral stenosis, who had been asymptomatic. He presents to the emergency room with complaints of mild exertional dyspnea and palpitations, present for the past 3 to 4 days. On arrival, he appears comfortable, with an O_2 saturation of 99% on room air. His pulse rate is 140 bpm and irregular. BP is 130/75 mmHg. Electrocardiogram reveals atrial fibrillation.

43. The above patient spontaneously converts to sinus rhythm. Which of the following are you *most* likely to recommend?

   a. Therapy with warfarin
   b. Percutaneous valvuloplasty
   c. Mitral valve replacement
   d. No change in therapy

Case 28

A 34-year-old woman presents to your office for evaluation because she had been on treatment with anorectic agents 5 years ago. She is asymptomatic at this time. She is now at her ideal body weight. On examination, she is in no acute distress. BP is 107/68 mmHg. Jugular venous pulsations appear normal. Chest is clear. Cardiac examination reveals a nondisplaced PMI. S_1 and S_2 are normal, with an appropriate physiologic split of S_2. P_2 is not loud. No S_3 or S_4 is heard. Auscultation is performed with the patient sitting, supine, and in the left lateral decubitus position. No murmur is heard.

44. What do you *most* likely recommend for this patient?

    a. Reassurance, with a repeat physical examination in 6 months

    b. Echocardiogram

    c. Stress test

    d. TEE

Case 29

A 50-year-old man presents for his first physical examination in several years. He notes that a murmur had been documented a number of years ago. He is entirely asymptomatic. On examination, he has a BP of 120/70 mmHg with a pulse rate of 58 bpm. Neck veins are not distended. Carotid upstrokes are brisk. Lungs are clear. Cardiac examination reveals a nondisplaced PMI. S_1 is soft; S_2 is normal (with a preserved A_2). An S_3 is heard. A III/VI holosystolic murmur is heard at the apex radiating to the base and carotids, which increases with handgrip.

Echocardiogram reveals myxomatous mitral valve disease with posterior leaflet prolapse and severe MR. The prolapse involves the P_2 (middle) segment and is severe. There is no calcification of the valve. End-systolic dimension is 3.0 cm; end-diastolic dimension is 5.6 cm. Ejection fraction is 65%. TR velocity is 2.9 m/s.

45. Which of the following would be most appropriate at this time?

    a. Referral for mitral valve replacement

    b. Consider elective mitral valve repair at a hospital where repair is performed with a high degree of success or if he wishes to defer surgery, follow up at 6 monthly intervals with echo

    c. The addition of an ACEI and follow-up in 2 years

    d. The addition of amiodarone to prevent atrial fibrillation

    e. Follow-up in 2 years without an echocardiogram

46. The above patient agrees to close medical follow-up. However, he does not present back to your office until 2 years later, now with complaints of dyspnea. A repeat echocardiogram reveals an ejection fraction of 45% with an end-systolic dimension of 4.7 cm. What do you recommend?

    a. Referral for mitral valve repair

    b. Start an ACEI and reassess in 3 months

    c. Mitral valve replacement

    d. Start a β-blocker and reassess in 3 months

Case 30

An 80-year-old man with severe AS is turned down for surgical AVR due to significant comorbidities. He is referred to you for consideration for transcatheter AVR.

47. Which of the following findings is considered a contraindication for this procedure?

    a. Calcified and tortuous femoral arteries

    b. The apex is not accessible

    c. Life expectancy <1 year

    d. A history of treated endocarditis

    e. Annulus size of 20 mm

Case 31

A 35-year-old man presents to your office for evaluation of valvular heart disease. He complains of shortness of breath with only modest amounts of exertion, as well as two-pillow orthopnea. He also complains of easy fatigability, as well as lower extremity edema and abdominal fullness. On examination, he is in no acute distress. He is normotensive. Jugular venous pressure is elevated, with a prominent *a* wave. The *v* wave is not easily discerned. S_1 is loud. S_2 is normal. A sound is heard in diastole, 0.07 milliseconds after S_2. A diastolic rumble is heard at the apex. A diastolic murmur is also heard along the left sternal border, which increases with inspiration. Mild hepatomegaly is present. There is 2+ peripheral edema.

48. What is your diagnosis?

a. Mitral stenosis

b. Mitral stenosis with tricuspid insufficiency

c. Mitral and tricuspid stenosis

d. Mitral stenosis and AS

e. Tricuspid stenosis

Case 32

An 80-year-old man presents to your office with complaints of chest tightness when climbing up a flight of stairs. His past medical history is unremarkable. On physical examination, he is in no acute distress. BP is 140/80 mmHg; pulse is 78 bpm and regular. Chest is clear. Carotid upstrokes are diminished. The PMI is sustained, but not displaced. A fourth heart sound is present. The second heart sound is diminished and single. A loud late-peaking systolic murmur is heard, loudest at the second intercostal space, radiating to the neck.

49. Which of the following would be a reasonable next step in this patient's management?

a. Stress sestamibi

b. Stress electrocardiogram

c. Cardiac catheterization

d. Prescribe prn SL (sublingual) NTG (nitroglycerin) and review back in one week

50. The above patient is found to have an aortic valve area of 0.7 cm² with a mean gradient of 60 mmHg. Following catheterization, he develops massive upper gastrointestinal bleeding. Endoscopy reveals a gastric ulcer with a bleeding vessel at its base. Cauterization is performed, which temporarily stops the bleeding. However, the bleeding recurs and urgent partial gastrectomy is recommended. He complains of chest pain during these bleeding episodes. What is the best course of action?

a. Proceed to AVR first.

b. Refer for percutaneous balloon valvuloplasty, followed by gastrectomy.

c. Start nitroprusside and proceed with gastric surgery.

d. Proceed with gastric surgery directly.

51. What valve would you recommend to an 80-year-old patient with severe symptomatic AS?

a. Bovine pericardial valve

b. Ball-and-cage mechanical valve

c. Bileaflet mechanical valve

d. Aortic homograft

Case 33

A 28-year-old man presents for evaluation of difficult to control hypertension. He initially denies any symptoms but on further questioning admits to some leg fatigue and weakness and cold feet. On examination his BP is 180/90 mmHg, heart rate is 77 bpm and regular. His radial pulses are easily palpable but his femoral pulses are weak and there is radiofemoral delay. An ejection systolic murmur is heard at the left upper sternal border that radiates to the intrascapular region. In addition, there is a soft continuous murmur heard throughout the precordium.

52. Based on your suspicion you order a CT aorta (Fig. 2.9). What is the most common associated lesion?

   a. ~5% of cases have a bicuspid aortic valve.

   b. ~50% of cases have mitral valve prolapse.

   c. ~50% of cases have a bicuspid aortic valve.

   d. ~5% of cases have an associated cleft mitral valve.

   e. This lesion is rarely associated with concomitant cardiac abnormalities.

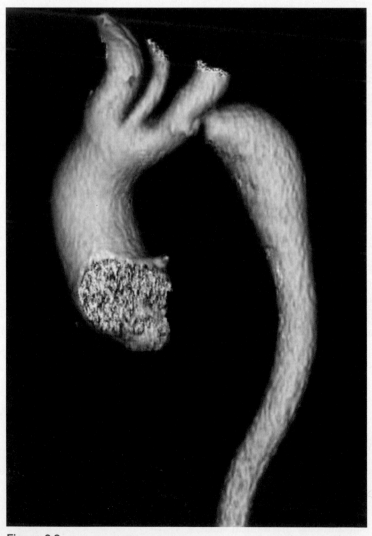

Figure 2.9

Case 34

A 65-year-old man with a history of rheumatoid arthritis (well controlled) presents for evaluation of a heart murmur. He notes some increase in fatigue and decrease in activity level over the past 2 years, but denies any specific complaints of dyspnea. He leads a rather sedentary lifestyle. On examination, he is 6-ft, 1-in. tall. BP is 150/50 mmHg. Heart rate is 80 bpm and regular. Carotid upstrokes are brisk with a rapid upstroke and decline. Apical impulse is displaced and hyperdynamic. S_1 and S_2 are normal. A decrescendo, nearly holodiastolic murmur is heard along the left sternal border, loudest with the patient sitting up. An echocardiogram is performed, which reveals a dilated LV (end-diastolic dimension of 6.8 cm and end-systolic dimension of 3.5 cm). Ejection fraction is 55%. There is significant aortic regurgitation.

53. What do you most likely recommend?

  a. Stress test

  b. Reassess with repeat echocardiogram in 6 months

  c. Start vasodilator therapy and reassess in 2 years

  d. Refer to surgery

54. He is started on a vasodilator and is seen back in 6 months. He reports no change in symptoms. A repeat echocardiogram demonstrates an end-diastolic dimension of 7.6 cm. Ejection fraction remains normal. What do you recommend now?

  a. Stress test

  b. Surgical intervention

  c. Increase vasodilators and reassess in 6 months

  d. MRI to assess LV volumes

Case 35

A 42-year-old woman, who underwent mitral valve replacement with a bileaflet tilting disk valve for rheumatic disease, presents to the emergency room with complaints of severe dyspnea. On examination, she has a BP of 120/60 mmHg. Heart rate is 83 bpm. Chest reveals bilateral crackles, one-third up. Cardiac examination reveals a nondisplaced PMI. Prosthetic clicks are muffled. A long diastolic rumble is heard at the apex. Her past medical history is otherwise unremarkable.

55. An echocardiogram is ordered on the above patient. Which of the following would you expect to see?

  a. Severe MR

  b. Mean gradient across the mitral prosthesis of 17 mmHg

  c. Pressure half-time of 80 milliseconds

  d. Ejection fraction of 20%

Case 36

A 26-year-old woman presents to your office for evaluation. She was told she had a murmur many years ago. She has a history of palpitations, but is otherwise asymptomatic. On examination, she is in no acute distress. Prominent v waves are noted in the JVP. Carotid upstrokes are normal. Chest is clear to auscultation. Cardiac examination reveals a nondisplaced PMI. Auscultation reveals a widely split first heart sound, with a loud second component that sounds like a click. A holosystolic murmur is heard at the right sternal border, which increases with inspiration. Hepatomegaly is present. An echocardiogram is performed (Fig. 2.10).

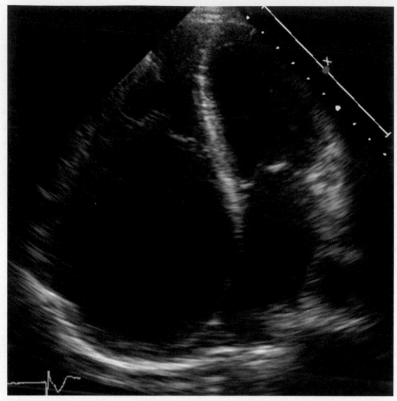

Figure 2.10

56. What is the most likely cause for her palpitations?

    a. Arrhythmias secondary to an accessory pathway

    b. AV nodal reentrant tachycardia

    c. Ventricular tachycardia

    d. Atrial fibrillation

    e. Anxiety

57. No intervention is performed for the above patient. She returns to your clinic 3 months later. She describes an episode of transient word-finding difficulty, which lasted for a number of seconds. This occurred while she was recovering from a fractured tibia. A CT scan was performed, which was negative. She is concerned that she may have a recurrence. What is the most appropriate next test for her?

    a. Echocardiography with saline contrast study

    b. Carotid Dopplers

    c. 24-hour ambulatory electrocardiographic monitoring

    d. Right heart catheterization with oxygen saturation run

Case 37

A 21-year-old man presents to your office for evaluation. He tells you that a murmur was noted a few days after birth. He is presently asymptomatic. On examination, he is normotensive. Pulse is 65 bpm and regular. Carotid upstrokes are normal. Chest is clear. Cardiac examination reveals a nondisplaced PMI. An RV lift is present. A systolic thrill is present in the suprasternal notch. A high-pitched sound is heard after S_1. A crescendo–decrescendo systolic murmur is heard at the left second intercostal space. A_2 is normal.

58. Which of the following would you expect to find on echocardiography?

    a. V_{max} across the aortic valve of 4 m/s

    b. V_{max} across the pulmonic valve of 4 m/s

c. A wide jet of mitral insufficiency

d. Flow reversal in the hepatic veins

59. The above patient returns 1 year later for follow-up. Which of the following is a definite indication for intervention?

   a. He tells you of an episode of syncope

   b. No symptoms, but RV to PA peak gradient of 30 to 39 mmHg

   c. No symptoms, but RV to PA peak gradient of 20 to 29 mmHg

   d. He has occasional feelings that his heart has extra beats

60. If intervention is recommended, what is the preferred treatment approach?

   a. Percutaneous valvuloplasty

   b. Ross procedure

   c. Mechanical valve

   d. Bioprosthetic valve

61. In the setting of AS with moderate insufficiency, which of the following methods would provide the most accurate estimate of aortic valve narrowing?

   a. Invasive hemodynamics, using the Gorlin formula

   b. Doppler echocardiography, using the continuity equation

   c. Pressure half-time

   d. Bernoulli equation

62. Which of the following valves has the lowest incidence of endocarditis?

   a. Mechanical valve

   b. Bioprosthetic valve

   c. Aortic homograft

   d. Stentless mitral valve

63. What is the most common cause of TR in an adult population?

   a. Rheumatic tricuspid disease

   b. Carcinoid

   c. Congenital abnormalities

   d. Pulmonary hypertension resulting from primary left-sided disease

   e. Myxomatous disease of the tricuspid valve

64. The most common organism seen in native valve endocarditis is what?

   a. *Streptococcus viridans*

   b. *Enterobacter faecalis*

   c. *Staphylococcus aureus*

   d. *Chlamydia pneumoniae*

   e. HACEK organisms

65. A patient presents with systemic embolic events 1 month after uncomplicated mitral valve replacement. He has been febrile for the past week. TEE demonstrates multiple echodensities on the valve ring. Blood cultures that are drawn are most likely to grow which of the following?

   a. *Streptococcus viridans*

   b. *Staphylococcus aureus*

   c. *Staphylococcus epidermidis*

   d. *E. faecalis*

   e. *Candida albicans*

ANSWERS

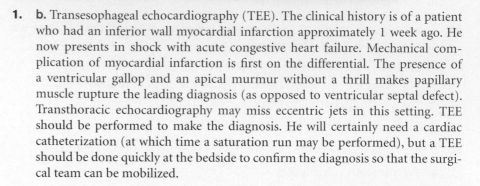

1. **b.** Transesophageal echocardiography (TEE). The clinical history is of a patient who had an inferior wall myocardial infarction approximately 1 week ago. He now presents in shock with acute congestive heart failure. Mechanical complication of myocardial infarction is first on the differential. The presence of a ventricular gallop and an apical murmur without a thrill makes papillary muscle rupture the leading diagnosis (as opposed to ventricular septal defect). Transthoracic echocardiography may miss eccentric jets in this setting. TEE should be performed to make the diagnosis. He will certainly need a cardiac catheterization (at which time a saturation run may be performed), but a TEE should be done quickly at the bedside to confirm the diagnosis so that the surgical team can be mobilized.

2. **b.** Posterior papillary muscle rupture as it has a single blood supply. The 3D reconstruction of the mitral valve shown here is orientated in the "surgeons view," looking down on the mitral valve from the left atrium with the aortic valve situated on top, the anterior mitral valve leaflet adjacent to it, and the posterior mitral valve leaflet inferiorly. We see a bulky mass (the posterior papillary muscle) protruding into the left atrium in systole. The middle panel (early diastole) clearly shows that the mass is attached to the posterior leaflet. The posterior papillary muscle has a single blood supply (usually the right coronary artery), while the anterior papillary muscle often has dual blood supply. For this reason, post infarction rupture of the posterior papillary muscle is more common.

3. **b.** She likely has more severe MR than is evident on the echocardiogram. Her examination is suggestive of severe MR. The echo confirms LV dilation and mitral leaflet pathology, which could be consistent. The eccentric nature of the jet suggests that it may have been underestimated by transthoracic imaging. A more definitive imaging procedure such as TEE will be helpful here.

4. **b.** Mitral valve surgery. The presence of mild LV dysfunction with LV dilation is a class I indication for surgery. TEE would be the next test of choice prior to surgery to confirm the severity and mechanism of MR and assess suitability for surgical repair. While exercise echo is reasonable in asymptomatic patients with severe MR to assess functional capacity the patient already has indications for surgery.

5. **c.** Stress echocardiogram, to assess for mitral pressures post stress. She has moderate mitral stenosis. The fact that she has stopped exercising may be a clue to the onset of symptoms. An assessment of functional capacity and post-stress mitral pressures would be useful in management There are insufficient data for immediate referral for intervention. Follow-up in a short period of time may not be unreasonable; however, 2 years is too long a period.

6. **a.** Consideration for percutaneous valvuloplasty. Her functional capacity is below average for her age. Her valve is favorable for percutaneous valvuloplasty (splittability score of 6) and she had a significant rise in PA pressures post stress. Ideally, the splittability index should be 8 or less for optimal results post balloon valvuloplasty. A increase in mean valve gradient of 15 mmHg with exercise is a class I indication by the American College of Cardiology (ACC)/American Heart Association (AHA) guidelines. A β-blocker would not be an unreasonable addition, but she should be followed more frequently than every 2 years. In addition, she does have class I indication for intervention. She has normal LV function and is in sinus rhythm—there is no role for digoxin in this setting. Valve replacement is considered only if the valve is deemed unsuitable for percutaneous valvuloplasty or surgical repair.

7. **b.** Carcinoid. The history and examination are consistent with tricuspid stenosis and regurgitation. (She has symptoms of fatigability from decreased cardiac output, signs, and symptoms of systemic venous congestion—hepatic distension and right upper quadrant pain, peripheral edema, and ascites. There is a diastolic murmur along the sternal border, which increases with inspiration, along with a prominent *a* wave in the JVP. In addition, she has a pansystolic murmur and a prominent *v* wave.) However, no evidence for mitral stenosis is noted on examination. Isolated rheumatic tricuspid stenosis is very rare. Thus, other causes for tricuspid stenosis should be considered. The second most common cause of tricuspid stenosis is the carcinoid syndrome. She also has bronchospasm and diarrhea, which go along with this diagnosis. She has a normal P_2, making primary pulmonary hypertension unlikely. Liver disease in and of itself would not produce elevation in the JVP.

8. **c.** Check lower extremity BP. He has a bicuspid aortic valve (an ejection sound is heard, along with a short systolic ejection murmur). There is an association between bicuspid aortic valves and coarctation of the aorta. Therefore, looking for discrepancy between the upper and lower extremity BP would be paramount.

9. **c.** Dobutamine echocardiogram. This is a patient presenting with low-gradient AS in the setting of LV dysfunction. It may be that the patient has severe AS, but the gradients are now low secondary to decreased stroke volume. However, the degree of AS may not be that significant, but because of decreased cardiac output, the continuity equation overestimates AS severity. In this setting, low-dose dobutamine echocardiography may be useful. With inotropic stimulation, an improvement in stroke volume and cardiac output may help to differentiate true severe AS from what has been labeled pseudo-AS. If true severe AS is not present, then valve area will increase. It would not be prudent to send such a patient to aortic valve surgery without performing such an evaluation. It would be necessary to exclude severe stenosis before proceeding with transplant evaluation. ACEI may be beneficial, but it would be important to proceed with the workup as above first. Afterload reduction would need to be introduced with very careful hemodynamic monitoring if true severe AS were in fact present. The use of dobutamine echocardiographic testing to evaluate low-gradient AS in the setting of LV dysfunction is a class IIa indication by ACC/AHA guidelines.

10. **a.** AVR. The patient has true, severe AS and although may have a higher potential complication rate with surgery is likely to benefit prognostically and symptomatically from surgery. Balloon aortic valvuloplasty has not been shown to improve survival without the addition of a more definitive procedure such as aortic valve surgery. It is only indicated for palliation or as a bridge to a more definitive procedure such as transcatheter aortic valve replacement (TAVR) or surgery.

11. **d.** Patient has a lack of contractile reserve but should still be considered for AVR. There are three possible outcomes to a low-dose dobutamine test in this situation: true AS, pseudo-AS, and absence of contractile reserve. As was the case in Question 10, there may be an increase in stroke volume (defined as ≥20% increase from baseline) associated with an increase in transvalvular gradients (mean gradient >40 mmHg) without a significant increase in aortic valve area (AVA) (AVA increase <0.2 cm^2) indicative of true AS. Conversely, in pseudo-AS the increase in stroke volume is associated with an increase in AVA without a significant change in gradients. Finally, absence of contractile reserve is defined as failure to increase the stroke volume by ≥20% from baseline. In this case, dobutamine does not help to differentiate between the former two scenarios. While there is a significantly higher mortality during the perioperative period in those with the absence of contractile reserve compared with true AS, for those that survive surgery their 5-year survival is significantly better than those treated with medical therapy alone. Therefore, surgery should be considered on an individual basis.

12. b. Addition of vasodilator therapy. The patient is asymptomatic with good functional capacity. He has a normal ejection fraction with a mildly dilated LV. Surgery is a class III indication (harmful) in this setting. Vasodilator therapy may have some benefit in this asymptomatic population with preserved ejection fraction and LV dilation, although this is not definite. This is a class IIb indication. However, he has systolic hypertension which is likely at least in part related to his aortic regurgitation, and vasodilator therapy is an optimal therapy for this. Observation alone would be reasonable, but such a patient should be followed at 6-month intervals initially and not every 3 years. There is no role for cardiac catheterization at this juncture.

13. a. <1%. From the available published literature, as summarized in the ACC/AHA consensus guidelines, the risk is about 0.2% per year in those asymptomatic patients with preserved LV function.

14. d. Referral for surgical intervention to repair or replace his aortic valve and to replace his ascending aorta. An aortic dimension >5.0 cm (or growth >0.5 cm per year) in a patient with a bicuspid aortic valve is a class I indication for surgery. The valve is often repairable in bicuspid valve associated with predominant aortic regurgitation assuming the mechanism is due to prolapse of the conjoint cusp, and there is no significant stenosis or calcification of the valve.

15. d. AVR with tricuspid valve repair if feasible. The mitral valve appears morphologically normal. After relief of the outflow tract obstruction, the MR will likely improve; therefore, mitral valve repair is not indicated. Tricuspid valve repair for moderate TR at the time of left-sided valve surgery is reasonable in the context of annular dilation and elevated PA pressures. This is a class IIb indication from the ACC/AHA guidelines but receives a class IIa recommendation from the European Society of Cardiology (2012). Tricuspid valve repair is favored over replacement.

16. a. 0.4 cm^2. The EROA based on the assumptions above is 0.4 cm^2 consistent with severe MR. The EROA is calculated using the abbreviated proximal isovelocity surface area (PISA) method as $r^2/2$ (r = radius of the PFCR). In this case, the radius is 0.9 cm; therefore, the EROA can be estimated as 0.4 cm^2.

17. b. 2+, moderate. Using the complete PISA method and calculating the regurgitant volume, the MR is determined to be only moderate in severity which is consistent with the brief duration of MR heard on physical examination. The complete method for calculating the EROA is $(2\pi r^2 \times AV)/V_{max}$ (AV: aliasing velocity; V_{max}: maximum velocity across the mitral valve); therefore, in this case the EROA = $(2\pi(0.9)^2 \times 38.5)/600 = 0.33$ cm^2. However, as we see from the continuous-wave Doppler signal, the MR only occurs in late systole consistent with mitral valve prolapse. The regurgitant volume is equal to EROA × VTI$_{MR}$ (VTI$_{MR}$ = velocity time integral of the mitral regurgitation), which in this case is = 0.33 × 100 = 33 mL consistent with 2+ MR. If we used the EROA from the abbreviated PISA method (0.4 cm^2), the regurgitant volume is 40 mL, which is still consistent with moderate MR.

18. a. Transesophageal echocardiogram. Left atrial and appendage thrombus should be excluded prior to proceeding with percutaneous valvuloplasty and is recommended by ACC/AHA guidelines to be performed prior to the procedure. Transthoracic echocardiography does not have sufficient sensitivity for this purpose. Documentation of atrial fibrillation by ambulatory monitoring may make the likelihood of finding a thrombus higher, but the transesophageal echocardiogram should be performed regardless. Routine surveillance for aortic calcification has no role in this setting. A nuclear perfusion study would not be necessary here (angiography can be performed if needed at the time of the procedure).

19. **a.** It is absolutely indicated. Given LV dysfunction (EF < 50%), this is a class I indication for surgery. There is no question as to the severity of the AS given the gradients and the aortic valve area; thus dobutamine echocardiography is not of value here.

20. **d.** The rate of mortality, for a patient with these findings, is higher compared with patients with severe AS and high gradients across the aortic valve but aortic valve surgery has resulted in better outcomes in these patients. This woman has paradoxical low-gradient, severe AS with preserved ejection fraction. Her clinical history, examination, and 2D imaging of the aortic valve are consistent with severe AS. She has a low indexed stroke volume (<35 mL/m^2), resulting in low gradients across the AV but the dimensionless index and AVA both are consistent with severe AS. When there is discordant echocardiographic data the accuracy of measurements should always be looked at again; however, in this case, the low gradients are consistent with low-stroke volume. There are currently no guidelines from the ACC or AHA on how to manage these patients; however, the recent 2012 European Society of Cardiology guidelines for valvular heart disease provide a class IIa recommendation for AVR in symptomatic patients with paradoxical low-gradient, severe AS with preserved ejection fraction. A number of studies have confirmed that the rate of mortality is higher in this cohort when compared with patients with severe AS and high gradients but surgery on the aortic valve is associated with significantly better outcomes.

21. **c.** Aortic root dimension. The patient clinically has severe AI. The murmur is loudest at the right sternal border, suggesting aortic root dilation as a potential cause of his AI. The presence of root dilation (≥5.5 cm) may lead to earlier surgery, hence is vital to know. The diastolic rumble is most likely an Austin Flint murmur and not concomitant mitral stenosis (no opening snap, S_1 not loud).

22. **a.** Cardiac catheterization with aortography. Clinically, the patient has severe aortic regurgitation. He is symptomatic. Consistent with this, the echocardiogram reveals a dilated LV with low normal systolic function. The degree of aortic regurgitation must be underestimated by this study. When there is such discrepancy, proceed with aortography to confirm aortic regurgitation severity and to assess coronaries prior to surgical referral. As he is symptomatic, continued observation and/or medical therapy is not the preferred treatment approach. β-Blockers, by prolonging the diastolic filling period, could actually increase regurgitant volume.

23. **a.** Transesophageal echocardiogram, emergent cardiac surgical consultation. The patient has a clinical presentation of severe acute AI (short diastolic murmur, soft S_1 from premature mitral valve closure, low output state, and pulmonary edema). In the context of chest pain, this scenario suggests aortic dissection until proven otherwise. The dissection flap likely involves the ostium of the right coronary artery, producing the inferior ST-segment elevation. Thrombolytics should not be used until dissection is ruled out. Even if there is no dissection, an intra-aortic balloon pump should not be used with severe AI. The augmented diastolic pressure worsens the severity of the insufficiency. MRI would also provide the diagnosis, but given the hemodynamic instability of the patient, a bedside TEE would be a safer and quicker option to arrive at the diagnosis.

24. **b.** No evidence for dysfunction. The physical examination does not suggest either stenosis or insufficiency. He appears to be in a high-output state, secondary to his febrile illness. As a result, the gradients are increased. The LVOT VTI is also increased, secondary to the increased cardiac output. The LVOT/aortic valve VTI ratio is the same in the two echocardiograms, which would speak against any significant obstruction.

25. **a.** TEE with surgical consultation. The clinical scenario, with a new first-degree AV block and acute aortic regurgitation, is highly suspicious for prosthetic valve abscess and possibly even partial dehiscence. A transesophageal echocardiogram should be

performed, but prompt surgical consultation should also be requested given the high suspicion for aortic root abscess and the onset of heart failure symptoms.

26. **c.** Repeat echocardiogram with planimetry of mitral valve area. With acute changes in atrial and ventricular compliance (as with valvuloplasty), the half-time is unreliable. Usually 72 hours or more is required after the procedure before the half-time can be used with reasonable reliability. Planimetry, if performed correctly, would provide a more reliable estimate of stenosis severity. Clinically, the patient seems to have had a good result (longer S_2–OS interval, shorter murmur). TEE rarely provides incremental data on mitral stenosis if the transthoracic images are reasonable.

27. **a.** Observation. The shunt is secondary to the valvuloplasty procedure where the interventionalist must perform an interatrial septal puncture in order to access the mitral valve. Most of these small shunts will close over the next 6 months without any intervention. The shunt is left to right by color. He has good O_2 saturation on room air, making any significant right-to-left shunting unlikely. Anticoagulation with an atrial septal defect/patent foramen ovale may be recommended in certain settings, however not indefinitely, given the good chance that the defect will close.

28. **b.** Antibiotic prophylaxis, with yearly office visits. He requires antibiotic prophylaxis with a prosthetic valve (by 2007 guidelines, prosthetic cardiac valves are an indication for subacute bacterial endocarditis prophylaxis prior to dental procedures). These patients still require close follow-up with complete evaluation on a yearly basis. Some advocate a 3-month period of warfarin therapy after bioprosthetic valve placement. He is now 4 months out, and has no other indications or a high-risk profile (LV dysfunction, prior embolic event, and atrial fibrillation); thus warfarin is no longer needed at this time. Similarly, there is no specific indication in this man for clopidogrel therapy.

29. **e.** No therapy at present but follow carefully with serial clinical and echo evaluation. Antibiotics are not recommended routinely for prophylaxis at the time of delivery for patients with valvular heart disease unless infection is suspected. If there is evidence of pulmonary congestion treatment with diuretics and afterload reduction with hydralazine is recommended but ACEIs are teratogenic and are absolutely contraindicated in pregnancy. Your patient is clinically euvolemic and therefore medical therapy need not be initiated. Surgery should only be performed if the mother's life is threatened due to the associated high fetal mortality rate (20% to 30%). Management will involve close follow-up and monitoring by her cardiologist and obstetrician and treatment only if her clinical situation deteriorates.

30. **a.** TEE. The echocardiogram reveals a normal-appearing aortic valve. Yet, the profile of the continuous-wave Doppler jet is more consistent with a fixed obstruction, as opposed to the dagger shape of dynamic obstruction. These findings are suggestive of the presence of a subvalvular membrane. TEE would be useful to better delineate this area and identify the membrane. The patient already has a 5-m jet in the absence of systolic anterior motion; therefore, it would not be prudent to use provocation with amyl nitrate. A stress echocardiogram would have no diagnostic value and may have some risk in the setting of symptomatic LVOT obstruction. One should always consider contamination with an MR signal; however, the physical examination is consistent with outflow tract obstruction and the continuous-wave Doppler signal begins after the QRS (after isovolumetric relaxation) consistent with outflow tract obstruction. The MR signal will begin earlier relative to the QRS (through isovolumetric contraction).

31. **c.** There is no clear role for aspirin therapy in such patients. If there is echocardiographic evidence for high-risk mitral valve prolapse (leaflet thickening, elongated chordae, left atrial enlargement, and LV dilation), aspirin therapy is considered a class IIb indication. Therapy is clearly recommended if there have been documented stroke or transient ischemic events.

32. b. Continue with vasodilator therapy and reassess in 6 months. By ACC/AHA guidelines, decline in ejection fraction following stress echocardiography by itself is not an accepted indication for referral to surgical intervention. Owing to the high afterload and the increase in afterload on exercise, a small-to-modest decline in ejection fraction (<10%) may still be consistent with well-compensated AI. This patient has normal resting ejection fraction and mildly dilated LV with excellent functional capacity.

33. b. Repeat the echocardiogram with amyl nitrate (Fig. 2.11). The physical examination is highly suggestive of hypertrophic cardiomyopathy (brisk, bisferiens carotid pulse, normal S_2, and murmur increasing with Valsalva and decreasing with handgrip). The patient may not have a significant resting gradient, but may have a significant provocable gradient. Generally, a transesophageal echocardiogram is not needed to make the diagnosis. Invasive hemodynamics with provocation would be useful, but angiography alone would not be sufficient.

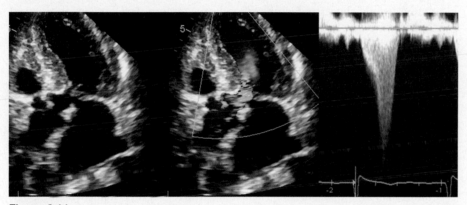

Figure 2.11

34. c. She will probably not need surgery on her mitral valve. MR secondary to systolic anterior motion of the mitral valve is related to hydrodynamic drag and Venturi effects on the anterior mitral valve. Often there are intrinsic mitral valve abnormalities that, in combination with septal hypertrophy, predispose to systolic anterior motion. Abnormal chordal attachments or hypermobile papillary muscles seen best on cardiac MRI may mandate chordae remodeling or papillary muscle reorientation; however, in this case the mitral valve apparatus is noted to be structurally normal. Relief of the hydrodynamic effects of a narrowed LVOT after myectomy will usually result in significant improvement in MR without further surgery. Before chest closure, careful assessment of MR should be done after the myectomy, usually with isoproterenol infusion, to ensure resolution.

35. b. Transesophageal echocardiogram. By examination, the patient has mitral insufficiency. The echocardiogram is consistent with this, with an elevated peak transmitral gradient. Pressure half-time is not prolonged; thus there does not appear to be any significant stenosis (gradients elevated owing to increased flow from regurgitant volume). A TEE would be the most useful to confirm the diagnosis. Fluoroscopy may identify partial dehiscence, but would not be helpful if there were a leak in the setting of a well-seated valve. There is no evidence for stenosis, where fluoroscopic evaluation of leaflet motion could be diagnostic. There is no clinical evidence for endocarditis.

36. a. Prominent closing click, soft and brief diastolic rumble. The bileaflet mechanical valves do not typically produce a loud opening sound, but do have prominent closing sounds. A brief diastolic rumble may be heard in a normally functioning prosthetic valve in the mitral position.

37. **b.** Prominent opening and closing clicks, soft and brief diastolic rumble. With the ball-and-cage valves, one would expect to hear the opening click as well.

38. **e.** Warfarin therapy with a target INR of 2.5 to 3.5 plus aspirin 75 to 100 mg. All patients with a mechanical valve require warfarin. The risk of thromboembolic events is higher for prosthetic valves in the mitral position; therefore, the recommended therapeutic range is higher than that for mechanical valves in the aortic position. The addition of low-dose aspirin (75 to 100 mg) further reduces the risk of thromboembolic event and reduces mortality from cardiovascular disease. Therefore, aspirin is recommended for all patients with valvular prostheses. Higher doses of aspirin have not been shown to be beneficial and increase the bleeding risk.

39. **a.** <2%. In the absence of symptoms, natural history studies would suggest a relatively low risk of sudden death.

40. **d.** >50%. He has a velocity across the aortic valve of >4 m/s. Observational studies would suggest a high likelihood of symptom development in the next 3 years.

41. **d.** Start ASA, 81 mg/day, and increase warfarin to achieve an INR of 2.5 to 3.5. ACC/AHA guidelines recommended an INR of 2.5 to 3.5 for patients with bileaflet tilting disk mechanical valves in the aortic position who have had a thromboembolic event, and who have atrial fibrillation, LV dysfunction, or a hypercoagulable state. Addition of low-dose ASA (75 to 100 mg) is a class I indication for all patients with mechanical heart valves, and those with the above risk factors and bioprosthetic valves.

42. **a.** Intravenous heparin. Since a small clot was present (without any obstruction to valve function) the patient would benefit from increased anticoagulant therapy. If he were to fail this, then the other alternatives could be considered, such as continuous infusion thrombolytic therapy. Such continuous therapy (although not bolus) could also be used as primary treatment. No established indications exist at this time for glycoprotein IIb/IIIa inhibitors in this clinical setting. It would not be advisable to proceed to reoperation just yet, in the absence of a large clot burden or obstruction to inflow. If treatment with heparin leads to clot resolution, then subsequent warfarin dosing should be increased to maintain INR in the 3.0 to 4.0 range.

43. **a.** Therapy with warfarin. He should be on warfarin. Valvuloplasty in this setting (onset of atrial fibrillation, in an otherwise asymptomatic patient) is a class IIb indication by current guidelines.

44. **a.** Reassurance, with a repeat physical examination in 6 months. If a thorough physical examination reveals no signs of cardiopulmonary disease and the patient has no symptoms, then reassurance and follow-up are all that are required. Echocardiography should be performed if obesity limits the physical examination or if signs or symptoms are present.

45. **b.** Consider elective mitral valve repair at a hospital where repair is performed with a high degree of success or if he wishes to defer surgery, follow up at 6 monthly intervals with echo. Referral for surgery is reasonable (class IIa indication) if chance of repair is >95%. There are no data to suggest a beneficial role for the addition of afterload-reducing agents in the absence of systemic hypertension (again by ACC/AHA guidelines). There is absolutely no role for the prophylactic use of amiodarone. Close clinical follow-up is reasonable, but repeat evaluation should not be deferred for 2 years. Guidelines use LV dimensions and ejection fraction to guide surgical intervention, even in the absence of symptoms. As such, these patients should have clinical reevaluation and echo every 6 months.

46. a. Referral for mitral valve repair. He is now symptomatic with depressed ejection fraction and a dilated LV. This is a class I indication for surgery. Valve repair as opposed to replacement is the preferred surgical treatment. Medical therapy may be needed as an adjunct, but is insufficient as the sole treatment.

47. c. Life expectancy <1 year. Life expectancy of <1 year, despite treatment of AS, is an absolute contraindication for TAVR. Severe peripheral artery disease precludes a transfemoral approach; however, the procedure may be done via a transapical approach, a transsubclavian approach, and even a transaortic approach. Severe pulmonary disease and an inaccessible apex preclude a transapical approach but the other approaches remain available. Active endocarditis is a contraindication to the procedure. The available valves are suitable for annular sizes between 19 and 29 mm.

48. c. Mitral and tricuspid stenoses. The loud S_1, opening snap, and apical diastolic rumble are features of mitral stenosis. The presence of the diastolic rumble along the sternal border, which increases with inspiration, along with the prominent a wave in the JVP and evidence of systemic venous congestion (hepatomegaly and peripheral edema) suggests that concomitant tricuspid stenosis is present as well.

49. c. Cardiac catheterization. By physical examination, the patient has severe AS (no A_2 of second heart sound, late-peaking murmur, and diminished carotid upstrokes). A stress test would not be appropriate in a patient with symptomatic AS. An echocardiogram would usually be the first step, but proceeding directly to catheterization to measure transvalvular gradients and assess coronary anatomy would be reasonable. SL NTG could have disastrous consequences in this setting. By reducing preload, it may precipitate syncope.

50. b. Refer for percutaneous balloon valvuloplasty, followed by gastrectomy. He has symptomatic critical AS. AVR, with concomitant need for anticoagulation while on cardiopulmonary bypass, is not an attractive first option. Proceeding directly to gastric surgery would carry high risk, given the ongoing symptoms. Valvuloplasty would be a reasonable bridge to lower risk from the noncardiac surgery.

51. a. Bovine pericardial valve. He is at an age where there is substantial durability of the bioprosthetic valve. He is at increased risk for anticoagulation; thus, mechanical valves would not be the valve of first choice. By history, he would not appear to need anticoagulation for any other indication. Homograft is not unreasonable, but there would not appear to be any hemodynamic or durability benefits for an 80-year-old patient, and its insertion requires a more difficult operation.

52. c. ~50% of cases have a bicuspid aortic valve. Coarctation of the aorta is suspected clinically and confirmed on a gated CT angiogram of the thoracic aorta. This lesion is frequently associated with concomitant congenital cardiac anomalies, the most frequent of which is a bicuspid aortic valve (occurs in ~50% to 85% of cases).

53. a. Stress test. The patient has significant aortic regurgitation with a dilated LV although not yet at the dimension that would be an indication for surgery in the absence of symptoms (his end-systolic dimension is <5.0 cm and end-diastolic dimension is <7.0 cm). He leads a sedentary lifestyle, and although he has no dyspnea, he does relate some equivocal symptom. A stress test would be useful to assess functional capacity and to objectively assess symptoms. If he were to develop symptoms at a low level of exercise, this may be an indication for surgical intervention. A vasodilator may be useful (class IIb indication with dilated LV), but he would need more frequent follow-up, given the LV dilation.

54. b. Surgical intervention. (Refer for surgery.) His ventricle has dilated even further. An end-diastolic dimension of >7.5 cm is a class IIa indication for surgery and is associated with an increased risk of sudden death, even in the absence of symptoms.

55. b. Mean gradient across the mitral prosthesis of 17 mmHg. The clinical presentation and examination are suggestive of prosthetic mitral stenosis (long diastolic rumble, muffled closing click, and clinical heart failure). The PMI is not displaced, so it is unlikely that she has significant LV dysfunction. There are no clinical signs of severe MR. Given the acute onset of symptoms, acute valvular thrombosis leading to valvular obstruction is high on the differential. If this were the case by ACC/AHA guidelines, reoperation would be the preferred treatment approach. If other comorbidities were prohibitive, thrombolytic therapy could be considered.

56. a. Arrhythmias secondary to an accessory pathway. The examination is highly suggestive of Ebstein anomaly (presence of TR, widely split first heart sound). The echocardiogram confirms this. Accessory pathways are frequently associated with this condition.

57. a. Echocardiography with saline contrast study. Ebstein anomaly is frequently associated with cardiac shunts (either patent foramen ovale, or atrial or ventricular septal defect). The setting of a TIA in someone who has been immobilized (such as with a fracture) raises the concern of paradoxical embolism of a venous thrombus to the systemic circulation.

58. b. V_{max} across the pulmonic valve of 4 m/s. The physical examination is consistent with pulmonic stenosis (presence of thrill, RV heave, ejection click, and crescendo-decrescendo murmur loudest over the pulmonic area). Normal carotid upstrokes and preserved A_2 make significant AS unlikely. The murmur is not consistent with a regurgitant murmur.

59. a. He tells you of an episode of syncope. The presence of exertional dyspnea, angina, syncope, or near-syncope are class I indications for intervention. For gradients between 30 and 39 mmHg, there is some divergence of opinion about the role of intervention (class IIb for gradients 30 to 39). There is no role for intervention in those with gradients <30 mmHg who have no symptoms. A peak-to-peak gradient >40 mmHg by catheterization is a class I indication for intervention, even in an asymptomatic patient.

60. a. Percutaneous valvuloplasty. This is the preferred treatment for young adults with pulmonic stenosis.

61. b. Doppler echocardiography, using the continuity equation. With significant insufficiency, the Gorlin formula becomes less reliable. Pressure half-time is not used to calculate aortic valve area, but does give a clue to the severity of the AI.

62. c. Aortic homograft. Mechanical and bioprosthetic valves have a similar incidence of endocarditis, which is higher than that seen for homografts. In the setting of acute bacterial endocarditis of a prosthetic aortic valve, homografts are the valve of first choice when surgery is indicated.

63. d. Pulmonary hypertension resulting from primary left-sided disease. The most common cause of tricuspid insufficiency is pulmonary hypertension that results from primary pathology on the left side of the heart. This includes aortic and mitral valvular diseases, as well as LV dysfunction from coronary artery disease or other cardiomyopathies.

64. a. *Streptococcus viridans* accounts for up to 50% of cases. *Staphylococcus aureus* is the next most common pathogen.

65. c. *Staphylococcus epidermidis.* This patient presents with early prosthetic valve endocarditis (within 2 months of surgery). This is usually acquired during the operation, and the skin species *Staphylococcus epidermidis* is the most frequent pathogen encountered. Late prosthetic valve endocarditis is similar to native valve endocarditis in terms of the spectrum of pathogens involved.

SUGGESTED READINGS

2014 AHA/ACC Guideline for the Management of Patients With Valvular Heart Disease: Executive Summary: A Report of the American College of Cardiology/American Heart Association Task Force on Practice Guidelines. Nishimura RA, Otto CM, Bonow RO, Carabello BA, Erwin JP 3rd, Guyton RA, O'Gara PT, Ruiz CE, Skubas NJ, Sorajja P, Sundt TM 3rd, Thomas JD. Circulation. 2014 Jun 10;129(23):2440–92. doi: 10.1161/CIR.0000000000000029.

Bonow RO, Lakatos E, Maron BJ, et al. Serial long-term assessment of the natural history of asymptomatic patients with chronic aortic regurgitation and normal left ventricular systolic function. *Circulation.* 1991;84(4):1625–1635.

Enriquez-Sarano M, Avierinos JF, Messika-Zeitoun D, et al. Quantitative determinants of the outcome of asymptomatic mitral regurgitation. *N Engl J Med.* 2005;352(9):875–883.

Holmes DR, Jr, Mack MJ, Kaul S, et al. 2012 ACCF/AATS/SCAI/STS expert consensus document on transcatheter aortic valve replacement: developed in collaboration with the American Heart Association, American Society of Echocardiography, European Association for Cardio-Thoracic Surgery, Heart Failure Society of America, Mended Hearts, Society of Cardiovascular Anesthesiologists, Society of Cardiovascular Computed Tomography, and Society for Cardiovascular Magnetic Resonance. *J Thorac Cardiovasc Surg.* 2012;144(3):e29–e84.

Ling LH, Enriquez-Sarano M, Seward JB, et al. Clinical outcome of mitral regurgitation due to flail leaflet. *N Engl J Med.* 1996;335(19): 1417–1423.

Otto CM, Burwash IG, Legget ME, et al. Prospective study of asymptomatic valvular aortic stenosis. Clinical, echocardiographic, and exercise predictors of outcome. *Circulation.* 1997;95(9):2262–2270.

Nishimura RA, Carabello BA, Faxon DP, et al. ACC/AHA 2008 guideline update on valvular heart disease: focused update on infective endocarditis: a report of the American College of Cardiology/American Heart Association Task Force on Practice Guidelines endorsed by the Society of Cardiovascular Anesthesiologists, Society for Cardiovascular Angiography and Interventions, and Society of Thoracic Surgeons. *J Am Coll Cardiol.* 2008;52(8):676–685.

Rosenhek R, Rader F, Klaar U, et al. Outcome of watchful waiting in asymptomatic severe mitral regurgitation. *Circulation.* 2006;113(18): 2238–2244.

Tandon A, Grayburn PA. Imaging of low-gradient severe aortic stenosis. *JACC Cardiovasc Imaging.* 2013;6(2):184–195.

Vahanian A, Alfieri O, Andreotti F, et al. Guidelines on the management of valvular heart disease (version 2012). *Eur Heart J.* 2012;33(19): 2451–2496.

chapter **3**

Acute Myocardial Infarction

Venu Menon • Bhuvnesh Aggarwal

QUESTIONS

1. Which one of the following statements is true regarding trends in incidence of acute coronary syndrome (ACS) in the United States?

   a. Percentage of ACS with ST-segment elevation myocardial infarction (STEMI) is declining.

   b. Percentage of ACS with non–ST-segment elevation myocardial infarction (NSTEMI) is declining.

   c. Percentage of ACS with unstable angina (UA) is increasing.

   d. Overall incidence of ACS is decreasing.

   e. All of the above.

2. Which of the following processes represents the dominant initiating event in the pathogenesis of an ACS?

   a. Plaque rupture

   b. Plaque erosion

   c. Platelet activation

   d. Venous stasis

   e. None of the above

3. What is the most important clinical predictor of 30-day mortality in a patient presenting with acute STEMI?

   a. Age

   b. Systolic blood pressure (BP)

   c. Heart rate

   d. Killip classification stage

   e. Location of myocardial infarction (MI)

4. Which of the following is a prodrug and requires bioactivation?

   a. Aspirin

   b. Clopidogrel

   c. Prasugrel

   d. Ticagrelor

   e. Both b and c

5. Which of the following statements regarding prasugrel is true?

  a. Prasugrel has faster onset of action when compared with clopidogrel.

  b. Unlike clopidogrel, prasugrel is not influenced by polymorphisms in cytochrome P450 enzyme pathway.

  c. Prasugrel provided no net mortality benefit when compared with clopidogrel in patients with ACS in the Trial to Assess Improvement in Therapeutic Outcomes by Optimizing Platelet Inhibition with Prasugrel–Thrombolysis in Myocardial Infarction (TRITON-TIMI)-38 trial.

  d. Prasugrel is contraindicated in patients with a prior history of transient ischemic attack (TIA)/stroke.

  e. All of the above.

6. A 72-year-old presents with sudden-onset chest pain at a local emergency department. He has a past medical history significant for hypertension, hyperlipidemia, and gastroesophageal reflux disease. On examination his BP is 95/60 mmHg and heart rate is 90 beats per minute and he is breathing at 90% on ambient air. He reports this is the first time he has had any episode of chest pain. His electrocardiogram (ECG) reveals ST elevation in V_1 to V_4. The nearest hospital with percutaneous coronary intervention (PCI) capability is 3 hours away. What is the next step in management?

  a. Perform fibrinolysis; administer unfractionated heparin, aspirin, and clopidogrel; and admit to hospital.

  b. Administer unfractionated heparin, aspirin, and clopidogrel and admit to hospital.

  c. Administer unfractionated heparin, aspirin, and clopidogrel followed by transfer to PCI-capable hospital.

  d. Computed tomography (CT) of the chest with intravenous contrast.

  e. Perform fibrinolysis; low-molecular-weight heparin (LMWH), aspirin, and clopidogrel; and transfer to the hospital for possible PCI.

7. The above patient is given intravenous tenecteplase and started on aspirin, clopidogrel, and unfractionated heparin. Thirty minutes into treatment his chest pain has now completely resolved. A repeat ECG shows complete resolution of the earlier noted ST elevation. What is the next step in management?

  a. Continue unfractionated heparin, aspirin, and clopidogrel and transfer to the nearest hospital with PCI capabilities.

  b. Admit to local hospital for observation.

  c. Discharge home with outpatient follow-up following a submaximal stress test.

  d. Discharge home with plan for possible angiography after 4 to 6 weeks.

  e. None of the above.

8. Which of the following is *true* for management of acute STEMI?

  a. The administration of aspirin has a much larger treatment effect than streptokinase.

  b. The administration of streptokinase has a much larger effect than aspirin.

  c. Streptokinase and aspirin each have a similar effect on outcome.

  d. When streptokinase and aspirin are used together, their effects are blunted.

  e. None of the above.

9. Which of the following is the mechanism of action of ticagrelor?

  a. Thromboxane inhibition

  b. Glycoprotein (GP) IIb/IIIa receptor blockade

  c. Adenosine diphosphate blockade

  d. Increase in cyclic adenosine monophosphate production

  e. Free radical scavenger

10. Which of the following is true regarding use of GP IIb/IIIa inhibitors in STEMI?

    a. Routine upstream use of GP IIb/IIIa inhibitors has been shown to reduce target vessel revascularization (TVR).

    b. Routine GP IIb/IIIa inhibitor use is associated with reduced incidence of recurrent MI.

    c. Routine GP IIb/IIIa inhibitor use is associated with increased risk of bleeding.

    d. Small-molecule GP IIb/IIIa inhibitor use has been shown to reduce 30-day mortality.

    e. Upstream use of GP IIb/IIIa inhibitors is given a class I indication in current American College of Cardiology (ACC)/American Heart Association (AHA) guidelines.

11. In the setting of primary angioplasty for acute MI, which of the following have stents been convincingly shown to do compared with balloon angioplasty alone?

    a. Decrease subsequent repeat TVR.

    b. Decrease long-term mortality.

    c. Decrease long-term MI risk.

    d. Decrease the incidence of heart failure.

12. Which of the following is *true* about reteplase in Global Use of Strategies to Open Occluded Coronary Arteries (GUSTO-III)?

    a. It had a significantly higher rate of stroke than alteplase.

    b. It significantly reduced mortality compared with alteplase.

    c. It significantly reduced mortality, but increased stroke compared with alteplase.

    d. It had similar rates of mortality compared with alteplase.

13. Which of the following statements is true regarding non–ST-segment elevation (NSTE)-ACS?

    a. NSTEMI has poorer prognosis than UA.

    b. Elevated troponin is associated with worse prognosis in NSTE-ACS.

    c. ST-segment deviation is associated with increased risk of long-term ischemic events.

    d. One in five patients with NSTEMI has normal ECG.

    e. All of the above.

14. A 46-year-old man presents to the emergency with complaints of sudden, severe chest pain radiating to his right arm. He admits to snorting crack cocaine 2 hours prior to the development of chest pain. His BP is 180/100 mmHg and heart rate is 96 per minute. An ECG done reveals downsloping ST depression and T-wave inversion in V_2 to V_4. What is the next best step in management?

    a. Administer aspirin, sublingual nitroglycerin, and intravenous metoprolol.

    b. Administer aspirin and sublingual nitroglycerin.

    c. Administer aspirin, sublingual nitroglycerin, and heparin.

    d. Administer activated charcoal.

15. The patient is started on aspirin, nitroglycerin, and intravenous heparin. He continues to have severe substernal chest pain. Repeat ECG is unchanged. Troponin T is borderline elevated to 0.04 ng/mL. What is the next best step in management?

    a. Activate the catheterization laboratory for emergent left heart catheterization.

    b. Administer diazepam and let the patient rest.

    c. Administer tissue plasminogen activator.

    d. Cycle cardiac biomarkers and monitor the patient.

    e. None of the above.

16. A 64-year-old man is brought to the emergency room for complaints of chest pressure, difficulty breathing, and palpitations. He has a past medical history of hypertension and type 2 diabetes and ischemic stroke and his home medications include metformin, glyburide, lisinopril, and aspirin. ECG on arrival reveals ST-segment elevation in leads I, avL and V_5 to V_6. Catheterization laboratory is activated and the patient is given 325 mg of aspirin and started on nitroglycerin drip. Which of the following additional therapies is currently indicated?

   a. Clopidogrel 300 mg, fondaparinux, and atorvastatin 80 mg

   b. Prasugrel 60 mg, unfractionated heparin, and atorvastatin 80 mg

   c. Ticagrelor 90 mg, unfractionated heparin, and atorvastatin 80 mg

   d. Clopidogrel 600 mg, bivalirudin drip, and atorvastatin 80 mg

   e. Both a and d are correct

17. Which of the following is true regarding adjunctive medical therapy in patients with acute MI receiving primary PCI?

   a. Routine intravenous β-blocker within 24 hours improves mortality.

   b. Intravenous angiotensin-converting enzyme inhibitor (ACEI) within 24 hours improves mortality.

   c. Mortality benefit with routine intravenous nitroglycerin is not established.

   d. Intravenous magnesium improves mortality when used as an adjunct to reperfusion.

18. Which of the following statements is incorrect with regard to acute MI?

   a. Primary PCI is associated with reduced rate of intracerebral hemorrhage as compared with fibrinolysis.

   b. If rapidly available, primary PCI provides a mortality benefit as compared with fibrinolysis.

   c. Primary PCI may be considered 12 hours after symptom onset in patients with signs of ongoing ischemia.

   d. Routine PCI of the totally occluded infarct-related artery should be avoided after 24 hours of presentation in hemodynamically stable patients without signs of ischemia.

   e. Fibrinolysis should be considered 12 hours after symptom onset in hemodynamically stable patients with signs of ongoing ischemia.

19. Which of the following is an absolute contraindication for use of fibrinolytics for acute MI?

   a. History of ischemic stroke

   b. Pregnancy

   c. Concomitant use of warfarin for another indication

   d. Suspected aortic dissection

   e. History of seizure disorder

   f. All of the above

20. Which of the statements is true regarding ventricular septal rupture (VSR) after acute MI?

   a. VSR is more common in men when compared with women.

   b. VSR is more likely after recurrent MI.

   c. Presence of collateral circulation in the infarct zone reduces risk of VSR.

   d. Fibrinolysis is associated with increased risk of VSR.

   e. VSR is more likely after anterior wall MI as compared with nonanterior wall MI.

21. An 82-year-old woman calls 911 after developing sudden-onset chest pain, nausea, and lightheadedness. An ECG done by emergency medical service (EMS) reveals 3-mm ST elevation in leads II, III, and aVF. The nearest catheterization laboratory is activated and the patient undergoes PCI to the right coronary artery (RCA) with drug-eluting stent. She is transferred to the intensive care unit (ICU) in stable condition after the procedure. Two days later, the patient develops sudden-onset lightheadedness and left-sided chest pain. Her vitals reveal BP of 115/60 mmHg, heart rate of 90 per minute and SaO_2 of 92% on ambient air. Physical examination reveals new systolic murmur at the left sternal border that radiates to the apex. An ECG done immediately reveals Q waves in leads II, III, and aVF. No new ST-T changes are noted. A stat bedside echocardiogram reveals basal septal VSR with left-to-right shunt and moderate mitral regurgitation. A pulmonary artery (PA) catheter is placed and shunt fraction (Q_p/Q_s) is calculated at 1.3. What is the next best step in management?

   a. Left heart catheterization with ventriculography for better assessment of septum

   b. Cardiac magnetic resonance imaging (MRI) to better assess the size of septal rupture

   c. Intravenous nitroprusside for afterload reduction

   d. Intra-aortic balloon pulsation (IABP) placement

   e. Urgent surgical repair

22. Which of the following statements is true regarding ventricular free wall rupture complicating acute MI?

   a. Incidence of ventricular free wall rupture is higher after fibrinolysis when compared with that after primary angioplasty.

   b. Ventricular free wall rupture usually presents with acute-onset signs and symptoms of cardiac tamponade, or sudden death.

   c. Type I rupture usually occurs within 24 hours of MI.

   d. All of the above.

23. Which of the following is true?

   a. Ventricular aneurysm is more common than ventricular pseudoaneurysm after MI.

   b. Most ventricular pseudoaneurysms resolve over time and require no specific therapy.

   c. Ventricular aneurysm is more common with inferior wall MI when compared with anterior MI.

   d. Ventricular pseudoaneurysm is more common with anterior wall MI as compared with inferior wall MI.

   e. All of the above.

24. A 63-year-old woman presents to the clinic after an episode of sudden transient left-sided vision loss. Symptoms lasted about 15 minutes with spontaneous resolution. Her past medical history is significant for an anterior MI 3 weeks ago treated with PCI with bare metal stent (BMS) to the left anterior descending artery (LAD). Other medical conditions include hypertension, type 2 diabetes mellitus, and hyperlipidemia. Current medications are aspirin, prasugrel, atorvastatin, metformin, and metoprolol. Physical examination is normal. There are no carotid bruits. Ophthalmologic examination is within normal limits. An ECG reveals sinus rhythm with persistent ST elevations in V_2 to V_4. What is the next step in management?

   a. Exercise stress test with nuclear imaging

   b. MRI of the brain with contrast

   c. Carotid ultrasound

    d. Left heart catheterization

    e. Transthoracic echocardiogram

25. A previously healthy and independently functional 77-year-old man is brought to the catheterization laboratory after developing sudden-onset chest pain radiating to the jaw and shortness of breath. ECG by EMS during transfer revealed ST elevation in V_2 to V_4 and leads I and aVL. The patient was in respiratory distress during transfer requiring emergent endotracheal intubation. His BP is 70/30 mmHg and heart rate is 110 per minute. Angiogram reveals fresh mural thrombus in proximal LAD, which is stented with BMS with resultant TIMI-2 flow. No significant disease is noted in the RCA and circumflex vessels. An echo reveals a left ventricular ejection fraction (LVEF) of 30% with no significant valvular pathology. He is subsequently transferred to the critical care unit (CCU) in critical condition. His current vital signs are as follows: BP 80/40 mmHg, HR 120 beats per minute, and SaO of 92% on 60% FiO_2. A PA catheter is placed. Which of the following readings is associated with worst prognosis in this patient?

    a. Pulmonary capillary wedge pressure (PCWP) 30, Cardiac Index (CI) 1.6

    b. PCWP 24, CI 3.2

    c. PCWP 10, CI 1.8

    d. PCWP 16, CI 2.4

26. What is the next step to be considered in the management of this patient?

    a. Consideration for advanced mechanical support

    b. IV nitroprusside

    c. Refer for urgent coronary artery bypass grafting (CABG)

    d. Repeat left heart catheterization

27. A 72-year-old woman is admitted to the hospital with acute STEMI. She has no other past medical history. She underwent BMS to the left circumflex artery with good subsequent flow. She is now free of chest pain and feels well. Echocardiogram revealed an estimated ejection fraction of 30%. In addition to aspirin and clopidogrel what other medications must be considered in the patient's discharge medication regimen?

    a. Atorvastatin, lisinopril, and carvedilol

    b. Atorvastatin, lisinopril, carvedilol, and warfarin

    c. Atorvastatin, lisinopril, carvedilol, and eplerenone

    d. Lisinopril, metoprolol, eplerenone, and niacin

28. The above patient had a brief (10 seconds) episode of nonsustained ventricular tachycardia (VT) at a rate of 180 beats per minute on the day of admission in the catheterization laboratory that spontaneously converted to sinus rhythm. What additional therapy is warranted for this patient?

    a. Amiodarone at the time of discharge

    b. Intravenous lidocaine in the hospital and amiodarone at discharge

    c. Only intravenous lidocaine in the hospital

    d. Implantable cardioverter–defibrillator (ICD) placement prior to discharge

    e. Cardiac Resynchronization Therapy with Defibrillator (CRT-D) device placement prior to discharge

    f. None of the above

29. A 45-year-old man presents to an emergency room with 30 minutes of crushing chest pain. The nearest catheterization laboratory is 45 minutes away and a decision to transfer for primary PCI is made. What is the optimal door in door out that has been associated with decreased mortality?

a. 60 minutes

b. 45 minutes

c. Within 120 minutes

d. Within 30 minutes

e. Within 24 hours

30. A 46-year-old man develops sudden chest pain and collapses to the ground. Bystander Cardio-Pulmonary Resuscitation (CPR) is immediately initiated. On EMS arrival 8 minutes later, he is noted to be in ventricular fibrillation and is promptly defibrillated. His ECG shows ST elevation in the inferior leads. The patient is comatose and is intubated for airway protection. Apart from performance of primary PCI which of the following actions is associated with mortality benefit?

a. Bolus of 2 L of normal saline

b. Intravenous lidocaine initiation to prevent recurrent arrest

c. Initiation of transvenous pacing to prevent polymorphic VT

d. Initiation of hypothermia protocol

e. Placement on Extracorporeal Membrane Oxygenation (ECMO)

31. An 85-year-old man presents with increasing intensity of his typical angina pain associated with shortness of breath. His ECG is unchanged from prior tracings. He has a history of established coronary artery disease and has previously refused revascularization. A decision is made to manage him conservatively. Which of the following interventions would be considered inappropriate?

a. Initiation of anticoagulation with fondaparinux

b. Treatment with clopidogrel 300 mg followed by 75 mg daily

c. Initiate treatment with prasugrel bolus 60 mg followed by 5 mg once daily

d. Increase the dosage of prior β-blocker therapy

e. Continue treatment with aspirin

32. Which of the following is not a direct thrombin inhibitor?

a. Bivalirudin

b. Argatroban

c. Hirudin

d. Dabigatran

e. Apixaban

33. Which of the following is *true* regarding pericarditis in acute MI?

a. Fibrinolysis has no effect on the incidence of pericarditis in MI.

b. Fibrinolysis reduces the incidence of pericarditis in MI.

c. Fibrinolysis increases the incidence of pericarditis in MI.

d. No data have examined this issue.

34. Which of the following are potential indications for IABP in the setting of acute MI?

a. Refractory ischemia despite intensive medical therapy

b. STEMI and secondary acute mitral regurgitation

c. STEMI and refractory polymorphic VT

d. STEMI and refractory cardiogenic shock

e. All of the above

35. A 66-year-old man presents to the emergency with complaints of on–off episodes of chest discomfort for the last 24 hours. Each episode lasts from 15 to 45 minutes and occurs at rest. He denies any history of similar pain in the past. He has a past medical history of hypertension, diabetes mellitus, and peripheral vascular

disease. He is an active smoker with 40 pack-year history. An ECG done reveals nonspecific ST-T wave changes. Troponin T is elevated at 0.62. He is taken to the catheterization laboratory and a 90% lesion is noted in first diagonal via a trans-femoral approach. He is treated with overlapping BMSs with subsequent TIMI-3 flow. He is transferred to CCU in stable condition. About 4 hours later, the patient develops hypotension with BP of 80/40 mmHg and heart rate of 110 per minute. There is no jugular venous distension. He is pale, diaphoretic, and dizzy. Cardiac auscultation is unchanged. A repeat ECG done is similar to admission ECG. No pericardial effusion is noted on a bedside echocardiogram. Which of the following is most likely to identify the cause of his current condition?

a. Repeat left heart catheterization

b. CT chest with contrast

c. CT abdomen without contrast

d. Chest X-ray

e. Bedside transesophageal echocardiography

36. A 48-year-old man presents to the emergency room agitated after abusing cocaine. His heart rate is 110 per minute, his BP is 200/120 mmHg, and an ECG shows ST elevation in the inferior leads. On examination he is diaphoretic with clear lung sounds. Auscultation is pertinent for a diastolic murmur at the base of the heart that accentuates with expiration. What is the appropriate next step for definitive diagnostic evaluation?

a. Performance of a CT pulmonary embolus protocol

b. Performance of a gated CT of the aorta

c. Activation of the catheterization laboratory for primary PCI

d. Initiation of intravenous heparin and load with ticagrelor

e. Performance of a two-dimensional echocardiogram at the bedside

37. A 78-year-old man calls 911 because he has sudden-onset chest pain. On EMS arrival he has a BP of 120/80 mmHg and a heart rate of 80 beats per minute. His lungs are clear to auscultation and he has a left ventricular (LV) S_4 noted. ECG done on the field confirms an anterior MI with ST elevation from V_1 to V_4. He is given an aspirin and a sublingual nitroglycerin and transfer is initiated. Within 5 minutes while en route his BP is noted to be 60 mmHg and a saline bolus is initiated. Cardiovascular examination is unchanged and no murmurs are noted. Which of the following scenarios may likely explain his observed hemodynamic deterioration?

a. Hypotension resulting from bleeding due to administration of aspirin

b. Right ventricular (RV) infarction

c. Anaphylaxis reaction from aspirin

d. Recent exposure to a phosphodiesterase 5 inhibitor

e. Massive pulmonary embolism

38. A 42-year-old mother is visiting her child who is undergoing chemotherapy in the Children's Hospital. She suddenly develops chest pain and is noted to be nauseous and diaphoretic. An ECG is performed (Fig. 3-1). On angiography, the coronaries are free of significant epicardial stenosis. A ventriculogram shows apical ballooning with an LVEF of 25%. The patient is admitted to the CCU. Which of the following statements will most likely define her clinical course?

a. She will likely require an ICD as LV function is unlikely to recover.

b. Her prognosis will likely be excellent with full recovery of LV function.

c. She is at risk for recurrent atherosclerotic ischemic events.

d. Indefinite anticoagulation with warfarin will be indicated.

e. She is at higher risk for a malignancy in the ensuing year.

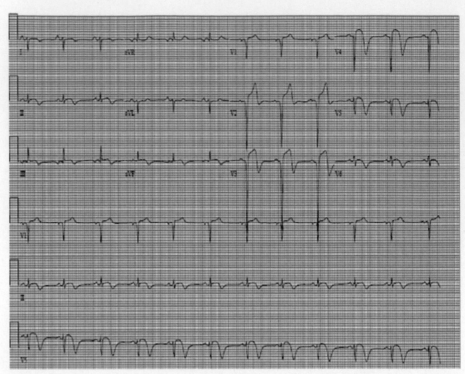

Figure 3.1

39. A 91-year-old man with a history of prior CABGx2 is brought from the nursing home with shortness of breath and hypotension. He is debilitated and has required 24/7 nursing care for activities of daily living. His ECG shows diffuse ST-segment depression, and he is noted to be in pulmonary edema. His heart rate is 110 per minute and his BP is 70/40 mmHg. He has a recent stroke 3 months prior and has stage 4 chronic kidney disease. History is also relevant for a diagnosis of prostate cancer with extensive metastasis to his spine. Which of the following is indicated?

   a. Discussion with the family explaining his poor prognosis and the near futility of escalating care
   b. Emergent catheterization and revascularization as indicated by anatomy
   c. Placement of an IABP for medical stabilization
   d. Plan for emergent dialysis
   e. Urgent oncology consultation to estimate his prognosis from his prostate cancer

40. A 64-year-old man presents with ST elevation and is taken for primary angioplasty (see Fig. 3-2). Identify the infarct-related artery?

   a. LAD
   b. Diagonal
   c. RCA
   d. Left Circumflex
   e. Obtuse marginal

41. A 45-year-old man is status post hip replacement. He develops sudden-onset shortness of breath. On examination, he is hypotensive with a BP of 80/40 mmHg. An ECG shows sinus tachycardia at 100 beats per minute with ST elevation in V_1 to V_2. A bedside echo is performed (Fig. 3-3). What is the most appropriate intervention?

   a. Activate catheterization laboratory to perform a primary PCI.
   b. Perform a CT angiogram to rule out a dissection.

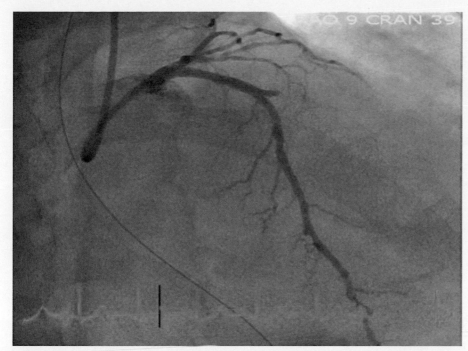

Figure 3.2

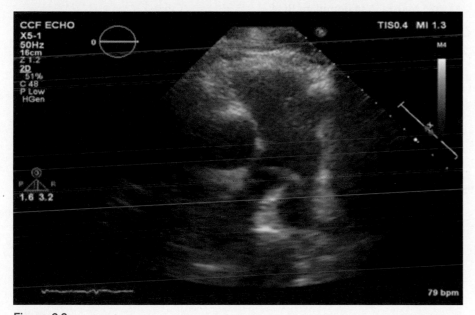

Figure 3.3

   c. Initiate intravenous heparin and assess risks and benefits of fibrinolysis.

   d. Perform a saline contrast study to assess right-to-left shunt.

   e. Initiate antibiotics and perform blood cultures.

42. A 75-year-old woman presented with shortness of breath and generalized malaise of 1-week duration. Her heart rate was 90 per minute and BP was 90/50 mmHg. Examination revealed rales in bilateral lung bases, an elevated jugular venous pulse, and a loud systolic murmur in the left parasternal area. An echo (Fig. 3-4) was performed. What is the likely infarct-related artery?

   a. Proximal LAD

   b. Distal LAD

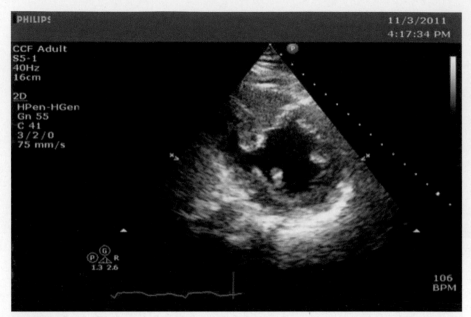

Figure 3.4

c. Obtuse marginal in a dominant circumflex

d. Mid-RCA in dominant RCA

e. Proximal nondominant RCA

43. A 42-year-old male nurse in a rural emergency room develops crushing chest pain 30 minutes after he smoked a cigarette during a break in his shift. An ECG (Fig. 3-5) is performed. What is the most appropriate intervention?

a. Load with clopidogrel 600 mg and initiate heparin for a diagnosis of NSTEMI ACS.

b. Load with prasugrel 60 mg once daily and transfer for primary PCI to a laboratory 4 hours away.

c. Treat with intravenous verapamil for vasospasm.

d. Initiate fibrinolytic therapy with reteplase with adjunctive treatment with aspirin and intravenous heparin.

e. Treat with intravenous metoprolol 5 mg three times.

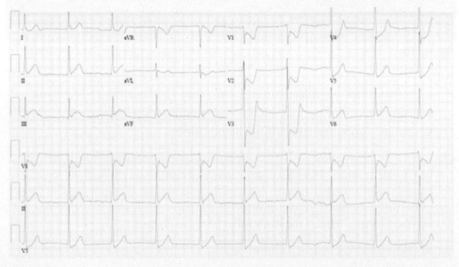

Figure 3.5

ANSWERS

1. **e.** All of the above. Based on data from national heart disease stroke statistics, while the incidence of overall ACS, STEMI, and NSTEMI has declined with time, the incidence of UA has been increasing in the last decade. The observed decline in the rate of UA is largely attributable to the availability of sensitive troponin assays that detect myocardial necrosis.

2. **a.** Plaque rupture. Plaque rupture is the dominating initiating event of acute MI. Rupture of the fibrous cap of the coronary atheroma exposes the underlying subendothelial matrix eventually leading to activation of platelets, thrombin generation, and final thrombus formation. While erosion of the plaque without rupture can lead to thrombus formation, it is not as frequent an event as plaque rupture and accounts for a third of MIs.

3. **a.** Age. Based on results of the large GUSTO-I trial the strongest predictor of mortality following STEMI is advanced age. In addition to age, other major predictors of poor prognosis on presentation include systolic BP <100 mmHg, heart rate >100 per minute, higher Killip classification stage, and anterior infarction.

4. **e.** Both b and c. Aspirin, clopidogrel, prasugrel, and ticagrelor are all antiplatelet agents. Aspirin irreversibly blocks the formation of thromboxane A_2 in platelets, producing an inhibitory effect on platelet aggregation. While clopidogrel and prasugrel are prodrugs that require hepatic bioactivation to their pharmacologically active metabolite, ticagrelor is phenotypically active and is not affected by hepatic metabolism.

5. **e.** All of the above are correct. Prasugrel has faster onset of action and potency of platelet inhibition when compared with clopidogrel. Unlike clopidogrel, prasugrel is not influenced by P-450 genetic polymorphisms. In the large, randomized TRITON-TIMI-38 trial, investigators compared prasugrel with clopidogrel in patients with ACS initiated following coronary angiography. While there was no difference in mortality, there was a reduction in composite of major adverse cardiovascular events primarily driven by reduction in nonfatal MI. A higher incidence of bleeding with prasugrel when compared with clopidogrel was noted. Post hoc analysis showed net harm in patients with prior history of TIA/stroke and prasugrel should be avoided in these patients.

6. **e.** Fibrinolysis; low-molecular-weight heparin (LMWH), aspirin, and clopidogrel; and transfer to hospital for possible PCI. This patient has acute STEMI. Current ACC/AHA guidelines recommend (class I) administration of fibrinolytic therapy (within 30 minutes) when there is an anticipated delay to performing primary PCI within 120 minutes of first medical contact. In addition to fibrinolysis, adjunctive antiplatelet therapy (aspirin 162 to 325 mg loading dose and clopidogrel 300 mg loading dose in patients aged <75 years) and antithrombotic therapy (weight-adjusted unfractionated heparin or LMWH) should be promptly initiated. Adjunctive LMWH in the setting of fibrinolysis was compared with heparin in the randomized ENTIRE-TIMI-23 trial. The study showed reduced ischemic events (death/recurrent MI) with LMWH when compared with unfractionated heparin at 30 days (4.4% versus 15.9%). The benefit of early routine angiography regardless of symptom status and hemodynamic stability has been confirmed in a number of clinical trials. As a result, transfer to a PCI hospital following lytic administration is encouraged.

7. **a.** Continue unfractionated heparin, aspirin, and clopidogrel and transfer to the nearest hospital with PCI capabilities. Repeat ECG reveals resolution of ST-segment elevation that likely indicates reperfusion. As previously stated, a significant proportion of patients receiving fibrinolysis may undergo reocclusion of the infarct artery. Therefore, it is reasonable to transfer patients to the nearest PCI-capable hospital (ACC/AHA class IIa recommendation). Angiography 3 to 24 hours after

fibrinolysis is now recommended in these subjects regardless of hemodynamic status. Discharge home after stress test and referral for delayed angiography are not preferred options for patients with acute STEMI treated with fibrinolysis.

8. **c.** Streptokinase and aspirin each have a similar effect on outcome. Based on results of International Studies of Infarct Survival (ISIS-2) trial from the fibrinolytic era, aspirin provides as much mortality benefit as streptokinase and the combination provides additive benefit in acute MI.

9. **c.** Adenosine diphosphate blockade. Ticagrelor reversibly blocks adenosine diphosphate receptors of subtype $P2Y_{12}$ on platelet cell membranes eventually leading to inhibition of platelet activation. Aspirin acts by a thromboxane inhibition and abciximab is a chimeric human monoclonal antibody that works by blockade of the activated GP II/IIIa receptor on the platelet surface.

10. **c.** Routine GP IIb/IIIa inhibitor use is associated with increased risk of bleeding. While prior studies documented benefits of routine intravenous GP IIb/IIIa in STEMI, the emergence of potent platelet adenosine diphosphate $P2Y_{12}$ receptor inhibitors sparked controversy regarding their additive benefit. Most subsequent trials demonstrated no clinical benefit with possible increased risk of bleeding with routine use of these agents in addition to dual oral antiplatelet therapy. A benefit for upstream GP IIb/IIIa inhibition was also not evident in the Early Glycoprotein IIb/IIIa Inhibition in Non–ST-Segment Elevation Acute Coronary Syndrome (EARLY ACS) and Acute Catheterization and Urgent Intervention Triage strategY (ACUITY) trials. Use of these agents is now reserved in the catheterization laboratory for patients undergoing high-risk PCI with high thrombus burden and for bailout.

11. **a.** Decrease subsequent repeat TVR. Stents decrease the rate of subsequent TVR compared with balloon angioplasty alone, but there is no favorable impact on TIMI-3 flow or mortality.

12. **d.** It had similar rates of mortality compared with alteplase. It had similar rates of mortality to alteplase. This noninferiority trial randomized over 15,000 patients with STEMI to intravenous alteplase or reteplase. The rates of mortality (11.20% and 11.06% at 1 year, respectively) and stroke were similar for reteplase and alteplase. The major advantage of reteplase was that it could be given as two boluses rather than as an infusion.

13. **e.** All of the above. Results from large TIMI registry indicate that biomarker elevation (NSTEMI) and ST-segment deviation on admission ECG carries poorer prognosis in patients with NSTE-ACS. In addition, one in five patients with NSTE-ACS may have normal or nonspecific changes on ECG.

14. **c.** Administer aspirin, sublingual nitroglycerin, and heparin. The patient has signs and symptoms suggestive of cocaine-induced ACS. The dominant underlying pathophysiologic factor in cocaine-induced ACS can be coronary spasm or thrombus formation caused by α-adrenergic stimulation. Atherosclerosis is also accelerated by cocaine use. This patient should be started on aspirin, sublingual nitroglycerin, and intravenous heparin. β-Blockers are contraindicated as they may allow unopposed α-adrenergic stimulation and have been associated with increased mortality.

15. **a.** Activate the catheterization laboratory for emergent left heart catheterization. The patient has persistent ischemia after initiation of antianginal therapy. He needs to be sent for emergent left heart catheterization. Intravenous benzodiazepine can temporarily relieve cocaine-induced chest pain but this patient has ischemic symptoms with ECG changes suggestive of ACS. Fibrinolytics have not been shown to be useful in cocaine-induced chest pain without evident thrombosis.

16. **d.** Clopidogrel 600 mg, bivalirudin drip, and atorvastatin 80 mg. This patient has acute MI. Current ACC/AHA guidelines mandate adjunctive medical therapy in

addition to aspirin, including loading dose of P2Y$_{12}$ receptor inhibitor (clopidogrel 600 mg, prasugrel 60 mg, or ticagrelor 180 mg) and anticoagulant therapy (unfractionated heparin or bivalirudin). Fondaparinux (a) should not be used as a sole anticoagulant to support primary PCI as it has been shown to increase catheter thrombosis. Prasugrel is contraindicated in patients with history of stroke.

17. **c.** Mortality benefit with routine intravenous nitroglycerin is not established. Although widely used, no randomized trial has established a mortality benefit with intravenous nitroglycerin. Intravenous ACE-I formulations have no proven benefit and were associated with increased mortality in Cooperative North Scandinavian Enalapril Survival Study (CONSENSUS 2). Routine intravenous β-blocker use within 24 hours also did not have any impact on mortality and led to higher rates of cardiogenic shock in the Clopidogrel and Metoprolol in Myocardial Infarction Trial/Second Chinese Cardiac Study (COMMIT/CCS-2) megatrial. No benefit with intravenous magnesium was noted in the National Heart, Lung and Blood Institute (NHLBI)-supported Myoblast Autologous Grafting in Ischemic Cardiomyopathy (MAGIC) trial.

18. **e.** Fibrinolysis should be considered 12 hours after symptom onset in hemodynamically stable patients with signs of ongoing ischemia. Fibrinolysis has not been shown to be useful and may even lead to harm after 12 hours of symptom onset in patients with STEMI. Two large, randomized trials (Late Assessment of Thrombolytic Efficacy (LATE) and Enhanced Myocardial Efficacy and Removal by Aspiration of Liberated Debris (EMERAS)) investigated the utility of late fibrinolysis in patients with STEMI and found no mortality benefit beyond 12 hours of symptom onset. Primary PCI is associated with reduced rate of intracerebral hemorrhage when compared with fibrinolysis. If rapidly available, primary PCI has been convincingly shown to reduce mortality when compared with fibrinolysis. Primary PCI may be considered 12 hours after symptom onset in patients with signs of ongoing ischemia. While primary PCI should be considered in patients with signs of ongoing ischemia 12 to 24 hours after symptom onset, routine PCI of the totally occluded infarct-related artery >24 hours after presentation in hemodynamically stable patients without signs of ischemia provides no additional benefit and may even be harmful. Delayed PCI (3 to 28 days after MI) of the occluded asymptomatic Infarct Related Artery (IRA) was evaluated in the randomized Occluded Artery Trial (OAT). While PCI did not reduce the occurrence of death, reinfarction, or heart failure, there was a trend toward excess reinfarction during long-term follow-up in stable patients.

19. **d.** Suspected aortic dissection. Suspected aortic dissection is an absolute contraindication for use of fibrinolysis. History of stroke, pregnancy, use of warfarin, and history of seizure disorders are all relative contraindications for fibrinolysis.

20. **c.** Presence of collateral circulation in the infarct zone reduces risk of VSR. VSR is more likely in women and after first MI. Fibrinolytic therapy is not associated with increased risk of VSR but may accelerate rupture in vulnerable subjects. VSR is equally likely after anterior or nonanterior wall MI.

21. **e.** Urgent surgical repair. This patient has VSR after acute MI. Although the shunt fraction is small, the rupture may rapidly progress in an unpredictable manner and lead to hemodynamic collapse and death. Although controversial, urgent surgical closure remains the treatment of choice. Vasodilators (nitroprusside) and IABP placements can reduce shunt fraction and increase forward flow and can be utilized in hemodynamically unstable patients as bridge to surgery. This patient is hemodynamically stable with a small shunt fraction.

22. **d.** All of the above. Acute ventricular free wall rupture usually presents with acute onset cardiac tamponade, pulsus paradoxus, and sudden death. It accounts for approximately 10% of mortality after MI. Fibrinolysis may increase risk and this potentially accounts for the "early hazard" with thrombolytic therapy as noted in the

randomized clinical trials. Type I rupture is a slit-like full-thickness rupture that is usually seen within the first 24 hours. It usually occurs in the border zone between the akinetic infarct-related segment and the adjacent hyperkinetic noninfarct zone.

23. **a.** Ventricular aneurysm is more common than ventricular pseudoaneurysm after MI. True ventricular aneurysm is more likely than pseudoaneurysm (contained rupture of LV free wall). While ventricular aneurysm is more likely with anterior MI, pseudoaneurysms occur more often after inferior wall MI. In contrast to patients with true aneurysms that are initially managed with medical therapy, pseudoaneurysms have a high risk of rupture and surgical therapy is recommended irrespective of size or presence/absence of symptoms.

24. **e.** Transthoracic echocardiogram. This patient presents with symptoms suggestive of TIA. He had a recent anterior wall MI. Persistent ST elevation in V_2 to V_4 suggests apical aneurysm that increases the risk of mural thrombus formation. Current symptoms suggest an embolic event secondary to LV mural thrombus. Echocardiogram must be done to confirm the diagnosis. Although the patient has persistent ST elevation on ECG, there are no clinical signs of recurrent ischemia and repeat left heart catheterization is not indicated.

25. **a.** Pulmonary capillary wedge pressure (PCWP) 30, confidence interval (CI) 1.6. This patient has acute STEMI complicated by cardiogenic shock. Cardiogenic shock is defined as evidence of ineffective tissue perfusion arising from cardiac dysfunction supported by the presence of a systolic BP <90 mmHg, PCWP >15 mmHg, and cardiac index <2.2 L/min/kg/m². Classic study performed in the pre-reperfusion era by Forrester risk stratified patients with cardiogenic shock based on PCWP and CI. Patients with both elevated PCWP and low CI have worst prognosis. In the GUSTO-I trial low cardiac output (and cardiac index) remained the strongest hemodynamic predictors of death in patients with cardiogenic shock.

26. **a.** Consideration for advanced mechanical support. Advanced mechanical support with IABP, ECMO, or TANDEM heart is indicated at this time. IABP reduces afterload, increases cardiac output, and reduces myocardial oxygen requirement by means of reduction in wall stress. The recently conducted Intra-aortic balloon counterpulsation in acute myocardial infarction complicated by cardiogenic shock (IABP SHOCK-II) trial failed to show a mortality benefit in this setting with IABP counterpulsation, as a result IABP support in the setting of shock is now downgraded to a IIa indication in the most recent ACC/AHA guidelines. Other supportive devices such as the TANDEM and Impella have been shown to provide superior hemodynamic support to IABP alone, although no clear benefits with regard to mortality have been noted. The patient described achieved satisfactory mechanical reperfusion and urgent CABG or repeat angiography is not indicated and nitroprusside would not be considered in this setting.

27. **c.** Atorvastatin, lisinopril, carvedilol, and eplerenone. Current guidelines in post reperfusion care include medical management for optimal risk factor control and treatment of myocardial dysfunction. High-potency statins (atorvastatin or rosuvastatin) and β-blockers are indicated in the absence of contraindications in all patients with STEMI. ACEIs are indicated in all patients after MI with ejection fraction <40% or anterior wall MI and aldosterone antagonists are indicated in patients with MI and ejection fraction <40% with clinical signs of heart failure.

28. **f.** None of the above. This patient had a brief episode of nonsustained VT in the setting of MI. Routine antiarrhythmic therapy with amiodarone or lidocaine is not indicated in patients with MI and brief, self-limited, and hemodynamically insignificant arrhythmias within 48 hours of symptoms. This patient has low ejection fraction and warrants consideration for a primary prophylaxis ICD based largely on the Multicenter Automatic Defibrillator Implantation Trial (MADIT II)

trial if ventricular function does not recover. Early use of ICD post MI was not associated with benefit in the Defibrillator in Acute Myocardial Infarction Trial (DINAMIT) and Immediate Risk Stratification Improves Survival (IRIS) trials. Patients with MI and low ejection fraction need to be reevaluated after 40 days on optimal medical therapy to determine candidacy for device therapy.

29. d. Within 30 minutes. Door in door out time in the setting of STEMI is the time from patient presentation to discharge from a non-PCI hospital to a PCI-capable hospital. A door in door out time of less than 30 minutes is associated with decrease in mortality.

30. d. Initiation of hypothermia protocol. Initiation of therapeutic hypothermia in post cardiac arrest patient has been shown to be associated with a significant mortality benefit. The patient is not in shock and administration of normal saline may lead to pulmonary edema. Prophylactic intravenous lidocaine in this setting has not been shown to have any clinical benefit and may lead to harm. The patient does not have polymorphic VT and there is no role for transvenous pacing in ischemically triggered polymorphic VT. While ECMO has been shown to be useful in patients with refractory cardiogenic shock, it is not indicated in a hemodynamically stable patient post cardiac arrest.

31. b. Treatment with clopidogrel 300 mg followed by 75 mg daily. This patient has UA and will likely rule in for an NSTEMI. Initiation of antiplatelet therapy with a bolus dose of clopidogrel 300 mg followed by 75 mg once daily is indicated based on the results of the Clopidogrel in Unstable Angina to Prevent Recurrent Events (CURE) trial. The use of prasugrel in the elderly is associated with increased risk of bleeding. In this patient who is not undergoing revascularization, the use of bolus dose prasugrel cannot be supported. In addition to antiplatelet therapy with aspirin, the patient also needs to be started on antithrombotic therapy (with unfractionated heparin, LMWH, or fondaparinux). Lastly, since he has refused revascularization, medical antianginal therapy should be maximized. Increasing β-blocker as tolerated is indicated.

32. e. Apixaban. Bivalirudin, argatroban, and hirudin are intravenous direct thrombin inhibitors and dabigatran is an oral direct thrombin inhibitor. Apixaban is an oral factor Xa inhibitor.

33. b. Fibrinolysis reduces the incidence of pericarditis in MI. Several studies, including Gruppo Italiano per lo Studio della Sopravvivenza nell'Infarto Miocardico (Italian) (GISSI 1), have examined this issue and found that fibrinolysis reduces the incidence of pericarditis in the setting of acute MI. Indeed, in the era of reperfusion therapy, the rate of both early and late pericarditis has decreased. Probably, by reducing infarct size, reperfusion decreases the incidence of pericarditis, which is more common with large MIs.

34. e. All of the above are acceptable indications for IABP use.

35. c. CT abdomen without contrast. The patient has signs and symptoms suggestive of massive retroperitoneal bleeding after left heart catheterization. Retroperitoneal bleeding is a common complication after left heart catheterization through femoral access. Patients present with anemia that may be hard to detect on clinical examination. CT abdomen without contrast is the test of choice to confirm bleeding. He has no signs of recurrent ischemia on ECG and as such repeat catheterization to look for stent thrombosis (a) is not indicated. Lack of elevated jugular venous pulse makes pulmonary embolism (b) or cardiac tamponade/acute mitral regurgitation (e) unlikely.

36. b. Performance of a gated CT of the aorta. This patient has acute aortic regurgitation and performance of gated CT aorta is urgently indicated. Development of a new diastolic murmur at the base of the heart that accentuates with expiration should raise suspicion of acute aortic regurgitation. Acute aortic regurgitation is usually secondary to endocarditis or acute ascending aortic dissection. Ascending aortic dissection can involve the coronary cusps leading to acute coronary dissection that can present with chest pain and ST elevations on ECG. Cocaine use is a major risk factor for acute aortic dissection. While nongated CT with pulmonary embolus protocol can often detect acute aortic detection, it is often associated with motion artifacts in the aortic root and is not the ideal test. The patient has a suspected acute aortic dissection, and activation of catheterization laboratory for revascularization or antiplatelet therapy is not indicated. Confirmation by the performance of a CT aorta followed by immediate surgical consultation appears warranted. While two-dimensional echo can often detect an aortic dissection flap, absence of the same does not rule out aortic dissection.

37. **d.** Recent exposure to a phosphodiesterase 5 inhibitor. This patient developed immediate hypotension after administration of nitroglycerin. Administration of nitrates in patients who have recently taken phosphodiesterase 5 inhibitors such as sildenafil acetate can lead to severe hypotension, circulatory collapse, and death. The patient is unlikely to develop massive hemorrhage within 5 minutes of aspirin load, and anaphylaxis in this setting is extremely uncommon. Administration of nitrates can cause profound hypotension in RV infarction but this patient has ST elevations in V_1 to V_4, suggesting anterior-apical wall MI.

38. **b.** Her prognosis will likely be excellent with full recovery of LV function. This patient has Takotsubo cardiomyopathy, also known as transient apical ballooning syndrome. This transient weakening of LV apex is often triggered by emotional stress, such as the death of a loved one, a breakup, or constant anxiety, and is most often seen in middle-aged women. Most patients achieve complete recovery within few months. There is no indication for ICD and there is no increased risk of atherosclerosis or malignancy. Routine anticoagulation with warfarin is not indicated in the absence of apical thrombus.

39. **a.** Discussion with the family explaining his poor prognosis and the near futility of escalating care is the ideal next step in this scenario. The patient presents with acute STEMI complicated by cardiogenic shock. The large randomized SHOCK trial did not show any benefit for a revascularization strategy in patients >75 years with cardiogenic shock. Data from multiple registries suggest that aggressive measures (IABP, heart catheterization, and revascularization) should be considered in patients with good baseline functional status, and such efforts are likely to be futile in this patient with poor functional status, extensive history of coronary artery disease, and multiple medical comorbidities.

40. **b.** Diagonal. The culprit infarct-related artery is the diagonal branch of LAD.

41. **c.** Initiate intravenous heparin and assess the risks and benefits of fibrinolysis. The echo shows a linear density in the main PA extending into the left PA. Findings are most consistent with a hemodynamically significant pulmonary embolism. Starting intravenous heparin and assessment for fibrinolysis are urgently indicated.

42. **d.** Mid RCA in dominant RCA. The echo shows a VSR in the basal inferoseptum. This area is usually supplied by the PDA. As a result, a dominant RCA infarction likely accounts for these changes.

43. **d.** Initiate fibrinolytic therapy with reteplase with adjunctive treatment with aspirin and intravenous heparin. The ECG shows significant anterior ST depression with upright T waves consistent with a true posterior current of injury. Although no benefit is noted with fibrinolytic therapy over placebo in randomized clinical trial, a benefit was noted in patients with true posterior injury defined as ST depression >2 mm in the anterior precordial leads. This patient is in the golden hour. Transfer to a remote location for PCI 4 hours later would be inappropriate.

chapter 4

Coronary Artery Disease

Baris Gencer • Debabrata Mukherjee • Marco Roffi

QUESTIONS

1. A 67-year-old man presents to the emergency room with increasing frequency of chest pain on exertion and one episode of rest pain lasting 15 minutes the day of admission. Other than for hypertension and hyperlipidemia his medical history is unremarkable. He quit smoking (1 pack a year for 20 years) 11 years ago. On physical examination he is afebrile, his pulse is 78 bpm, and his blood pressure is 138/76 mmHg. Cardiac and pulmonary auscultations are unremarkable. His current medications include aspirin, metoprolol, ramipril, and atorvastatin. The electrocardiogram (ECG) at admission reveals deep T-wave inversion in the precordial leads and no pathologic Q waves. You admit the patient to the hospital and start intravenous (IV) unfractionated heparin (UFH) and nitroglycerine. The first available serum troponin I level is 1.4 µg/L (upper limit of normal, 0.09 µg/L). Cardiac echocardiography shows an anterior and apical hypokinesia with mildly depressed left ventricular function. The next step in his management would be

   a. low-level exercise stress ECG next morning.

   b. to continue IV heparin and nitroglycerin, increase β-blocker, and add a calcium antagonist until completely free of chest pain for 24 hours, then discharge home.

   c. coronary angiography within 48 hours followed by percutaneous intervention/surgical revascularization if indicated.

   d. dobutamine echocardiogram or myocardial perfusion scan within 48 hours.

   e. continue IV heparin and nitroglycerin, increase β-blocker, and add a calcium antagonist until completely free of chest pain for 24 hours, then transfer to a cardiac rehabilitation program.

2. A 57-year-old man presenting with unstable angina (UA) was successfully treated with percutaneous coronary intervention (PCI) of a significant lesion of the right coronary artery (RCA) in the presence of a normal left ventricular ejection fraction (LVEF). He is referred for cardiac rehabilitation program. What is the expected benefit?

   a. Reduced risk of stent restenosis

   b. Lower rate of hospital readmission

   c. Reduction in maximal $\dot{V}O_2$

   d. Higher event rate related to exercise

   e. Reduced risk of stent thrombosis

3. A 66-year-old man with stable angina at low exertion level was investigated with coronary angiography that showed an isolated significant lesion (70%) of the ostium and mid-portion of the left main coronary artery in the presence of a normal left ventricular function. What is the correct statement regarding the recommended approach?

  a. Heart team discussion between the interventional cardiologist and the cardiac surgeon to select the best treatment option is the recommended approach.

  b. Coronary artery bypass grafting (CABG) is the recommended approach for all patients with left main disease.

  c. PCI is the recommended approach for all patients with left main disease.

  d. A calculation of the Society of Thoracic Surgeons (STS) and SYNTAX (Synergy between PCI with TAXUS and Cardiac Surgery) scores is not recommended at this stage.

  e. The choice of treatment is independent of the clinical presentations (stable angina or acute coronary syndromes [ACSs]).

4. A 58-year-old man with coronary artery disease (CAD) and severe chronic obstructive pulmonary disease (COPD) with forced expiratory volume in the first second of expiration (FEV_1)/forced vital capacity <0.74 with FEV_1 <40% predicted had stenting of the mid-left anterior descending artery (LAD) 10 months prior to admission with a 3.0 mm × 24 mm bare metal stent (BMS). He presents now with recurrent angina despite intensified medical treatment, and coronary angiography reveals a severe and diffuse in-stent restenosis (ISR). A reasonable next therapeutic option would be

  a. plain balloon angioplasty.

  b. coronary artery bypass surgery.

  c. drug-eluting stent (DES) implantation (stent-in-stent).

  d. medical therapy.

  e. brachytherapy.

5. A 66-year-old man had in the last few months sporadic episodes of chest pain on exertion. His cardiovascular (CV) risk factors included diabetes, hypertension, and hypercholesterolemia. He had no other comorbidity. Coronary angiography revealed a lesion of 60% of the RCA in addition to multiple nonsignificant plaques affecting the three coronary arteries. The fractional flow reserve (FFR) of the RCA (0.0.85) and LVEF were normal. What is the recommended treatment for this patient?

  a. CABG is the first recommended approach as the risk of surgical procedure is low.

  b. PCI is the first recommended approach as the SYNTAX score is low.

  c. Perform an additional imaging (myocardial perfusion scan or magnetic resonance [MR] perfusion scan) in addition to optimal medical management.

  d. Guideline-directed medical therapy is the first recommended approach.

  e. Repeat coronary angiography after 6 months to exclude disease progression in addition to optimal medical management.

6. A 58-year-old male smoker treated for hypertension complained about chest pain on exertion in the preceding 4 weeks. To investigate the clinical symptoms, you performed a stress perfusion cardiac magnetic resonance showing hypoperfusion during IV administration of adenosine. Which area of the myocardium is more vulnerable to hypoperfusion?

  a. Subepicardium

  b. Mid-myocardium

  c. Subendocardium

  d. Pericardium

  e. All of the above

7. A 73-year-old man presents to the emergency room with severe mid-sternal chest discomfort. He appears anxious and in distress. His heart rate is 66 bpm, blood pressure is 92/68 mmHg, and respiratory rate is 14. There is marked jugular venous distention. Cardiac auscultation is unremarkable and the lungs are clear. ECG reveals 2-mm ST-segment elevation in leads II, III, and aVF. The most likely diagnosis is

   a. acute pericarditis.

   b. acute aortic dissection.

   c. pneumothorax.

   d. inferior wall myocardial infarction (MI) with right ventricular infarction.

   e. pneumonia.

8. A 65-year-old hypertensive man was hospitalized for non-ST-segment-elevation myocardial infarction (NSTEMI). The clinical examination shows a fourth heart sound (S_4). What is expected to be found at the echocardiography?

   a. Reduction in left ventricular compliance

   b. Rapid deceleration of transmitral flow during protodiastolic filling of the left ventricle

   c. Increased inflow into the left ventricle

   d. Reduced left ventricular systolic function

   e. Aortic sclerosis

9. A 66-year-old man known for diabetes mellitus treated with oral glucose lowering medications presents with UA. Coronary angiography reveals a three-vessel disease: 70% mid-LAD lesion, complex, long, and calcified; 70% focal proximal left circumflex artery (LCX) stenosis; and 70% focal mid-RCA lesion. A hybrid coronary revascularization was proposed. All the following statements are correct regarding hybrid coronary revascularization, with the exception of one.

   a. Hybrid revascularization is defined as the planned combination of surgical and percutaneous revascularization (typically left internal mammary artery [LIMA]-to-LAD and PCI of ≥1 additional vessel).

   b. Hybrid revascularization is reasonable in patients with limitations to traditional CABG, such as heavily calcified proximal aorta.

   c. Hybrid revascularization is reasonable in patients with lack of suitable graft conduit.

   d. Hybrid revascularization is reasonable in patients with unfavorable LAD artery for PCI.

   e. Hybrid revascularization mandates surgical and percutaneous revascularization during the same procedure.

10. A 57-year-old female smoker presents to the emergency department for an ongoing new typical chest pain lasting 30 minutes. The physical examination is unremarkable and she is hemodynamically stable. The ECG reveals T inversion in II, III, and aVF leads. Which of the following biomarker elevation has been associated with an improved benefit of ticagrelor therapy over clopidogrel in patients hospitalized with ACS?

    a. Ultrasensible C-reactive protein

    b. Interleukin-6

    c. High-sensitive troponin T (Hs-TnT)

    d. D-dimers

    e. Lactate dehydrogenase

11. A 58-year-old man known for a metabolic syndrome shows increasing frequency of chest pain on exertion in the preceding 2 weeks. Resting ECG did not show significant abnormalities. Which of the exercise parameters are associated with adverse prognosis?

a. Duration of symptom-limiting exercise <5 METs (metabolic equivalents)

b. Failure to increase systolic blood pressure ≥120 mmHg, or a sustained decrease ≥10 mmHg, or below rest levels, during progressive exercise

c. ST-segment depressions ≥2 mm

d. Angina pectoris at low exercise workloads

e. All of the above

12. A 58-year-old man presented stable chest pain on moderate effort exertion in the preceding 12 months. The medical history is relevant for hypertension and hyperlipidemia. His current treatment includes lisinopril, atorvastatin, metoprolol, and aspirin. He is addressed for coronary angiography that showed a 70% to 90% lesion of the LCX successfully treated with PCI with a placement of a DES. The LVEF was normal. What was the expected benefit of a PCI over a medical therapy?

a. Decrease of total mortality

b. Decrease of CV mortality

c. Decrease of MI

d. Decrease of heart failure events

e. No improvement of any of the mentioned endpoints

13. The same patient was investigated with stress imaging before and after PCI to assess the extension of myocardial ischemia. Which of the following statements is correct regarding the benefit of PCI over medical therapy in this setting?

a. A greater reduction in the extension of residual myocardial ischemia

b. A greater resolution of angina episodes

c. An increased benefit of ischemia reduction in patients with extensive ischemic areas at baseline

d. A greater improvement in symptoms

e. All of the above

14. A 63-year-old man has been successfully treated with percutaneous coronary revascularization for a stable angina pectoris. His low-density lipoprotein cholesterol (LDL-C) value was 143 mg/dL. Which of the following statement is incorrect regarding the impact of prescribing intensive lipid-lowering therapy (e.g., 80 mg atorvastatin daily) compared with less intensive therapy (e.g., 10 mg atorvastatin daily)?

a. Higher LDL-C level reduction

b. Significant absolute risk reduction of major adverse cardiovascular events (MACE) of ~2% over 5 years

c. Significant relative risk reduction of MACE of ~20% over 5 years

d. Increased incidence of persistent liver aminotransferase levels of 1%

e. Significant reduction of overall mortality

15. A 67-year-old man is treated with PCI. Which of the following statement is not correct regarding periprocedural anticoagulation?

a. An anticoagulant should be administered to all patients undergoing PCI.

b. Administration of IV UFH is useful in patients undergoing PCI.

c. An additional dosage of IV enoxaparin should be administered at the time of PCI to patients who received the last subcutaneous dose of enoxaparin 12 hours or more prior to PCI.

d. The appropriate diagnostic test to check for the level of anticoagulation with UFH during PCI is the activated clotting time.

e. Fondaparinux might be used as the sole anticoagulant to support PCI.

16. A 65-year-old male hypertensive smoker benefited from primary PCI of the RCA for inferior STEMI. Which of the following statements is not correct regarding secondary prevention in this patient?

   a. Medically supervised cardiac rehabilitation programs are recommended.

   b. Blood pressure should be controlled with a goal of <140/90 mmHg.

   c. Statin therapy should be uptitrated to achieve an LDL-C <70 mg/dL

   d. Smoking cessation program should be proposed.

   e. Even in the absence of symptoms, routine periodic stress testing is indicated.

17. A 60-year-old male patient was treated 2 years earlier with PCI and the implantation of BMS in the LAD for NSTEMI. He complains about recurrent worsening exertional chest pain in the last week. Coronary angiography reveals ISR. What are the predisposing factors for BMS restenosis?

   a. Diabetes

   b. Increasing stent length

   c. Increasing stent number

   d. Decreasing stent diameter

   e. All of the above

18. A 60-year-old healthy colleague on no medication with an LDL-C level of 123 mg/dL and High-sensitivity C-reactive protein (hs-CRP) level >2.0 mg/L asked to you whether he should take rosuvastatin 20 mg a day. Which of the following statements is incorrect regarding JUPITER trial?

   a. Rosuvastatin 20 mg/day reduced LDL-C levels by 50%.

   b. Rosuvastatin 20 mg/day significantly decreased the incidence of MI.

   c. Rosuvastatin 20 mg/day reduced hs-CRP by 37%.

   d. Rosuvastatin 20 mg/day did not significantly decrease the incidence of stroke.

   e. Rosuvastatin 20 mg/day significantly increased the incidence of physician-reported diabetes.

19. A 65-year-old man with diabetes presented typical chest pain on exertion in the previous 2 months. Coronary angiography revealed significant complex multivessel coronary disease (SYNTAX score, 34). What is the expected benefit of a revascularization with CABG versus PCI?

   a. CABG is associated with a reduction of death only.

   b. CABG is associated with a reduction of stroke only.

   c. CABG is associated with a reduction of death and of MI, but not of stroke.

   d. CABG is associated with a reduction of all following individual endpoints: stroke, myocardial infraction, and death.

   e. CABG is associated with a reduction of MI only.

20. A 41-year-old male smoker was admitted for STEMI and quitted smoking after hospitalization. Which of the following statements is incorrect regarding smoking cessation?

   a. Smoking cessation reduces the relative risk of total mortality by >30% over a mean follow-up of 5 years.

   b. Smoking cessation reduces the relative risk of nonfatal MI by >30% over a mean follow-up of 5 years.

   c. More than 70% of patients quit smoking after ACS.

   d. Smoking cessation counseling program is effective to help smokers to quit smoking.

   e. Smoking cessation counseling program should be proposed during hospital stay and continued after discharge.

21. Six hours after the start of chest pain, a 55-year-old diabetic man was admitted to the emergency department for anterior STEMI with hemodynamic instability (cold extremities, heart rate of 110 bpm and blood pressure of 85/50 mmHg) and severe reduced LVEF (25% to 30%) estimated by echocardiography. What is the correct statement regarding the decision to perform an emergent revascularization versus an initial medical stabilization according to the SHOCK trial?

    a. Significant reduction of mortality with early revascularization compared with intensive medical therapy at 30 days
    b. No significant difference of mortality with early revascularization compared with intensive medical therapy at 30 days
    c. Significant reduction with intensive medical therapy compared with early revascularization at 30 days
    d. Significant reduction of mortality with early revascularization compared with intensive medical therapy at 6 months
    e. Answers b and d are correct

22. A 63-year-old man known for chronic kidney disease (CKD) due to long-term uncontrolled hypertension is hospitalized for elective coronary angiography. Which of the following statements is not correct?

    a. Patients with CKD undergoing cardiac catheterization should receive adequate preparatory hydration.
    b. In patients with CKD, the volume of contrast should be minimized.
    c. Administration of *N*-acetyl-cysteine is useful for the prevention of contrast-induced acute kidney injury (AKI).
    d. Contrast-induced AKI is one of the leading causes of hospital-acquired AKI.
    e. In elective cases, patients should be assessed for risk of contrast-induced AKI before coronary angiography.

23. A 45-year-old man benefited from primary PCI for STEMI. The adjunctive antithrombotic therapy consisted of aspirin, heparin, and abciximab. The addition of abciximab is associated with

    a. no significant difference in the risk of stroke.
    b. a significant increase in the risk of stroke.
    c. a significant decrease in the risk of stroke.
    d. a significant decrease of nonhemorrhagic stroke only.
    e. a significant increase of hemorrhagic stroke only.

24. A 65-year-old diabetic man known for a multivessel coronary disease underwent revascularization with CABG. What is the target LDL-C that should be aimed?

    a. 160 mg/dL
    b. 130 mg/dL
    c. 100 mg/dL
    d. 70 mg/dL
    e. 50 mg/dL

25. A 62-year-old man was hospitalized for an NSTEMI and underwent invasive strategy with DES-based PCI. Which of the following statements about antiplatelet therapy is wrong?

    a. Patients not on aspirin should be given nonenteric aspirin 325 mg before PCI.
    b. After PCI, use of aspirin should be continued indefinitely.
    c. Additional aspirin (81 to 325 mg) is recommended in all patients on chronic aspirin therapy before PCI.

d. A loading dose of a $P2Y_{12}$ receptor inhibitor should be given to patients undergoing PCI with stenting at the latest after completion of PCI (e.g., clopidogrel 600 mg, prasugrel 60 mg, and ticagrelor 180 mg).

e. In patients receiving a stent (BMS or DES) during PCI for ACS, $P2Y_{12}$ receptor inhibitor should be given for 12 months.

26. A 50-year-old white female nonsmoker without history of cardiovascular disease (CVD) and treated only with ramipril for hypertension was hospitalized for UA. The ECG revealed T inversion in the lateral leads. The medical student who admitted the patient asks you what is the proportion of patients that undergo coronary angiography for ACS who have nonsignificant CAD.

a. <5%

b. 10% to 15%

c. 20% to 30%

d. 25% to 35%

e. 30% to 40%

27. A 59-year-old man was successfully treated with PCI for NSTEMI. During the procedure, the patient received bivalirudin. Due to closure device failure, the patient suffered a major bleeding at the access site difficult to control with manual compression and you are in need of reversing the anticoagulation. Your treatment of choice is

a. fresh frozen plasma.

b. prothrombin complex.

c. epsilon aminocaproic acid.

d. protamine.

e. vitamin K.

28. A 63-year-old man presents typical chest pain at moderate exertion in the preceding month and he is admitted to the hospital for coronary angiography. While considering the best access for the procedure, which of the following statements is not correct regarding a radial vascular access?

a. The radial vascular access may be useful to decrease access site complications.

b. The radial vascular access is preferred in patients with coagulopathy.

c. The radial vascular access is preferred in patients with morbid obesity.

d. The radial vascular access is preferred in patients with an elevated INR.

e. The radial vascular access is more frequently performed in the United States than in Europe.

29. Which of the following conditions does not justify immediate coronary angiography and, if needed, revascularization?

a. A 57-year-old man presenting with typical chest pain lasting 60 minutes up to emergency department arrival. As cardiologist on call you are called in immediately and when you see the patient, his pain has virtually disappeared while ECG shows 2-mm ST-segment elevation in the inferior leads.

b. A 60-year-old diabetic man known for previous coronary disease presenting with not better defined chest discomfort lasting for 10 hours and currently decreasing in intensity, pulmonary edema, and 3-mm ST-segment elevation in the anterior leads on ECG in the absence of Q waves.

c. A 65-year-old man known for CAD complaining of progressive shortness of breath since 1 week. At admission, no ongoing chest pain with stable hemodynamic status but bibasilar rales at lung auscultation. The ECG revealed ST-segment elevation as well as Q waves in the anterior leads.

d. A 70-year-old man presenting to the emerging department with on–off chest pain in the preceding 20 hours. Upon your arrival he has mild chest pain and on ECG 2-mm ST elevation in the lateral leads in the absence of Q waves.

e. A 68-year-old diabetic man presenting to the emerging department with chest pain lasting 4 hours, hypotension, and tachycardia and on ECG 3-mm ST-segment elevation in the anterior and lateral leads.

30. A 76-year-old man with no prior cardiac history presents to the emergency department with acute retrosternal chest pain. He had a single episode of chest pain lasting 4 hours 5 days ago. At that time he did not seek medical attention. Physical examination reveals a slightly confused diaphoretic patient, with heart rate of 95 bpm, blood pressure of 76/42 mmHg, and cold extremities. He is able to lie flat, the lungs are clear, and the jugular veins are distended even if the upper part of the body is raised at 45°. On cardiac auscultation a loud systolic murmur is audible, while on ECG Q waves associated with ST-segment elevation are detected in the inferior leads. The most likely diagnosis is

a. severe left ventricular failure.

b. ventricular septal defect.

c. acute mitral regurgitation.

d. right ventricular infarction.

e. cardiac rupture.

31. Considering the suspected diagnosis for the patient described in the previous question, what is the next diagnostic step?

a. Cardiac enzymes

b. Chest X-ray

c. Transesophageal echocardiography

d. Immediate coronary angiography

e. Transthoracic echocardiography

32. While considering surgery for the patient described in the previous two questions, the most effective cardiac unloading treatment for him is

a. fluid resuscitation.

b. β-blockers.

c. mechanical ventilation with positive end-expiratory pressure.

d. vasopressors.

e. intra-aortic balloon pump.

33. A 66-year-old man with a history of diabetes was referred for coronary angiography. The procedure showed complex multivessel disease. Which of the following statements justify the use of DES over BMS?

a. Patient with diabetes mellitus

b. Long coronary lesions

c. Multifocal coronary lesions

d. Small vessel disease

e. All of the above

34. A 63-year-old male smoker with no history of CVD and a treatment for hypertension complains of typical chest pain on exertion the preceding 2 months without any aggravation. He is scheduled for coronary angiography in 7 days. In the meantime, you should start the following antiplatelet treatment(s):

a. Low-dose aspirin daily

b. Clopidogrel 75 mg daily without loading dose

   c. A loading dose of clopidogrel 300 mg followed by 75 mg daily should be given

   d. A loading dose of ticagrelor 180 mg followed by 2 × 90 mg/day should be given

   e. No antiplatelet therapy needed prior to coronary angiography

35. A 66-year-old man with intermediate probability of ischemic heart disease is scheduled for stress testing. Which of the following strategies is not recommended?

   a. Exercise ECG if able to exercise and ECG interpretable

   b. Exercise echocardiography if able to exercise but uninterpretable ECG

   c. Pharmacologic stress with nuclear myocardial perfusion imaging if able to exercise and ECG interpretable

   d. Exercise stress with nuclear myocardial perfusion imaging if able to exercise but uninterpretable ECG

   e. Pharmacologic stress with cardiac MR imaging if unable to exercise and interpretable ECG

36. A 65-year-old man with hypercholesterolemia, diabetes, and hypertension presents new, worsening, typical angina symptoms. The angiogram (Fig. 4.1) shows

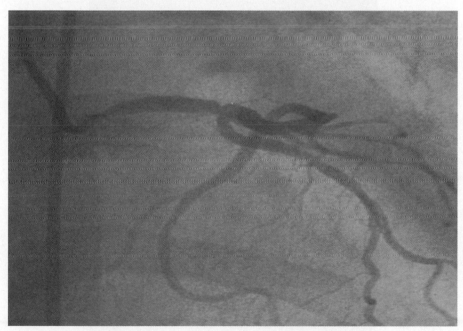

Figure 4.1

   a. occluded LAD.

   b. occluded left circumflex coronary artery.

   c. severe ostial and moderate distal left main trunk stenosis.

   d. normal coronary arteries.

   e. normal RCA.

37. A 64-year-old man with stable ischemic heart disease (SIHD) wants to know whether he is at high risk for mortality. Which of the following clinical and exercise testing data are useful to predict the risk?

   a. Typical angina symptoms

   b. Diabetes

c. ST-segment depression during exercise

d. Proportion of predicted METs achieved

e. All of the above

38. A 48-year-old woman presents with congestive heart failure. The etiology of her heart failure based on the coronary angiogram (Fig. 4.2) is

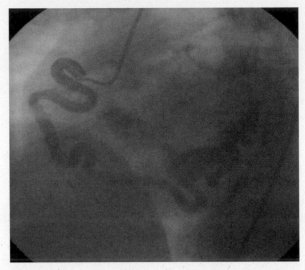

Figure 4.2

a. severe CAD.

b. arteriovenous fistula.

c. aortic regurgitation.

d. absent RCA.

e. coronary perforation.

39. A 72-year-old man known with a history of coronary heart disease presents typical chest pain. During the transport to the PCI center, the patient had two episodes of ventricular fibrillation requiring electrical reanimation. ECG shows inferolateral ST depression. What does the angiography show (Fig. 4.3)?

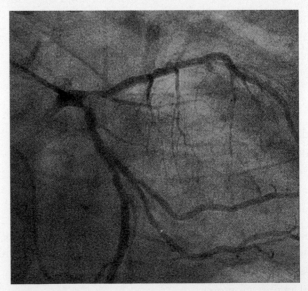

Figure 4.3

a. Lesions at bifurcation

b. Stenosis of the ostium of the LCX

c. Stenosis of the ostium of the LAD

d. Stenosis of the distal left main trunk

e. All of the above

40. During coronary angioplasty of the RCA, this 72-year-old patient developed sharp chest pain with rapid development of hypotension and tachycardia. The etiology based on Figure 4.4 is

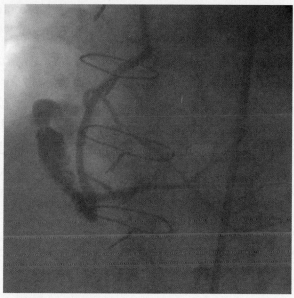

Figure 4.4

a. abrupt closure of the RCA.

b. dissection of the RCA.

c. perforation of the RCA.

d. allergic reaction.

e. distal embolization of an atherosclerotic plaque.

41. For which clinical situation is coronary angiography not recommended in patients with SIHD?

a. Risk assessment in patients with SIHD not candidates for revascularization because of comorbidities

b. Risk assessment in patients with SIHD who have preserved LV function and low-risk criteria on noninvasive testing

c. Risk assessment in patients who are at low risk according to clinical criteria and have not undergone noninvasive risk testing

d. Risk assessment in asymptomatic patients with no evidence of ischemia on noninvasive testing

e. All the mentioned clinical situations do not justify coronary angiography in the initial phase of patient management

42. A 66-year-old man with diabetes with no hypertension but end-stage renal failure treated with hemodialysis in the last 15 years presents with worsening dyspnea and suspicion of ischemia at the stress imaging. What are the most characteristic findings relating to the coronary arteries to be found at angiography?

a. Tortuous coronary vessels

b. Calcified coronary arteries

c. Ectatic coronary arteries

d. Coronary arteries with anomalous origins

e. Normal coronary arteries (symptoms caused by small vessel disease)

43. A 65-year-old man with SIHD wants to optimize secondary prevention. Which of the following statements does not apply?

a. Smoking cessation and avoidance of exposure to environmental tobacco smoke at work and home should be encouraged.

b. Patients should be screened for depression and treated when indicated.

c. Treatment with clopidogrel is reasonable when aspirin is contraindicated.

d. Dipyridamole is not recommended as antiplatelet therapy for patients with SIHD.

e. Acupuncture might be used for the purpose of improving symptoms of patients with SIHD.

44. A 74-year-old man was hospitalized for a subacute MI. He presented 1 week prior to admission one episode of chest pain lasting 3 hours but he did not seek medical attention. The ECG at admission revealed deep Q waves and persisting ST-segment elevation in the anterior leads. The angiography showed a total occlusion of the proximal left anterior ascending coronary artery. Which statement about the benefit of revascularization in this particular patient does apply?

a. PCI reduces the occurrence of death.

b. PCI reduces the occurrence of reinfarction.

c. PCI reduces the occurrence of heart failure.

d. CABG should be preferred to PCI.

e. PCI does not reduce the occurrence of death, reinfarction, or heart failure.

45. A 60-year-old man with a history of PCI 3 years previously asks for your advice with respect to his pharmacologic treatment. He is asymptomatic and his CV risk factors include smoking, hypertension, hypercholesterolemia, and impaired glucose tolerance. His medications include aspirin, atorvastatin, metoprolol, metformin, and lisinopril. His friend told him that clopidogrel should be added to his regimen. What is the correct statement about that suggestion in this particular patient?

a. There is no significant benefit associated with clopidogrel plus aspirin as compared with placebo plus aspirin in reducing the incidence of the primary endpoint of MI, stroke, or death from CV causes.

b. There is a significant benefit associated with clopidogrel plus aspirin as compared with placebo plus aspirin in reducing the incidence of the primary endpoint of MI, stroke, or death from CV causes.

c. The rate of severe or moderate bleeding is not significantly greater with clopidogrel and aspirin compared with aspirin alone.

d. The rate of severe or moderate bleeding is significantly greater with clopidogrel and aspirin compared with aspirin alone.

e. Answers a and d are correct.

46. A 60-year-old woman was discharged after an MI. Pharmacologic secondary prevention with antiplatelet agents, statins, β-blockers, and angiotensin-converting enzyme inhibitors is associated with

a. significant reduction in recurrent angina but no mortality benefit.

b. significant survival advantage.

c. no significant clinical benefit.

d. significant reduction in recurrent hospitalization but no mortality benefit.

e. significant survival advantage only in patients treated with PCI.

47. A 55-year-old man presents since 3 months typical chest pain at moderate exertion. The angiography revealed single-vessel disease. An optimal therapy has been started; what is the benefit of a treatment with PCI of the culprit lesion?

  a. PCI would reduce the risk of death, MI, or other major CV events when added to optimal medical therapy (OMT).

  b. PCI may reduce the episodes of angina in the presence of moderate-to-severe ischemia at stress single-photon emission computed tomography (SPECT) but not the risk of death, MI, or other major CV events when added to OMT.

  c. PCI would not reduce the risk of death, MI, angina episodes, or other CV events when added to OMT.

  d. The benefit of revascularization in patients with stable angina and ischemia detected on SPECT is independent of the extent of ischemia.

  e. Selective ischemia-driven PCI approach should be avoided, as thus not improved clinical outcomes.

48. A 67-year-old man known for hypertension and hypercholesterolemia presented significant ST elevation in inferoposterior leads during the treadmill test. The angiogram shows (Fig. 4.5)

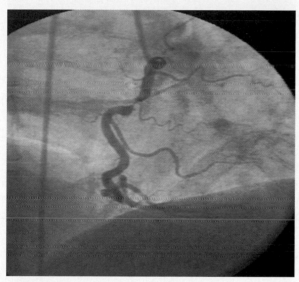

Figure 4.5

  a. severe LCX stenosis.

  b. severe left main trunk stenosis.

  c. severe LAD stenosis.

  d. severe RCA stenosis.

  e. no significant coronary artery stenosis.

49. A 66-year-old man hospitalized for an NSTEMI was successfully treated with DES for a subtotal lesion of the proximal LAD. What is the recommended minimal duration of dual antiplatelet therapy according to the 2011 American College of Cardiology (ACC)/American Heart Association (AHA) guidelines on PCI?

  a. 1 month

  b. 3 months

  c. 6 months

  d. 12 months

  e. 24 months

50. A 54-year-old man known for smoking and hypertension is admitted to the emergency department with an NSTEMI. Echocardiography reveals abnormalities in the acute lateral wall motion. The angiogram (Fig. 4.6) shows

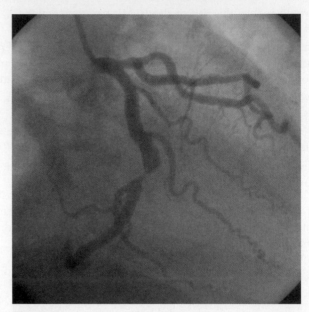

Figure 4.6

a. severe LCX stenosis.

b. severe left main trunk stenosis.

c. severe LAD stenosis.

d. severe RCA stenosis.

e. no significant coronary artery stenosis.

51. A 75-year-old man has been treated 1 month ago with a DES in the proximal LAD for ACS. At that time he did not mention that he was supposed to require surgery for debilitating knee arthritis. Which of the following statements is correct?

a. The recent implantation of a DES is not problematic as long as aspirin can be continued during surgery.

b. The recent implantation of DES is not problematic as long as clopidogrel can be continued during surgery.

c. The recent implantation of DES is not problematic as long as aspirin and clopidogrel can be continued during surgery.

d. Discontinuation of dual antiplatelet therapy followed by noncardiac surgery in the first few weeks following stent implantation is associated with increased ischemic cardiac events with both DES and BMS.

e. Discontinuation of dual antiplatelet therapy followed by surgery in the first few weeks following stent implantation is problematic with DES but not BMS.

52. A 66-year-old woman had a second-generation DES implantation after an acute MI. What is the correct statement?

a. To prevent DES late thrombosis, dual antiplatelet therapy with aspirin and clopidogrel is recommended for 3 years.

b. Based on the results of the CHARISMA (Clopidogrel for High Atherothrombotic Risk and Ischemic Stabilization Management, and Avoidance) trial, aspirin and clopidogrel should be administered for at least 2 years in patients with an acute coronary event, independently of the implantation of a DES.

c. At 1 year, clopidogrel may be discontinued but if the patient is on low-dose aspirin, the dose of aspirin has to be increased to 325 mg/day.

d. In patients who have already suffered a stent thrombosis dual antiplatelet therapy may be extended long term, although currently there are no data to support this strategy.

e. Following DES implantation, aspirin should be discontinued at 12 months and clopidogrel administered indefinitely.

53. A 60-year-old man known for current smoking is admitted to the emergency department for prolonged typical chest pain. The 12-lead ECG is shown in Figure 4.7. What is the most likely finding at the coronary angiography?

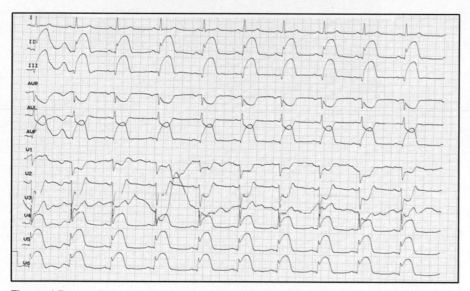

Figure 4.7

a. Occlusion of the first marginal branch of the left circumflex coronary artery
b. Occlusion of the proximal left anterior descending coronary artery
c. Occlusion of the dominant RCA
d. Occlusion of the left main trunk
e. Occlusion of the first diagonal branch

54. A 37-year-old man known for obesity felt typical chest pain while playing tennis accompanied by nausea, dyspnea, and sudations. The ECG shows ST-segment elevation. He is immediately admitted to the catheterization laboratory (Fig. 4.8). What is the underlying pathology?

a. Thrombotic occlusion of the left main trunk
b. Anomalous origin of the left main trunk
c. Dissection of the left main trunk
d. Vasospasm of the left main trunk
e. None of the above

55. A 58-year-old man known for hypertension and smoking suffered chest pain and dyspnea in the previous 48 hours. He consulted emergency department for persisting symptoms. The rest 12-lead ECG at admissions is shown in Figure 4.9. What is the diagnosis?

a. Takotsubo cardiomyopathy
b. Pericarditis
c. Anterior subacute MI

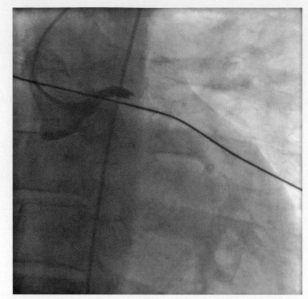

Figure 4.8

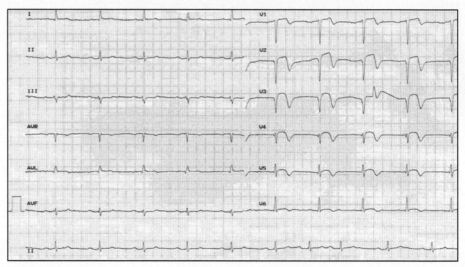

Figure 4.9

d. Cardiomyopathy hypertrophic obstructive

e. Hypertensive heart disease

56. A 28-year-old male smoker presented after wakeup typical inaugural chest pain. The 12-rest ECG at admission is shown in Figure 4.10. He is transferred immediately to the catheterization laboratory. What is the most likely finding?

a. Occlusion of a large diagonal branch

b. Occlusion of the left anterior descending coronary artery

c. Occlusion of the left circumflex coronary artery

d. Occlusion of the RCA

e. Normal coronary angiogram

57. A 69-year-old man known for hypertension and diabetes consulted emergency department for typical chest pain. The ECG did not show significant changes. Troponins were elevated (1.4 μg/L). Coronary angiography (Fig. 4.11) shows

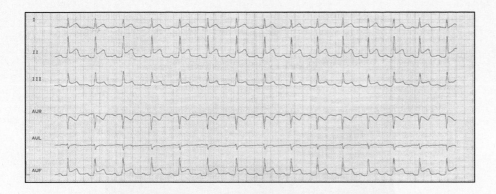

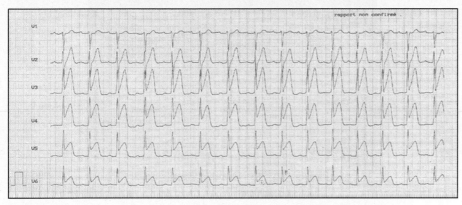

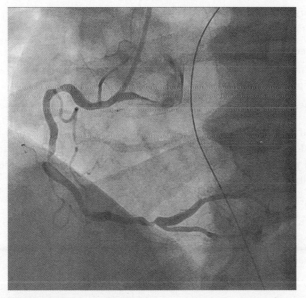

Figure 4.10

Figure 4.11

a. no significant lesion of the RCA.

b. perforation of the mid-portion of the RCA.

c. anomalous origin of the RCA.

d. visible thrombus in the mid-portion of the RCA.

e. dissection of the mid-portion of the RCA.

58. A 41-year-old overweight heavy-smoker construction worker presented with chest pain while on the job associated with diaphoresis and dyspnea. In the field, no ECG could be obtained due to the extreme diaphoresis. In the ambulance, the patient developed hypotension, bradycardia, and subsequently asystole. Under cardiopulmonary resuscitation he was transferred to the cardiac catheterization laboratory and circulation was reestablished using extracorporeal membrane oxygenation. Subsequently, coronary angiography (Fig. 4.12) shows

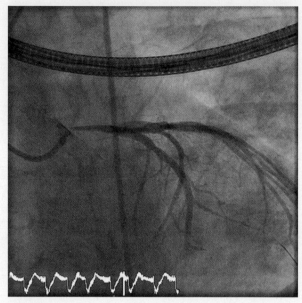

Figure 4.12

   a. subtotal occlusion of the left main trunk.

   b. aortic dissection.

   c. anomalous origin of the left main trunk.

   d. left main trunk stenosis equivalent (i.e., severe stenosis of the left anterior descending coronary artery and left circumflex).

   e. severe aortic stenosis.

59. A 61-year-old man known for diabetes, hypercholesterolemia, hypertension, and a history of PCI with stenting of the mid-left anterior descending coronary artery 10 years earlier presents with worsening typical angina on exertion and a positive stress test. Coronary angiography (Fig. 4.13) shows

   a. ISR of the left descending coronary artery.

   b. significant stenosis of LCX.

   c. stenosis of the ostium of the left main trunk.

   d. normal coronary arteries.

   e. none of the above.

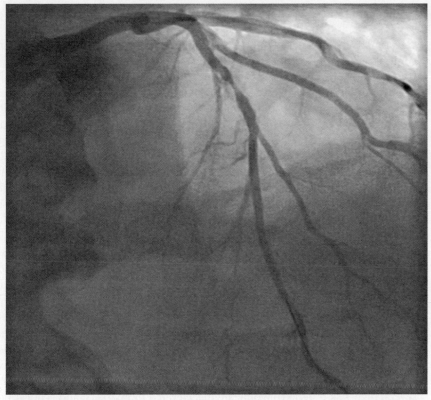

Figure 4.13

ANSWERS

1. **c.** Coronary angiography within 48 hours followed by percutaneous intervention/ surgical revascularization if indicated. There is continued debate as to whether a routine, early invasive strategy is superior to a conservative strategy for the management of UA and NSTEMI. A pooled analysis of randomized controlled trials with 5,467 patients compared the impact of routine invasive (RI) strategy with selective invasive (SI) strategy: Over 5 years, 14.7% of patients randomized to an RI strategy experienced CV health or nonfatal MI versus 17.9% in the SI strategy (hazard ratio [HR]: 0.81; 95% confidence interval [CI]: 0.71 to 0.93; $P = 0.002$). However, the largest absolute effect was mainly observed in higher-risk patients (11.1%).[1] Another meta-analysis using data from eight trials (3,075 women and 7,075 men) compared early invasive versus conservative treatment strategies in women and men with UA and NSTEMI and reported comparable odds ratio (OR) for reducing MACE (death, MI, and rehospitalization for ACS) of 0.81 (95% CI: 0.65 to 1.01) in women and 0.73 (95% CI: 0.55 to 0.98) in men. In contrast, an invasive strategy was not associated with a significant reduction in low-risk (biomarker-negative) women.[2] The 2012 ACC/AHA guidelines for the management of patients with unstable angina/non-ST-elevation myocardial infarction recommend an early invasive strategy (i.e., diagnostic angiography with intent to perform revascularization) in patients who have refractory angina or hemodynamic or electrical instability, and in those initially stabilized who have an elevated risk of clinical events.[3] Table 4.1 lists patients at elevated risk and in whom invasive strategy is preferred based on the ACC/AHA 2011 guidelines. Our patient has several high-risk criteria (ongoing angina, elevated biomarkers, and echocardiographic abnormalities). TIMI (Thrombolysis in Myocardial Infarction) risk score revealed 5 points (26% risk at 14 days of MACE) and GRACE (Global Registry of Acute Cardiac Events) risk score showed a high risk of mortality.

2. **b.** Lower rate of hospital readmission. Belardinelli et al. addressed the effects of exercise training (ET) on functional capacity and quality of life (QOL) in patients who received percutaneous transluminal coronary angioplasty (PTCA) or coronary stenting (CS). The authors studied 118 consecutive patients with CAD (mean age 57 ± 10 years) who underwent PTCA or CS on one (69%) or two (31%) native epicardial coronary arteries. Patients were randomized into two matched groups. Group T ($n = 59$) was exercised three times a week for 6 months at 60% of peak VO_2. Group C ($n = 59$) was the control group. Only patients in the active group had significant improvements in peak VO_2 (26%, $P <0.001$) and QOL (26.8%, $P = 0.001$ versus C). The angiographic restenosis rate was unaffected by ET (T: 29%; C: 33%, $P =$ not significant). However, residual diameter stenosis was lower in trained patients (−29.7%, $P = 0.045$). In patients with angiographic restenosis, thallium uptake improved only in group T (19%, $P <0.001$). During the follow-up (33 ± 7 months), trained patients had a significantly lower event rate than controls (11.9% versus 32.2%; risk ratio [RR]: 0.71; 95% CI: 0.60 to 0.91; $P = 0.008$) and a lower rate of hospital readmission (18.6% versus 46%; RR: 0.69; 95% CI: 0.55 to 0.93; $P <0.001$). Moderate ET improved functional capacity and QOL after PTCA or CS. During the follow-up, trained patients had fewer events and a lower hospital readmission rate than controls, despite an unchanged restenosis rate.[4] The 2011 ACC/AHA guidelines for PCI recommend (class I, evidence A) medically supervised exercise programs to patients after PCI, particularly for moderate- to high-risk patients for whom supervised ET is warranted.[5] Participation in cardiac rehabilitation is associated with significant reductions in all-cause mortality (OR 0.80; 95% CI: 0.68 to 0.93)[6] in several community-based surveys and meta-analyses.[6-8]

3. **a.** Heart team discussion between the interventional cardiologist and the cardiac surgeon to select the best treatment option is the recommended approach.

TABLE 4-1 Selection of Initial Treatment Strategy: Invasive Versus Conservative Strategy

Preferred Strategy	Patient Characteristics
Invasive	Recurrent angina or ischemia at rest or with low-level activities despite intensive medical therapy
	Elevated cardiac biomarkers (TnT or TnI)
	New or presumably new ST-segment depression
	Signs or symptoms of HF or new or worsening mitral regurgitation
	High-risk findings from noninvasive testing
	Hemodynamic instability
	Sustained ventricular tachycardia
	PCI within 6 mo
	Prior CABG
	High risk score (e.g., TIMI, GRACE)
	Reduced left ventricular function (LVEF 40%)
Conservative	Low risk score (e.g., TIMI, GRACE)
	Patient or physician preference in the absence of high-risk features

TnT, troponin T; TnI, troponin I; HF, heart failure; PCI, percutaneous coronary intervention; CABG, coronary artery bypass grafting; GRACE, Global Registry of Acute Cardiac Events; TIMI, Thrombolysis in Myocardial Infarction; LVEF, left ventricular ejection fraction.

Adapted from Anderson JL, Adams CD, Antman EM, et al. ACC/AHA 2007 guidelines for the management of patients with unstable angina/non-ST-elevation myocardial infarction: a report of the American College of Cardiology/American Heart Association Task Force on Practice Guidelines (writing committee to revise the 2002 guidelines for the management of patients with unstable angina/non-ST-elevation myocardial infarction) developed in collaboration with the American College of Emergency Physicians, the Society for Cardiovascular Angiography and Interventions, and the Society of Thoracic Surgeons endorsed by the American Association of Cardiovascular and Pulmonary Rehabilitation and the Society for Academic Emergency Medicine. *J Am Coll Cardiol.* 2007;50:e1–e157.

The 2011 AHA/ACC guidelines for PCI recommend the heart team approach (class I, evidence C) for the revascularization of patients with unprotected left main trunk disease.[5] Several trials used protocols that involve a multidisciplinary approach.[9,10] The heart team is composed of an interventional cardiologist and a cardiac surgeon and aims at (1) reviewing patients' medical history, (2) determining the approach of revascularization (PCI versus CABG), and (3) discussing with the patient the options of revascularization. The guidelines endorse a heart team approach in patients with unprotected left main CAD and/or complex CAD in whom the optional strategy is not straightforward. Because the STS score and the SYNTAX score predict clinical outcomes, their use is often useful in making revascularization decisions.[11,12]

4. **c.** Drug-eluting stent (DES) implantation (stent-in-stent). In the randomized trial TAXUS V ISR (treatment of De Novo Coronary Disease Using a Single Paclitaxel-Eluting Stent trial), the slow-release, polymer-based, paclitaxel-eluting stent was found to be not only noninferior to β-source vascular brachytherapy but also superior in terms of reducing clinical and angiographic restenosis at 9 months after treatment of bare-metal ISR lesions. Because of both greater acute gain and less late loss, luminal dimensions were significantly larger with paclitaxel-eluting stents compared with brachytherapy in the injury zone, at the distal edge, and over

the entire analysis segment. Proximal edge luminal dimensions were also numerically larger with the paclitaxel-eluting stent.[13] Similarly, the Sirolimus-Eluting Stent with Vascular Brachytherapy for the Treatment of In-Stent Restenosis (SISR) trial demonstrated a marked reduction in target vessel failure with the sirolimus-eluting stent, driven predominantly by a reduction in the rate of target vessel revascularization.[14] Based on available data and the severity of the patient's COPD, DES implantation is the best option for this patient with BMS restenosis. Brachytherapy is no longer available except in a few research centers.[15]

5. **d.** Guideline-directed medical therapy is the first recommended approach. In the COURAGE (Clinical Outcomes Utilizing Revascularization and Aggressive Drug Evaluation) trial, 2,287 patients with stable CAD were randomized to undergo PCI and medical therapy or to medical therapy alone. The primary outcome was death from any cause and nonfatal MI during a follow-up of 2.5 to 7.0 years. The cumulative event rates were 19.0% in the PCI group and 18.5% in the medical therapy group ($P = 0.62$). As an initial management strategy, PCI did not reduce the risk of death, MI, or other MACE in the COURAGE trial.[16] About 314 patients were enrolled in the nuclear substudy of the COURAGE study to perform serial stress imaging. The addition of PCI to medical therapy improved ischemia reduction in patients with significant ischemia at baseline.[17] A recent meta-analysis of 10 randomized controlled trials (6,752 patients) comparing PCI with medical therapy in stable CAD did not detect significant differences in PCI versus CABG; the relative risk (RR) for all-cause mortality was 0.97 (95% CI: 0.84 to 1.12), CV mortality RR 0.91 (95% CI: 0.70 to 1.12), MI RR 1.09 (95% CI: 0.92 to 1.29), or angina relief RR 1.10 (95% CI: 0.97 to 1.26).[18] According to the AHA/ACC guidelines CABG or PCI should not be performed to improve symptoms or survival in patients with CAD with one or more coronary stenoses who do not meet anatomic ($\geq$70% non-left main stenosis diameter), physiologic (FFR >0.80, no or mild ischemia on noninvasive testing) criteria for revascularization and involve only LCX or RCA, or subtend only a small area of viable myocardium.[5] The multiple meta-analyses comparing PCI versus medical therapy in patients with SIHD showed that PCI reduced the incidence of angina, but has not been demonstrated to improve survival or lower the long-term risk of MI in stable patients.[17,19] Our patient does not have criteria for coronary revascularization, and the first-line therapy should be an aggressive medical therapy.

6. **c.** Subendocardium. The subendocardium is most susceptible to ischemic damage. Although the mechanisms of subendocardial ischemia remain to be fully defined, they are clearly associated with the transmural distribution of intramyocardial systolic pressures. Even though almost all the myocardium is perfused in diastole, a reduction of diastolic perfusion pressure or duration will result in subendocardial ischemia.[11] The abnormal subendocardial perfusion in patients with cardiac syndrome X (typical angina, abnormal exercise test results, and normal coronary arteries) has been described with CV MR imaging during the IV administration of adenosine.[20]

7. **d.** Inferior wall myocardial infarction (MI) with right ventricular infarction. The association of inferior wall MI on ECG and elevated jugular venous pressure with clear lungs is suggestive of additional right ventricular infarction. Tall *c–v* waves of tricuspid regurgitation may be evident in patients with necrosis or ischemia of the right ventricular papillary muscles.

8. **a.** Reduction in left ventricular compliance. An S_4 is frequently present in patients with acute MI and is related to auricular contraction and ventricular compliance reduction during ventricular filling.[21] Rapid deceleration of transmitral flow during protodiastolic filling of the left ventricle and increased inflow into the left ventricle are responsible for the third heart sound (S_3). A systolic ejection murmur is suggesting for aortic sclerosis.

9. e. Hybrid revascularization mandates surgical and percutaneous revascularization during the same procedure. According to the ACC/AHA PCI guidelines, hybrid coronary revascularization is defined as the planned combination of LIMA-to-LAD artery grafting and PCI of ≥1 non-LAD coronary arteries and intended to combine the advantages of CABG (i.e., durability of the LIMA graft) and PCI. Hybrid revascularization is particularly suitable in patients with limitations to traditional CABG (e.g., heavily calcified proximal aorta, lack of graft conduits, or a non-LAD coronary artery unsuitable for bypass but amenable to PCI) and situations in which PCI of the LAD artery is not feasible (e.g., excessive tortuosity or calcification, complex bifurcation lesion, and very long lesion). The procedure may be performed in one operative setting or as a staged procedure. CABG before PCI is preferred.[5] Preliminary reports suggest that this approach is feasible and safe,[22] but randomized data are lacking.

10. c. High-sensitive troponin T (Hs-TnT). In the PLATO (Platelet Inhibition and Patient Outcomes) trial, 9,946 patients presented with non-ST-elevation ACS: 5,357 were revascularized and 4,589 managed conservatively. High-sensitive elevated Hs-TnT (>14.0 ng/L) have been described to predict substantial benefit (reduction rate of CV death, MI, and stroke) of ticagrelor over clopidogrel in patients who were revascularized or treated conservatively, while no apparent was observed in those who had normal Hs TnT.[23]

11. e. All of the above. Patients with extensive and severe CAD are more likely to present abnormal exercise ECG results.[24] Early onset of angina, ischemic ST depression ≥2 mm, downsloping ST segment starting at <5 METs, involving ≥5 leads and persisting ≥5 minutes into recovery, and fall in blood pressure at low exercise are all associated with adverse prognosis.

12. e. No improvement of any of the mentioned endpoints. The COURAGE trial enrolled 2,287 patients with significant CAD to an initial strategy: (1) PCI and OMT or (2) OMT only. There were no significant differences between the PCI group and the medical therapy group in the composite of death, MI, and stroke (HR: 1.05; 95% CI: 0.87 to 1.27), and hospitalization for ACS (HR: 1.07; 95% CI: 0.84 to 1.37) or MI (HR: 1.13; 95% CI: 0.89 to 1.43). The authors concluded that as initial management strategy in patients with stable CAD, PCI did not reduce the risk of death, MI, or other MACE when added to OMT.[16] According to the 2011 ACC/AHA PCI guidelines, revascularization should not be performed to improve survival in patients with SIHD with one or more coronary artery stenoses that are not anatomically significant, or involve only the LCX or RCA, or subtend only a small area of viable myocardium.[5]

13. e. All of the above. In the COURAGE patients, 314 were enrolled in the substudy of myocardial perfusion SPECT performed before treatment and 6 to 18 months after randomization. At follow-up, the reduction in ischemic myocardium was greater with PCI + OMT than with OMT (−2.7% versus −0.5%, $P <0.0001$). The patients with PCI + OMT exhibited significant ischemia reduction (33% versus 19%, $P = 0.0004$), especially those patients with moderate-to-severe myocardial ischemia at baseline (78% versus 52%, $P = 0.007$).[17] The 2012 AHA/ACC guidelines for PCI mentioned in patients with stable ischemic coronary heart disease a benefit of angina reduction and symptom improvement with PCI versus OMT; however, PCI has not been demonstrated to improve survival in stable patients.[5]

14. b. Significant absolute risk reduction of major adverse cardiovascular events (MACE) of ~2% over 5 years. The 2012 ACC/AHA guidelines for the management of SIHD recommend the prescription of moderate or high dose of a statin therapy in addition to lifestyle changes (class I, evidence A).[25] The Treating to New Targets (TNT) study randomized 10,001 patients with stable coronary heart disease and LDL >130 mg/dL to receive atorvastatin 10 or 80 mg daily. The mean LDL-C was 2.0 mmol/L during the treatment with 80 mg of atorvastatin, whereas it was 2.6 mmol/L during the treatment with 10 mg of atorvastatin. About 8.7% of patients in the group with intensive lipid-lowering therapy and 10.9% in the group with moderate lipid-lowering therapy presented MACE during a median follow-up of 4.9 years, representing a significant absolute reduction in the rate of MACE of 2.2% and a 22% relative reduction in risk. There was no difference between both treatment groups in the overall mortality.[26]

15. **e.** Fondaparinux might be used as the sole anticoagulant to support PCI. The 2011 ACCF/AHA PCI guidelines made the following recommendations regarding anticoagulant therapy during the procedure. Following recommendations are class I: (1) All patients undergoing PCI should receive an anticoagulant to prevent thrombus formation during the procedure; (2) the administration of IV UFH is a useful standard therapy in patients undergoing PCI; (3) an additional dose of 0.3 mg/kg IV enoxaparin should be administered at the time of PCI to patients who have received fewer than two therapeutic subcutaneous doses (e.g., 1 mg/kg) or received the last subcutaneous enoxaparin dose 8 to 12 hours before PCI; and (4) for patients undergoing PCI, bivaluridin is useful as an anticoagulant with or without prior treatment with UFH. In contrast, fondaparinux should not be used as the sole anticoagulant to support PCI.[5] An additional anticoagulant with anti-IIa activity should be administered because of the risk of catheter thrombosis. Fondaparinux is an indirect factor Xa inhibitor, but no effect on thrombin (IIa). The use of fondaparinux alone was associated with thrombus catheter formation and therefore the anticoagulant with anti-IIa should be used during PCI.[27]

16. **e.** Even in the absence of symptoms, routine periodic stress testing is indicated. According to the 2011 AHA/ACC PCI and 2011 AHA/ACC secondary prevention guidelines, the following interventions and targets are strongly recommended in patients with CHD to reduce morbidity and mortality: (1) to refer to a medically supervised cardiac rehabilitation program post discharge, (2) to manage lipid-lowering treatment for an LDL-C target <70 mg/dL, (3) to control blood pressure with the goal of <140/90 mmHg, and (4) to advise patients for complete smoking cessation. Conversely, there is no proven benefit or indication for routine periodic stress testing in patients after PCI, and thus, it is not indicated.[24]

17. **e.** All of the above. The clinical situations associated with higher risk of BMS restenosis have been defined by the 2011 AHA/ACC PCI guidelines as follows: (1) left main disease, (2) small vessels, (3) ISR, (4) bifurcations, (5) diabetes, (6) long lesions, (7) multiple lesions, and (8) saphenous vein grafts. The ISR of BMS presented by the patient should be treated with DES,[5] as sirolimus- or paclitaxel-eluting stents are superior to balloon angioplasty.[28] The use of DES over BMS had decreased the incidence of ISR by over 70%.[13,28]

18. **b.** Rosuvastatin 20 mg/day significantly decreased the incidence of MI. The JUPITER trial randomized 17,802 men and women without CVD presenting an LDL-C lower than 130 mg/dL, but high levels of hs-CRP, to rosuvastatin, 20 mg daily, or to placebo. Rosuvastatin reduced LDL-C levels by 50% and hs-CRP levels by 37%. The primary endpoint outcome was a composite of MI, stroke, arterial revascularization, hospitalization for UA, or death from CVD. The study was interrupted after 1.9 years at interim analyses because of a significant decrease for primary outcome (HR: 0.56; 95% CI: 0.46 to 0.69). HR for MI was 0.46, 95% CI (0.30 to 0.70), and HR for stroke was 0.52, 95% CI (0.34 to 0.79). In the adverse events section, the physician-reported diabetes was more frequent in the rosuvastatin group ($n = 270$) than in the placebo group ($n = 216$, $P = 0.01$); the difference in the median glycated hemoglobin value was minimal (5.9% versus 5.8%, respectively, $P = 0.001$).[29]

19. **c.** CABG is associated with a reduction of death and of MI, but not of stroke. The future Revascularization Evaluation in Patients with Diabetes Mellitus: Optimal Management of Multivessel Disease (FREEDOM) trial randomized 1,900 patients with diabetes and multivessel CAD to a revascularization strategy with (1) CABG or (2) PCI. The primary outcome was defined as death from any cause, nonfatal MI, or nonfatal stroke. The primary outcome rate at 5 years was 26.6% in the PCI group and 18.7% in the CABG group. The benefit of CABG was observed in reduction of death ($P = 0.049$) and MI ($P < 0.001$) rates, but stroke was more frequent in the CABG group than the PCI group (5.2% versus 2.4%, $P = 0.03$).[30]

20. **c.** More than 70% of patients quit smoking after ACS. About 50% to 70% of smokers continue to smoke after an ACS,[31] despite the fact that smokers who quit smoking have a 36% reduction in the risk of mortality and 32% in the risk of recurrent nonfatal MI in comparison with continuing smokers over a mean follow-up of 5 years.[32] Smoking cessation intervention is a major target of secondary prevention of CVD and should be one of the priorities of clinicians providing care to such patients. Given the large benefits of smoking cessation, promotion of smoking cessation is the most effective intervention to reduce morbidity and mortality in smokers with CHD.[32] Unfortunately smoking receives less attention from cardiologists than other CV risk factors,[33] and many smokers with CHD are unable to quit smoking without assistance. Based on a systemic review, several studies found a beneficial effect on smoking cessation rates through a smoking cessation intervention that started in hospital and continued in the ambulatory setting.[31]

21. **e.** Answers b and d are correct. The leading cause of death in patients hospitalized for acute MI is cardiogenic shock. The SHOCK investigators conducted a randomized trial to evaluate early revascularization in patients with cardiogenic shock. Patients with shock caused by left ventricular failure complicating MI were randomly assigned to emergency revascularization (152 patients) or initial medical stabilization (150 patients). Revascularization was accomplished by either CABG or angioplasty. Intra-aortic balloon counterpulsation was performed in 86% of the patients in both groups. The primary endpoint was mortality from all causes at 30 days. Six-month survival was a secondary endpoint. The mean age of the patients was 66 ± 10 years; 32% were women and 55% were transferred from other hospitals. The median time to the onset of shock was 5.6 hours after infarction, and most infarcts were anterior in location. Ninety-seven percent of the patients assigned to revascularization underwent early coronary angiography, and 87% underwent revascularization; only 2.7% of the patients assigned to medical therapy crossed over to early revascularization without clinical indication. Overall mortality at 30 days (primary endpoint) did not differ significantly between the revascularization and medical therapy groups (46.7% and 56.0%, respectively; difference, −9.3%; 95% CI for the difference, −20.5% to 1.9%; $P = 0.11$). However, at 6 months mortality was lower in the revascularization group than in the medical therapy group (50.3% versus 63.1%, $P = 0.027$).[34]

22. **a.** Patients with CKD undergoing cardiac catheterization should receive adequate preparatory hydration. The 2011 ACC/AHA PCI guidelines made recommendations regarding contrast-induced AKI. Contrast-induced AKI is considered one of the most frequent causes of iatrogenic AKI. Risk factors for developing contrast-induced AKI are hypotension, intra-aortic balloon pump, congestive heart failure, CKD, diabetes, age >75 years, anemia, and volume of contrast.[35] The following recommendations are of class I for the prevention of AKI: (1) Patients should be assessed for risk of contrast-induced AKI before PCI; (2) patients undergoing catheterization with contrast media should receive adequate preparatory hydration; and (3) in patients with CKD (creatinine clearance <60 mL/min), the volume of contrast media should be minimized. However, the administration of *N*-acetyl-cysteine is not useful for the prevention of contrast-induced AKI and is not recommended based on the results of several randomized controlled trials.[36]

23. **a.** No significant difference in the risk of stroke. Abciximab, a potent inhibitor of the platelet glycoprotein IIb/IIIa receptor, reduces thrombotic complications in high-risk patients undergoing PCI in the setting of ACS compared with a regimen of aspirin and UFH. Akkerhuis et al. combined analysis of data from 8,555 patients undergoing PCI assigned to receive a bolus and infusion of abciximab ($n = 5,476$) or matching placebo ($n = 3,079$). No significant difference in stroke rate was observed between patients assigned abciximab ($n = 22$ [0.40%]) and those assigned placebo ($n = 9$ [0.29%]; $P = 0.46$). The rate of nonhemorrhagic stroke was 0.17% in patients treated with abciximab and 0.20% in patients treated with placebo (difference: −0.03%; 95% CI: −0.23% to 0.17%), and the rates of hemorrhagic stroke were 0.15% and 0.10%, respectively (difference: 0.05%; 95% CI: −0.11% to 0.21%). Abciximab in addition to aspirin and heparin does not increase the risk of stroke in patients undergoing PCI.[39]

24. **d.** 70 mg/dL. For patients with established CAD, LDL-lowering therapies significantly reduce the risk of MACE and yield highly favorable cost-effectiveness ratios. In high-risk persons, the recommended LDL-C goal is <100 mg/dL. An LDL-C goal of <70 mg/dL is a therapeutic option on the basis of available clinical trial evidence, especially for patients at very high risk. Diabetic patients with established advanced CAD, like the mentioned patient, should be considered at very high risk for MACE and qualify for the ambitious target of LDL <70 mg/dL.[42]

25. **c.** Additional aspirin (81 to 325 mg) is recommended in all patients on chronic aspirin therapy before PCI. The 2011 AHA/ACC PCI guidelines recommend the use of antiplatelet therapy before PCI.[5] Aspirin reduced ischemic CV events after PCI[37,38] and should be given at least 2 hours before PCI after which aspirin has to be continued indefinitely.[39] In addition to aspirin, a loading dose of $P2Y_{12}$ receptor inhibitor might be given to patients undergoing PCI with stenting.[40-42] Options include clopidogrel 600 mg, prasugrel 60 mg, or ticagrelor 180 mg. The duration of $P2Y_{12}$ receptor inhibitor after stent implantation (BMS or DES) for ACS should be of at least 12 months.[43,44] Options include clopidogrel 75 mg daily, prasugrel 10 mg daily, and ticagrelor 90 mg twice daily. In patients receiving DES for a non-ACS indication, clopidogrel 75 mg daily should be given for 12 months if patients are not at high risk for bleeding.[45] In patients receiving BMS for a non-ACS indication, clopidogrel should be given for a minimum of 1 month and ideally up to 12 months.[44] A benefit of additional aspirin in patients on chronic aspirin undergoing PCI has never been demonstrated.

26. **c.** 20% to 30%. A proportion of patients who present with suspected ACS are found to have insignificant CAD during coronary angiography. Of the 5,767 patients with non-ST-segment-elevation ACS who were enrolled in the Platelet Glycoprotein IIb/IIIa in Unstable Angina: Receptor Suppression Using Integrilin (Eptifibatide) Therapy (PURSUIT) trial and who underwent inhospital angiography, 88% had significant CAD (any stenosis >50%), 6% had mild CAD (any stenosis >0% to ≤50%), and 6% had no CAD (no stenosis identified). Overall, 12% of the patients had nonsignificant CAD.[44] Patients with nonsignificant CAD were more likely to be women, non-white, younger, nondiabetic, nonhypercholesterolemic, without history of CVD, without ST-segment changes, but with more T-wave inversion compared with patients with significant CAD. Based on the profile of the patient admitted, her probability of having nonsignificant CAD is >12%.

27. **b.** Prothrombin complex. Bivaluridin is a naturally occurring anticoagulant secreted by the salivary glands of the leech *Hirudo medicinalis*. It is a potent and specific anticoagulant and exerts its action by binding directly to the active

catalytic site of thrombin. Unlike heparin, it does not require a cofactor (anti-thrombin) and does not appear to cause immune-mediated thrombocytopenia. It is also a more potent inhibitor of platelet function than heparin, probably because of a direct inhibitory effect on thrombin. Unlike heparin, which is readily neutralized by protamine or platelet factor 4, a specific agent useful in reversing the effects of bivalirudin is unavailable. Irani et al. demonstrated the first clinical experience, suggesting benefit from prothrombin complex concentrate in neutralizing the effect of r-hirudin. Although the specific mechanism of action remains unclear, the generation of additional thrombin probably plays a role. Also, epinephrine-induced platelet aggregation in hirudinized platelet-rich plasma is restored by addition of prothrombin complex concentrate, most probably by additional thrombin generation. Adverse effects of prothrombin complex concentrate include intravascular thrombosis, particularly in patients with liver disease and possible viral hepatitis. As the product contains some activated clotting factors (II, VII, IX, and X) and has thrombogenic potential, it should be used as a last resort, especially in patients with liver disease. Clinical experience suggests that prothrombin complex concentrate in a dose of 25 to 30 UI/kg can be considered for patients with life-threatening hemorrhage caused by bivalirudin.[45]

28. e. The radial vascular access is more frequently performed in the United States than in Europe. Radial site access is used more frequently in Europe and Canada than in the United States.[46] The 2011 AHA/ACC PCI guidelines recommend radial artery access to decrease access site complications.[5] In fact, it has been demonstrated that radial access, compared with femoral access, decreases the rate of access-related bleeding and complications.[47] Its utility is more pronounced in patients at higher risk for bleeding or vascular access complications such as in patients with coagulopathy, anticoagulated, or morbid obesity.

29. c. A 65-year-old man known for CAD complaining of progressive shortness of breath since 1 week. At admission, no ongoing chest pain with stable hemodynamic status but bibasilar rales at lung auscultation. The ECG revealed ST-segment elevation as well as Q waves in the anterior leads. The 2011 AHA/ACC PCI guidelines elaborated indication of PCI in patients with STEMI.[5] Primary PCI should be performed in patients within 12 hours of onset of STEMI, within 90 minutes of the first medical contact in patients presenting to a hospital with PCI capabilities and within 120 minutes of the first medical contact in patients presenting to a hospital without PCI capabilities ("systems goal").[48–50] Primary PCI should be performed in patients with STEMI who are candidates for primary PCI, who develop severe heart failure or cardiogenic shock irrespective of time delay,[34,51] and who had clinical and/or ECG evidence for ongoing ischemia between 12 and 24 hours after symptom onset.[52] Delayed PCI in patients with STEMI is reasonable in patients with infarct artery reocclusion or demonstrating ischemia on invasive testing.[53] PCI of hemodynamically significant stenosis in patent infarct artery greater than 24 hours after STEMI might be considered as part of an invasive strategy (class of recommendations IIb).[54,55] PCI of a totally occluded infarct artery greater than 24 hours after STEMI should not be performed in asymptomatic patients with one- or two-vessel disease if patients are hemodynamically stable and do not present evidence of severe ischemia (class III).[56]

30. d. Right ventricular infarction. Rupture of the interventricular septum is one of the mechanical complications of MI, less frequent than left free wall rupture.[57] It occurs in general 3 to 5 days after acute MI. An increase in risk is observed in patients with occlusion of LAD wrapping the distal inferior wall and inferior septum (inferior MI with large anterior MI). The ECG findings of the interventricular septum rupture are typical for ST elevation and Q waves in the inferior leads II, III, and aVF.[58] Clinically, the patients present a rapid onset of hemodynamic compromise characterized by hypotension, biventricular failure, and a new harsh, loud, holosystolic murmur best heard at the lower left sternal border.[59]

31. **d.** Immediate coronary angiography. The septal defect and the associated turbulent transseptal flow can be visualized by a transthoracic echocardiography using color flow Doppler imaging.[60] The addition of Doppler to echocardiography improves significantly the sensitivity of the examination demonstrating the transseptal turbulent flow and diastolic–systolic turbulences in the right ventricle.

32. **c.** Mechanical ventilation with positive end-expiratory pressure. The timing of surgical repair with post-MI ventricular septal rupture is controversial. In patients with cardiogenic shock, a fatal prognosis is inevitable in the absence of urgent surgical treatment. First, stabilization with an intra-aortic balloon pump counterpulsation, inotropic agents, diuretics, and, if tolerated, vasodilators is attempted.[61] This is followed by cardiac catheterization to define the coronary anatomy and then surgical repair.

33. **e.** All of the above. The 2011 ACC/AHA PCI guidelines assessed the risk–benefit profile for the use of BMS versus DES. DES is preferred to BMS when high risk of stent restenosis is present with BMS. The clinical situations associated with higher risk of restenosis are (1) left main disease, (2) small vessels, (3) ISR, (4) bifurcations, (5) diabetes, (6) long lesions, (7) multiple lesions, and (8) saphenous vein grafts. All the criteria mentioned above increased the risk of restenosis, suggesting the use of DES over BMS.[5]

34. **a.** Low-dose aspirin daily. The patient will have coronary angiography for a high suspicion of SIHD. Until the angiogram is performed, he should be treated with optimal medical treatment including aspirin, statins, control of blood pressure (β-blockers/angiotensin converting), and additional medical therapy for the relief of symptoms (β-blockers, calcium channel blockers, long-acting nitrates, or sublingual nitroglycerin).[25] The efficacy of clopidogrel pretreatment compared with the administration in the catheterization laboratory is controversial.[62] There is no evidence to give prasugrel or ticagrelor in patients with SIHD.

35. **c.** Pharmacologic stress with nuclear myocardial perfusion imaging if able to exercise and interpretable ECG. Patients with intermediate pretest probability of CAD are those who most benefit from stress testing to improved diagnostic accuracy. The choice of stress test depends on two questions: Is the patient able to exercise? Is the resting ECG interpretable?[25] The ACC/AHA SIHD guidelines recommend standard exercise ECG testing for interpretable ECG and at least moderate physical functioning or no disabling comorbidity (level of evidence A, class I).[63] Exercise with nuclear myocardial perfusion imaging or echocardiography is recommended for patients with an intermediate to high pretest probability of ischemic heart disease who have an uninterpretable ECG and at least moderate physical activity functioning or no disabling comorbidity.[64,65] Pharmacologic stress with cardiac MR can be useful for patients with an intermediate to high pretest probability who have an uninterpretable ECG and at least moderate physical functioning or no disabling comorbidity.[66] Pharmacologic stress with nuclear myocardial perfusion imaging, echocardiography, or cardiac MR is not recommended for patients who have an interpretable ECG and at least moderate physical functioning or no disabling comorbidities.[67]

36. **c.** Severe ostial and moderate distal left main trunk stenosis. The coronary angiography shows severe ostial and moderate distal left main trunk stenosis.

37. **e.** All of the above. The 2012 AHA/ACC guidelines on SIHD[25] recommend using a nomogram to predict the risk of death in patients with SIHD.[68] This score is based on following clinical and exercise testing variables: age, male gender, typical angina, diabetes, cigarette smoking, hypertension, proportion of predicted

METs achieved, ST-segment depression, test-induced angina, abnormal heart rate recovery, and frequent ventricular ectopy during recovery.

38. b. Arteriovenous fistula. The coronary angiography reveals large coronary AV fistula involving the RCA. Patient underwent surgical ligation of the fistula with resolution of her symptoms.

39. e. All of the above. The coronary angiography shows a bifurcation lesion involving the distal left main trunk as well as the ostium of the left anterior descending and left circumflex coronary arteries.

40. c. Perforation of the RCA. The coronary angiography demonstrates extravasation of contrast caused by perforation of the RCA.

41. e. All the mentioned clinical situations do not justify coronary angiography in the initial phase of patient management. According to 2012 AHA/ACC SIHD guidelines,[25] coronary angiography is not recommended as an initial testing strategy to assess risk in the following clinical situations (class III, no benefit): (1) patients with SIHD who elect not to undergo revascularization or who are not candidates for revascularization because of comorbidities or individual preferences; (2) patients with SIHD who have preserved left ventricular function and low-risk criteria on noninvasive testing; (3) low risk according to clinical criteria and who have not undergone noninvasive risk testing; and (4) asymptomatic patients with no evidence of ischemia on noninvasive testing.

42. b. Calcified coronary arteries. Patients with long-standing terminal nephropathy have frequently severely calcified vessels including the coronary arteries.[69] Qualitative analysis of the coronary arteries showed significantly more calcified plaques of coronary arteries in patients with end-stage renal failure. Plaques of nonuremic patients were mostly fibroatheromatous, while coronary plaques in patients with end-stage renal failure were characterized by increased media thickness and marked calcification. Deposition of calcium within the plaques may contribute to the high event rate in uremic patients.

43. e. Acupuncture might be used for the purpose of improving symptoms of patients with SIHD. According to 2012 AHA/ACC SIHD guidelines,[25] acupuncture should not be used for the purpose of improving symptoms or reducing CV risk in patients with SIHD (class III, no benefit). Smoking cessation and avoidance of exposure to environmental tobacco smoke at work and home should be encouraged (class I), dipyridamole is not recommended as antiplatelet therapy for patients with SIHD (class III, no benefit), treatment with clopidogrel is reasonable when aspirin is contraindicated in patients with SIHD (class I), and it is reasonable to consider screening SIHD patients for depression and to refer or treat when indicated (class IIa).

44. e. PCI does not reduce the occurrence of death, reinfarction, or heart failure. The Occluded Artery Trial (OAT) study showed high rates of procedural success with PCI and sustained patency but no clinical benefit during an average 3-year follow-up with respect to death, reinfarction, or heart failure.[56] There was, in fact, a trend toward excess nonfatal reinfarction when routine PCI was performed in stable patients who were found to have occlusion of the infarct-related artery 3 to 28 days after MI. A strategy of CABG was not tested in the OAT.

45. e. Answers a and d are correct. In the CHARISMA trial of 15,603 patients with established stable atherothrombotic disease or at high risk for such disease, there was no significant benefit associated with clopidogrel plus aspirin as compared with placebo plus aspirin in reducing the incidence of the primary endpoint of MI, stroke, or death from CV causes. Clopidogrel was associated with a significant increase in the rate of moderate bleeding.[70]

46. b. Significant survival advantage. A cohort study of approximately 1,400 patients demonstrated that the use of combination evidence-based medical therapies was independently and strongly associated with lower 6-month mortality in patients with ACSs.[71] Furthermore, there was a gradient of benefit across the different TIMI risk groups with higher-risk patients obtaining higher absolute benefit.[72] The 2013 AHA/ACCA STEMI guidelines[73] recommend (1) indefinitely aspirin 81 to 325 mg daily maintenance dose after PCI (class I), (2) β-blockers should be continued after hospitalization for all patients with STEMI and with no contraindications to their use (class I), (3) angiotensin-converting enzyme inhibitors are reasonable for all patients with STEMI and no contraindications to their use (class IIa and class I if presence of reduced LVEF), and (4) high-intensity statin therapy should be initiated or continued in all patients with STEMI and no contraindications to its use.

47. b. PCI may reduce the episodes of angina in the presence of moderate-to-severe ischemia at stress single-photon emission computed tomography (SPECT) but not the risk of death, MI, or other major CV events when added to optimal medical therapy. The COURAGE trial compared OMT alone or in combination with PCI as an initial management strategy in patients with stable CAD. Although the addition of PCI to OMT reduced the prevalence of angina, especially in case of moderate-to-severe ischemia detected by SPECT, it did not reduce long-term rates of death, nonfatal MI, and hospitalization for ACSs.[16]

48. d. Severe RCA stenosis. Coronary angiography shows severe mid-RCA stenosis explaining the inferior ischemia.

49. d. 12 months. The 2011 AHA/ACC PCI guidelines recommend the continuation of aspirin indefinitely (class I) and the duration of $P2Y_{12}$ inhibitor after stent implantation as follows: (1) BMS or DES during PCI for ACS, at least 12 months; (2) DES for a non-ACS indication, at least 12 months if patients are not at high risk for bleeding; and (3) BMS for a non-ACS indication, a minimum of 1 month, and ideally up to 12 months (unless the patient is at increased risk for bleeding).[5]

50. a. Severe LCX stenosis. The coronary angiography of the left circulation shows severe mid-left circumflex coronary artery stenosis.

51. e. Discontinuation of dual antiplatelet therapy followed by surgery in the first few weeks following stent implantation is problematic with DES but not BMS. In patients scheduled for noncardiac surgery in the year following PCI, the implantation of DESs should be avoided. Accordingly, one of the most frequent predisposing conditions to DES thrombosis is the (partial or complete) discontinuation of dual antiplatelet therapy because of urgent or elective noncardiac surgery.[74] Although preliminary data suggest that continuation of dual antiplatelet therapy during surgery, if feasible, may be protective of DES thrombosis, no recommendation can be made at this time. Conceptually, the potential for stent thrombosis remains because of the intrinsic prothrombotic state related to surgery. Perioperative thrombosis of BMS implanted shortly prior to noncardiac surgery have been described and associated with prohibitive morbidity and mortality. Therefore, whenever possible, noncardiac surgery should be postponed for at least 6 weeks following implantation of a BMS and 6 to 12 months following DES implantation.

52. d. In patients who have already suffered a stent thrombosis dual antiplatelet therapy may be extended long term, although currently there are no data to support this strategy. Currently, there are no data to support an extension of dual antiplatelet therapy beyond 12 months. Nevertheless, in selected patients at high risk for stent thrombosis, aspirin and clopidogrel may be administered for a longer period of time. The CHARISMA trial[70] did show a benefit of prolonged aspirin and clopidogrel therapy over aspirin only in the secondary prevention setting, but did not specifically address the PCI population. According to the 2011 AHA/ACC PCI, continuation of $P2Y_{12}$ inhibitor after stent implantation for ACS should be at least 12 months.[5]

53. **e.** Occlusion of the first diagonal branch. The ECG showed inferoposterolateral STEMI. Coronary angiography showed a thrombotic occlusion of mid-portion of the dominant RCA.

54. **a.** Thrombotic occlusion of the left main trunk. The coronary angiography shows thrombotic occlusion of the left main trunk artery. This lesion has been treated with thromboaspiration and implantation of a DES.

55. **c.** Anterior subacute MI. ECG reveals ST elevation of anterolateral fields. Due to persisting chest pain, the patient has been investigated with angiography. The ventriculography showed occlusion of the mid-portion of the left anterior descending coronary artery treated with thromboaspiration and implantation of a BMS. The image of the thrombus extracted is shown in Figure 4.14.

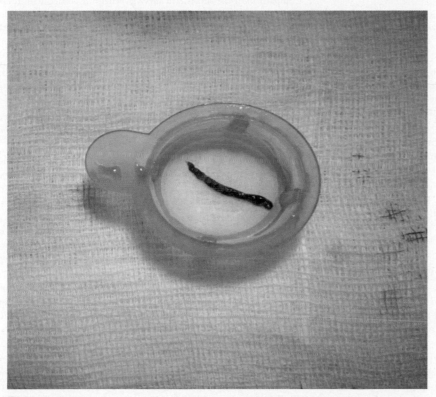

Figure 4.14

56. **b.** Occlusion of the left anterior descending coronary artery. The coronary angiography showed an occlusion of the proximal left anterior descending coronary artery. The fact that the vessel perfused the apex including the inferoapical portion of the left ventricles explains the ST elevations in the anterior and inferior leads.

57. **d.** Visible thrombus in the mid-portion of the RCA. The coronary angiography showed a subtotal stenosis of the mid-RCA followed by a filling defect compatible with a large thrombus. The thromboaspiration was successfully performed and the lesion was subsequently treated with stenting.

58. **a.** Subtotal occlusion of the left main trunk. Coronary angiography showed subtotal occlusion of the left main trunk and the lesion was treated with stenting. Ventriculography showed a severely reduced LVEF (15%) under a mechanical chest compression system. The patient did not recover and subsequently died.

59. **a.** ISR of the left descending coronary artery. Coronary angiography shows a ISR of the mid-left anterior descending coronary artery.

REFERENCES

1. Fox KA, Clayton TC, Damman P, et al. Long-term outcome of a routine versus selective invasive strategy in patients with non-ST-segment elevation acute coronary syndrome a meta-analysis of individual patient data. *J Am Coll Cardiol.* 2010;55(22):2435–2445.

2. O'Donoghue M, Boden WE, Braunwald E, et al. Early invasive vs conservative treatment strategies in women and men with unstable angina and non-ST-segment elevation myocardial infarction: a meta-analysis. *JAMA.* 2008;300(1):71–80.

3. Jneid H, Anderson JL, Wright RS, et al. 2012 ACCF/AHA focused update of the guideline for the management of patients with unstable angina/non-ST-elevation myocardial infarction (updating the 2007 guideline and replacing the 2011 focused update): a report of the American College of Cardiology Foundation/American Heart Association Task Force on practice guidelines. *Circulation.* 2012;126(7):875–910.

4. Belardinelli R, Paolini I, Cianci G, Piva R, Georgiou D, Purcaro A. Exercise training intervention after coronary angioplasty: the ETICA trial. *J Am Coll Cardiol.* 2001;37(7):1891–1900.

5. Levine GN, Bates ER, Blankenship JC, et al. 2011 ACCF/AHA/SCAI Guideline for percutaneous coronary intervention: executive summary: a report of the American College of Cardiology Foundation/American Heart Association Task Force on practice guidelines and the society for cardiovascular angiography and interventions. *Circulation.* 2011;124(23):2574–2609.

6. Taylor RS, Brown A, Ebrahim S, et al. Exercise-based rehabilitation for patients with coronary heart disease: systematic review and meta-analysis of randomized controlled trials. *Am J Med.* 2004;116(10):682–692.

7. Goel K, Lennon RJ, Tilbury RT, Squires RW, Thomas RJ. Impact of cardiac rehabilitation on mortality and cardiovascular events after percutaneous coronary intervention in the community. *Circulation.* 2011;123(21):2344–2352.

8. Witt BJ, Jacobsen SJ, Weston SA, et al. Cardiac rehabilitation after myocardial infarction in the community. *J Am Coll Cardiol.* 2004;44(5):988–996.

9. Kim YH, Park DW, Kim WJ, et al. Validation of SYNTAX (Synergy Between PCI with Taxus and Cardiac Surgery) score for prediction of outcomes after unprotected left main coronary revascularization. *JACC. Cardiovasc Interv.* 2010;3(6):612–623.

10. Feit F, Brooks MM, Sopko G, et al. Long-term clinical outcome in the Bypass Angioplasty Revascularization Investigation Registry: comparison with the randomized trial. BARI Investigators. *Circulation.* 2000;101(24):2795–2802.

11. Morice MC, Serruys PW, Kappetein AP, et al. Outcomes in patients with de novo left main disease treated with either percutaneous coronary intervention using paclitaxel-eluting stents or coronary artery bypass graft treatment in the Synergy Between Percutaneous Coronary Intervention with TAXUS and Cardiac Surgery (SYNTAX) trial. *Circulation.* 2010;121(24):2645–2653.

12. Shahian DM, O'Brien SM, Normand SL, Peterson ED, Edwards FH. Association of hospital coronary artery bypass volume with processes of care, mortality, morbidity, and the Society of Thoracic Surgeons composite quality score. *J Thorac Cardiovasc Surg.* 2010;139(2):273–282.

13. Stone GW, Ellis SG, Cannon L, et al. Comparison of a polymer-based paclitaxel-eluting stent with a bare metal stent in patients with complex coronary artery disease: a randomized controlled trial. *JAMA.* 2005;294(10):1215–1223.

14. Holmes DR Jr, Teirstein P, Satler L, et al. Sirolimus-eluting stents vs vascular brachytherapy for in-stent restenosis within bare-metal stents: the SISR randomized trial. *JAMA.* 2006;295(11):1264–1273.

15. Mukherjee D, Moliterno DJ. Brachytherapy for in-stent restenosis: a distant second choice to drug-eluting stent placement. *JAMA.* 2006;295(11):1307–1309.

16. Boden WE, O'Rourke RA, Teo KK, et al. Optimal medical therapy with or without PCI for stable coronary disease. *N Engl J Med.* 2007;356(15):1503–1516.

17. Shaw LJ, Berman DS, Maron DJ, et al. Optimal medical therapy with or without percutaneous coronary intervention to reduce ischemic burden: results from the Clinical Outcomes Utilizing Revascularization and Aggressive Drug Evaluation (COURAGE) trial nuclear substudy. *Circulation.* 2008;117(10):1283–1291.

18. Thomas S, Gokhale R, Boden WE, Devereaux PJ. A meta-analysis of randomized controlled trials comparing percutaneous coronary intervention with medical therapy in stable angina pectoris. *Can J Cardiol.* 2013;29(4):472–482.

19. Hachamovitch R, Hayes SW, Friedman JD, Cohen I, Berman DS. Comparison of the short-term survival benefit associated with revascularization compared with medical therapy in patients with no prior coronary artery disease undergoing stress myocardial perfusion single photon emission computed tomography. *Circulation.* 2003;107(23):2900–2907.

20. Panting JR, Gatehouse PD, Yang GZ, et al. Abnormal subendocardial perfusion in cardiac syndrome X detected by cardiovascular magnetic resonance imaging. *N Engl J Med.* 2002;346(25):1948–1953.

21. Williams ES. Chapter 25: The fourth heart sound. In: Hurst JW, ed. *Clinical Methods: The History, Physical, and Laboratory Examinations,* 3rd ed. Boston, MA: Butterworths; 1990:129–130.

22. Reicher B, Poston RS, Mehra MR, et al. Simultaneous "hybrid" percutaneous coronary intervention and minimally invasive surgical bypass grafting: feasibility, safety, and clinical outcomes. *Am Heart J.* 2008;155(4):661–667.

23. Wallentin L, Lindholm D, Siegbahn A, et al. Biomarkers in relation to the effects of ticagrelor compared with clopidogrel in non-ST-elevation acute coronary syndrome patients managed with or without in-hospital revascularization: a substudy from the prospective randomized Platelet Inhibition and Patient Outcomes (PLATO) trial. *Circulation.* 2014;129(3):293–303.

24. Gibbons RJ, Balady GJ, Bricker JT, et al. ACC/AHA 2002 guideline update for exercise testing: summary article: a report of the American College of Cardiology/American Heart Association Task Force on Practice Guidelines (Committee to Update the 1997 Exercise Testing Guidelines). *Circulation.* 2002;106(14):1883–1892.

25. Fihn SD, Gardin JM, Abrams J, et al. 2012 ACCF/AHA/ACP/AATS/PCNA/SCAI/STS Guideline for the diagnosis and management of patients with stable ischemic heart disease: a report of the American College of Cardiology Foundation/American Heart Association Task Force on Practice Guidelines, and the American College of Physicians, American Association for Thoracic Surgery, Preventive Cardiovascular Nurses Association, Society for Cardiovascular Angiography and Interventions, and Society of Thoracic Surgeons. *J Am Coll Cardiol.* 2012;60(24):e44–e164.

26. LaRosa JC, Grundy SM, Waters DD, et al. Intensive lipid lowering with atorvastatin in patients with stable coronary disease. *N Engl J Med.* 2005;352(14):1425–1435.

27. Yusuf S, Mehta SR, Chrolavicius S, et al. Comparison of fondaparinux and enoxaparin in acute coronary syndromes. *N Engl J Med.* 2006;354(14):1464–1476.

28. Kastrati A, Mehilli J, von Beckerath N, et al. Sirolimus-eluting stent or paclitaxel-eluting stent vs balloon angioplasty for prevention of recurrences in patients with coronary in-stent restenosis: a randomized controlled trial. *JAMA.* 2005;293(2):165–171.

29. Ridker PM, Danielson E, Fonseca FA, et al. Rosuvastatin to prevent vascular events in men and women with elevated C-reactive protein. *N Engl J Med.* 2008;359(21):2195–2207.

30. Farkouh ME, Domanski M, Sleeper LA, et al. Strategies for multivessel revascularization in patients with diabetes. *N Engl J Med.* 2012;367(25):2375–2384.

31. Rigotti NA, Munafo MR, Stead LF. Smoking cessation interventions for hospitalized smokers: a systematic review. *Arch Intern Med.* 2008;168(18):1950–1960.

32. Critchley JA, Capewell S. Mortality risk reduction associated with smoking cessation in patients with coronary heart disease: a systematic review. *JAMA.* 2003;290(1):86–97.

33. Cardiologists should be less passive about smoking cessation. *Lancet.* 2009;373(9667):867.

34. Hochman JS, Sleeper LA, Webb JG, et al. Early revascularization in acute myocardial infarction complicated by cardiogenic shock. SHOCK investigators. Should we emergently revascularize occluded coronaries for cardiogenic shock. *N Engl J Med.* 1999;341(9):625–634.

35. Mehran R, Aymong ED, Nikolsky E, et al. A simple risk score for prediction of contrast-induced nephropathy after percutaneous coronary intervention: development and initial validation. *J Am Coll Cardiol.* 2004;44(7):1393–1399.

36. Acetylcysteine for prevention of renal outcomes in patients undergoing coronary and peripheral vascular angiography: main results from the randomized Acetylcysteine for Contrast-induced nephropathy Trial (ACT). *Circulation.* 2011;124(11):1250–1259.

37. Jolly SS, Pogue J, Haladyn K, et al. Effects of aspirin dose on ischaemic events and bleeding after percutaneous coronary intervention: insights from the PCI-CURE study. *Eur Heart J.* 2009;30(8):900–907.

38. Popma JJ, Berger P, Ohman EM, Harrington RA, Grines C, Weitz JI. Antithrombotic therapy during percutaneous coronary intervention: the Seventh ACCP Conference on Antithrombotic and Thrombolytic Therapy. *Chest.* 2004;126(3 Suppl):576S–599S.

39. Baigent C, Blackwell L, Collins R, et al. Aspirin in the primary and secondary prevention of vascular disease: collaborative meta-analysis of individual participant data from randomised trials. *Lancet.* 2009;373(9678):1849–1860.

40. Yusuf S, Zhao F, Mehta SR, Chrolavicius S, Tognoni G, Fox KK. Effects of clopidogrel in addition to aspirin in patients with acute coronary syndromes without ST-segment elevation. *N Engl J Med.* 2001;345(7):494–502.

41. Wiviott SD, Braunwald E, McCabe CH, et al. Prasugrel versus clopidogrel in patients with acute coronary syndromes. *N Engl J Med.* 2007;357(20):2001–2015.

42. Wallentin L, Becker RC, Budaj A, et al. Ticagrelor versus clopidogrel in patients with acute coronary syndromes. *N Engl J Med.* 2009;361(11):1045–1057.

43. Patrono C, Baigent C, Hirsh J, Roth G. Antiplatelet drugs: American College of Chest Physicians Evidence-Based Clinical Practice Guidelines (8th Edition). *Chest.* 2008;133(6 Suppl):199S–233S.

44. Steinhubl SR, Berger PB, Mann JT 3rd, et al. Early and sustained dual oral antiplatelet therapy following percutaneous coronary intervention: a randomized controlled trial. *JAMA.* 2002;288(19):2411–2420.

45. Brar SS, Kim J, Brar SK, et al. Long-term outcomes by clopidogrel duration and stent type in a diabetic population with de novo coronary artery lesions. *J Am Coll Cardiol.* 2008;51(23):2220–2227.

46. Rao SV, Cohen MG, Kandzari DE, Bertrand OF, Gilchrist IC. The transradial approach to percutaneous coronary intervention: historical perspective, current concepts, and future directions. *J Am Coll Cardiol.* 2010;55(20):2187–2195.

47. Jolly SS, Yusuf S, Cairns J, et al. Radial versus femoral access for coronary angiography and intervention in patients with acute coronary syndromes (RIVAL): a randomised, parallel group, multicentre trial. *Lancet.* 2011;377(9775):1409–1420.

48. Lambert L, Brown K, Segal E, Brophy J, Rodes-Cabau J, Bogaty P. Association between timeliness of reperfusion therapy and clinical outcomes in ST-elevation myocardial infarction. *JAMA.* 2010;303(21):2148–2155.

49. Terkelsen CJ, Sorensen JT, Maeng M, et al. System delay and mortality among patients with STEMI treated with primary percutaneous coronary intervention. *JAMA.* 2010;304(7):763–771.

50. Aguirre FV, Varghese JJ, Kelley MP, et al. Rural interhospital transfer of ST-elevation myocardial infarction patients for percutaneous coronary revascularization: the Stat Heart Program. *Circulation.* 2008;117(9):1145–1152.

51. Wu AH, Parsons L, Every NR, Bates ER. Hospital outcomes in patients presenting with congestive heart failure complicating acute myocardial infarction: a report from the Second National Registry of Myocardial Infarction (NRMI-2). *J Am Coll Cardiol.* 2002;40(8):1389–1394.

52. Schomig A, Mehilli J, Antoniucci D, et al. Mechanical reperfusion in patients with acute myocardial infarction presenting more than 12 hours from symptom onset: a randomized controlled trial. *JAMA.* 2005;293(23):2865–2872.

53. Erne P, Schoenenberger AW, Burckhardt D, et al. Effects of percutaneous coronary interventions in silent ischemia after myocardial infarction: the SWISSI II randomized controlled trial. *JAMA.* 2007;297(18):1985–1991.

54. Stenestrand U, Wallentin L. Early revascularisation and 1-year survival in 14-day survivors of acute myocardial infarction: a prospective cohort study. *Lancet.* 2002;359(9320):1805–1811.

55. Alter DA, Tu JV, Austin PC, Naylor CD. Waiting times, revascularization modality, and outcomes after acute myocardial infarction at hospitals with and without on-site revascularization facilities in Canada. *J Am Coll Cardiol.* 2003;42(3):410–419.

56. Hochman JS, Lamas GA, Buller CE, et al. Coronary intervention for persistent occlusion after myocardial infarction. *N Engl J Med.* 2006;355(23):2395–2407.

57. Figueras J, Alcalde O, Barrabes JA, et al. Changes in hospital mortality rates in 425 patients with acute ST-elevation myocardial infarction and cardiac rupture over a 30-year period. *Circulation.* 2008;118(25):2783–2789.

58. Hayashi T, Hirano Y, Takai H, et al. Usefulness of ST-segment elevation in the inferior leads in predicting ventricular septal rupture in patients with anterior wall acute myocardial infarction. *Am J Cardiol.* 2005;96(8):1037–1041.

59. Reeder GS. Identification and treatment of complications of myocardial infarction. *Mayo Clinic Proceedings. Mayo Clin Proc.* 1995;70(9):880–884.

60. Smyllie JH, Sutherland GR, Geuskens R, Dawkins K, Conway N, Roelandt JR. Doppler color flow mapping in the diagnosis of ventricular septal rupture and acute mitral regurgitation after myocardial infarction. *J Am Coll Cardiol.* 1990;15(6):1449–1455.

61. Crenshaw BS, Granger CB, Birnbaum Y, et al. Risk factors, angiographic patterns, and outcomes in patients with ventricular septal defect complicating acute myocardial infarction. GUSTO-I (Global Utilization of Streptokinase and TPA for Occluded Coronary Arteries) Trial Investigators. *Circulation.* 2000;101(1):27–32.

62. Widimsky P, Motovska Z, Simek S, et al. Clopidogrel pre-treatment in stable angina: for all patients > 6 h before elective coronary angiography or only for angiographically selected patients a few minutes before PCI? A randomized multicentre trial PRAGUE-8. *Eur Heart J.* 2008;29(12):1495–1503.

63. Shaw LJ, Mieres JH, Hendel RH, et al. Comparative effectiveness of exercise electrocardiography with or without myocardial perfusion single photon emission computed tomography in women with suspected coronary artery disease: results from the What Is the Optimal Method for Ischemia Evaluation in Women (WOMEN) trial. *Circulation.* 2011;124(11):1239–1249.

64. Fleischmann KE, Hunink MG, Kuntz KM, Douglas PS. Exercise echocardiography or exercise SPECT imaging? A meta-analysis of diagnostic test performance. *JAMA.* 1998;280(10):913–920.

65. Garber AM, Solomon NA. Cost-effectiveness of alternative test strategies for the diagnosis of coronary artery disease. *Ann Intern Med.* 1999;130(9):719–728.

66. Nandalur KR, Dwamena BA, Choudhri AF, Nandalur MR, Carlos RC. Diagnostic performance of stress cardiac magnetic resonance imaging in the detection of coronary artery disease: a meta-analysis. *J Am Coll Cardiol.* 2007;50(14):1343–1353.

67. Underwood SR, Shaw LJ, Anagnostopoulos C, et al. Myocardial perfusion scintigraphy and cost effectiveness of diagnosis and management of coronary heart disease. *Heart.* 2004;90(Suppl 5):v34–v36.

68. Lauer MS, Pothier CE, Magid DJ, Smith SS, Kattan MW. An externally validated model for predicting long-term survival after exercise treadmill testing in patients with suspected coronary artery disease and a normal electrocardiogram. *Ann Intern Med.* 2007;147(12):821–828.

69. Schwarz U, Buzello M, Ritz E, et al. Morphology of coronary atherosclerotic lesions in patients with end-stage renal failure. *Nephrol Dial Transplant.* 2000;15(2):218–223.

70. Bhatt DL, Fox KA, Hacke W, et al. Clopidogrel and aspirin versus aspirin alone for the prevention of atherothrombotic events. *N Engl J Med.* 2006;354(16):1706–1717.

71. Mukherjee D, Fang J, Chetcuti S, Moscucci M, Kline-Rogers E, Eagle KA. Impact of combination evidence-based medical therapy on mortality in patients with acute coronary syndromes. *Circulation.* 2004;109(6):745–749.

72. Mukherjee D, Fang J, Kline-Rogers E, Otten R, Eagle KA. Impact of combination evidence based medical treatment in patients with acute coronary syndromes in various TIMI risk groups. *Heart.* 2005;91(3):381–382.

73. O'Gara PT, Kushner FG, Ascheim DD, et al. 2013 ACCF/AHA guideline for the management of ST-elevation myocardial infarction: a report of the American College of Cardiology Foundation/American Heart Association Task Force on Practice Guidelines. *Circulation.* 2013;127(4):e362–e425.

74. Schouten O, van Domburg RT, Bax JJ, et al. Noncardiac surgery after coronary stenting: early surgery and interruption of antiplatelet therapy are associated with an increase in major adverse cardiac events. *J Am Coll Cardiol.* 2007;49(1):122–124.

chapter 5

Pharmacology

Alexander Kantorovich • Michael A. Militello • Jodie M. Fink

QUESTIONS ● ● ● ●

Pharmacokinetics and Pharmacodynamics

1. P. M. is admitted to the coronary intensive care unit (ICU) with atrial fibrillation (AFib) and rapid ventricular rate. After controlling the ventricular rate with metoprolol, it is decided to initiate procainamide by intravenous (IV) infusion. P. M. weighs 80 kg. How much of a loading dose would be required to target a level of 8 μg/L? The average steady-state volume of distribution (V_d) for procainamide is 2 L/kg. The bioavailability of the IV formulation is 100%, whereas the oral (PO) form is only 83%.

   a. 1,000 mg
   b. 1,300 mg
   c. 1,500 mg
   d. 1,700 mg

2. L. M. has been receiving digoxin 0.25 mg PO tablets daily. Her serum drug level is 1.8 ng/mL. She is no longer able to take PO medications and needs to receive digoxin IV. By what percentage do you need to decrease the dose to maintain the current digoxin level?

   a. 10%
   b. 25%
   c. 40%
   d. 50%

3. What two pharmacokinetic parameters alter the half-life of medications?

   a. Loading dose and clearance
   b. Absorption and clearance
   c. V_d and clearance
   d. Absorption and V_d

4. What is the relationship between drug concentration and pharmacologic effect known as?

   a. Pharmacokinetics
   b. Pharmacogenetics
   c. Pharmacology
   d. Pharmacodynamics

5. Each line in Figure 5.1 represents a β-blocker in development. Which β-blocker is the most potent?

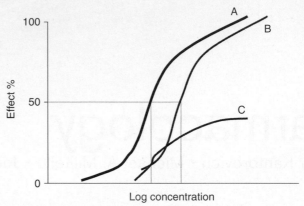

Figure 5.1 • Relationship between drug concentration and effect.

    a. A

    b. B

    c. C

    d. Potency cannot be determined from the above graph

6. Ethanol alters the metabolism of warfarin. Two types of ethanol abuse are chronic ethanol abuse and binge ethanol drinking. How do these types of ethanol use alter warfarin metabolism? Chronic ethanol use _____ and binge ethanol drinking _____.

    a. decreases warfarin metabolism, increases warfarin metabolism

    b. decreases warfarin metabolism, decreases warfarin metabolism

    c. increases warfarin metabolism, decreases warfarin metabolism

    d. increases warfarin metabolism, increases warfarin metabolism

7. Which of the following drugs can significantly increase digoxin concentrations?

    a. Amiodarone

    b. Metoprolol

    c. Simvastatin

    d. Fenofibrate

Angiotensin-Converting Enzyme (ACE) Inhibitors

8. Which of the following statements is *true* with regard to ACE inhibitors?

    a. Mortality benefit in heart failure (HF) patients is a class effect with ACE inhibitors, and all are Food and Drug Administration (FDA) approved for this indication.

    b. ACE inhibitor dose is negligible in HF with regard to mortality benefit.

    c. Sodium depletion is an important factor in the development of renal insufficiency associated with ACE inhibitors.

    d. ACE inhibitor–associated potassium retention is related to the increase in feedback that leads to aldosterone release.

β-Blockers

9. Match the properties with the associated β-blocking agents.

    1. Pindolol   i. α-Blockade

    2. Propranolol   ii. Intrinsic sympathomimetic activity (ISA)

3. Labetalol   iii. Membrane-stabilizing activity

4. Bisoprolol   iv. β_1-Selectivity

  a. (1) iv; (2) ii; (3) iii; (4) i

  b. (1) iii; (2) i; (3) ii; (4) iv

  c. (1) ii; (2) iii; (3) i; (4) iv

  d. (1) ii; (2) iv; (3) iii; (4) i

Calcium Channel Blockers (CCBs)

10. By which of the following mechanisms do diltiazem and verapamil slow ventricular rate in patients with AFib?

  a. They decrease the conduction velocity within the atrioventricular (AV) node.

  b. They decrease the refractory period of nodal tissue.

  c. They stimulate vagal tone.

  d. They prolong the refractory period of atrial tissue.

11. Which of the following CCBs is indicated in patients presenting with a subarachnoid hemorrhage?

  a. Verapamil

  b. Diltiazem

  c. Isradipine

  d. Nimodipine

Diuretics

12. Which of the following loop diuretics is a *not* a sulfonamide and can, therefore, be given to a patient with a sulfonamide allergy?

  a. Ethacrynic acid

  b. Bumetanide

  c. Torsemide

  d. Furosemide

13. True or False: Conivaptan is indicated for the treatment of hyponatremia for patients with underlying HF.

  a. True

  b. False

Inotropic Agents

14. How does digoxin improve myocardial contractility?

  a. Inhibition of the Na^+/K^+-adenosine triphosphatase

  b. Inhibition of the breakdown of cyclic adenosine monophosphate (cAMP)

  c. Increases intracellular K^+, leading to the opening of calcium channels

  d. Directly stimulates calcium release from the sarcoplasmic reticulum

15. F. F. is a 75-year-old man with a history of HF and AFib and was initiated on amiodarone and warfarin. He has been treated for many years with captopril, furosemide, potassium, amlodipine, and digoxin. After 3 days in the hospital, the patient was sent home. One week after discharge, he developed nausea, vomiting, confusion, and symptomatic ventricular tachycardia (VT). His serum digoxin concentration was 3.9 ng/mL and serum potassium level was 5.8 mmol/L. The rhythm was treated with lidocaine, and the patient is now having episodes of nonsustained VT with a blood pressure (BP) of 80/40 mmHg during each episode. What should be your next course of action?

  a. Discontinue the amiodarone and digoxin and observe.

  b. Discontinue the digoxin and administer digoxin-specific antibodies.

   c. Decrease the dose of digoxin.

   d. Discontinue digoxin and observe.

16. N. M. is a 75-year-old woman with a long-standing history of HF secondary to viral cardiomyopathy. She presents to the outpatient clinic for routine follow-up. On examination, she was short of breath and reported increasing orthopnea. She was admitted to the ICU for right heart catheterization. Initial readings show a cardiac index of 1.8 L/min/m^2, elevated pulmonary capillary wedge pressure (25 mmHg), and high pulmonary pressures (72/45 mmHg). Her initial BP was 105/55 mmHg, and she had a heart rate of 105 beats per minute (bpm). Home medications include captopril, spironolactone, metoprolol XL, and furosemide. Which of the following inotropic agents would be most appropriate?

   a. Dopamine

   b. Dobutamine

   c. Milrinone

   d. Isoproterenol

Anticoagulation

17. Which of the following statements is *true* regarding vitamin K administration?

   a. Subcutaneously administered vitamin K exhibits the same bioavailability as oral or IV vitamin K

   b. IV vitamin K is superior at lowering the INR than oral vitamin K at similar doses

   c. IV vitamin K works faster to lower the INR than oral vitamin K at similar doses

   d. Rates of anaphylaxis are similar between oral and IV administration of vitamin K

18. Which of the following agents bind only to factor Xa?

   a. Enoxaparin

   b. Fondaparinux

   c. Bivalirudin

   d. Unfractionated heparin (UFH)

19. A. F. is a 52-year-old man with a history of AFib, transient ischemic attacks, hypertension (HTN), and rheumatic heart disease. The recommendations from the Sixth American College of Chest Physicians (ACCP) Consensus Conference on Antithrombotic Therapy suggest that this patient be initiated on _____ for antithrombotic therapy because of AFib.

   a. aspirin, 81 mg daily

   b. aspirin, 325 mg daily

   c. warfarin, with a target goal international normalized ratio (INR) of 2.5

   d. warfarin, with a target goal INR of 3.5

20. The patient above is going to be electively cardioverted. What is the timing of PO anticoagulant therapy?

   a. Warfarin with a target INR of 3.5 for 4 weeks before cardioversion and continued for 6 weeks after cardioversion

   b. Warfarin with a target INR of 3.5 for 3 weeks before cardioversion and continued for 6 weeks after cardioversion

   c. Warfarin with a target INR of 2.5 for 3 weeks before cardioversion and continued for 4 weeks after cardioversion

   d. Warfarin with a target INR of 2.5 for 6 weeks before cardioversion and continued for 6 weeks after cardioversion

21. Heparin must first bind to _____ to exert its anticoagulant activity.

   a. antithrombin

   b. thrombin

   c. factor X

   d. protein C

22. J. M. was initiated on heparin and was given a 5,000-unit bolus. Five minutes after the loading dose of heparin, she began to have bloody emesis, and her systolic pressure dropped to 80 mmHg. How much protamine will she require?

   a. 25 mg

   b. 50 mg

   c. 75 mg

   d. 100 mg

23. Patients who develop heparin-induced thrombocytopenia have an in vitro cross-reactivity with low-molecular-weight heparin (LMWH) by what percent?

   a. 90% to 100%

   b. 60% to 70%

   c. 25% to 45%

   d. 5% to 10%

24. A patient with a recent history of heparin-associated antibodies presents with new-onset symptomatic AFib and requires anticoagulation. Other significant past medical history includes severe renal failure secondary to long-standing HTN. The patient's baseline serum creatinine is 4 mg/dL, with an estimated creatinine clearance of 10 mL/min. Which of the following choices is the best initial therapy?

   a. Lepirudin, 0.4 mg/kg bolus, then 0.15 mg/kg/h

   b. Lepirudin, 0.2 mg/kg bolus, then 0.15 mg/kg/h

   c. Argatroban, 2 µg/kg/min

   d. Enoxaparin, 1 mg/kg SC daily

Antiplatelet Agents

25. What is the maximum dose of aspirin that can be concomitantly administered with ticagrelor?

   a. 81 mg

   b. 100 mg

   c. 162 mg

   d. 325 mg

26. All of the following are differences between clopidogrel and ticagrelor except?

   a. Time to maximum platelet inhibition after bolus administration

   b. Number of metabolic enzyme activations to active drug

   c. Irreversible versus reversible effect at the $P2Y_{12}$ receptor

   d. The number of days to discontinue therapy prior to CABG

27. Respiratory diseases should be closely monitored with the use of which of the following antiplatelet agents?

   a. Clopidogrel

   b. Prasugrel

   c. Ticagrelor

   d. Eptifibatide

28. Which of the following side effects differentiate ticlopidine from clopidogrel?

   a. Diarrhea

   b. Rash

   c. Neutropenia

   d. Thrombotic thrombocytopenic purpura

29. By which of the following mechanisms do clopidogrel and ticlopidine exert their antiplatelet effects?

   a. Cyclo-oxygenase inhibitor

   b. Glycoprotein IIb/IIIa inhibitor

   c. Adenosine diphosphate (ADP) inhibitor

   d. Direct thrombin inhibitor

30. Which of the following glycoprotein IIb/IIIa inhibitors has the highest incidence of severe thrombocytopenia?

   a. Tirofiban

   b. Abciximab

   c. Eptifibatide

   d. The incidence is not different between the different agents

31. Which of the following glycoprotein IIb/IIIa inhibitors has the shortest half-life but the longest duration of therapy?

   a. Tirofiban

   b. Eptifibatide

   c. Abciximab

   d. Lamifiban

Antiarrhythmic Agents

32. Dronedarone use is contraindicated in which patient population?

   a. Post-acute myocardial infarction

   b. Severe renal impairment

   c. NYHA class IV heart failure

   d. 1st degree AV block

33. Y.K is a 65-year-old male with symptomatic paroxysmal atrial fibrillation and heart failure recently admitted to the hospital for decompensation. The decision has been made to restore sinus rhythm and utilize antiarrhythmic therapy for rhythm control. Which of the following antiarrythmic agents is most appropraite to use in this patient for rhythm control?

   a. Dofetalide

   b. Dronedarone

   c. Flecanide

   d. Quinidine

34. Which of the following agents is effective for converting AFib to sinus rhythm and for maintaining sinus rhythm after it is restored?

   a. Digoxin

   b. Amiodarone

   c. Diltiazem

   d. Propranolol

35. M. G., a 50-year-old man, collapsed at home after shoveling his sidewalk. His son initiated cardiopulmonary resuscitation immediately, and an emergency medical service was called. When the squad arrived, it was determined that M. G. was in ventricular fibrillation (VF), and he was cardioverted with 200, 300, and 360 J. Epinephrine was given, and M. G. was shocked again. M. G. was still in VF. It was decided to initiate antiarrhythmic therapy. Choose the most appropriate agent from the list below.

   a. Lidocaine
   b. Amiodarone
   c. Procainamide
   d. Bretylium

Acute Coronary Syndromes

36. G. M. is a 45-year-old man presenting with a non-ST-segment-elevation myocardial infarction (MI). His creatinine clearance is estimated to be 30 mL/min. You would like to initiate eptifibatide. Which of the following doses would be the best choice?

   a. Loading dose of 180 μg/kg and a maintenance of 2 μg/kg/min
   b. Loading dose of 90 μg/kg/min and a maintenance dose of 2 μg/kg/min
   c. Loading dose of 180 μg/kg and a maintenance dose of 1 μg/kg/min
   d. Loading dose of 90 μg/kg/min and a maintenance dose of 1 μg/kg/min

37. M. M. is a 39-year-old man with an inferior wall non-ST-segment-elevation MI. He has a history of poorly controlled HTN and diabetes mellitus (DM). You initiate aspirin, clopidogrel, and atorvastatin. His baseline serum creatinine is 3.4 mg/dL and you estimate his creatinine clearance to be 25 mL/min. What dose of enoxaparin would you choose?

   a. 1 mg/kg every 12 hours
   b. 1 mg/kg daily
   c. Enoxaparin is not indicated at this time
   d. Fondaparinux is safer to use in M. M.

38. B. B. is a 77-year-old man who presents with typical chest pain and pressure. He has ST elevations in lead V_{2-4}. He is 80 kg with a serum creatinine of 0.7 mg/dL with an estimated creatinine clearance of 75 mL/min. You initiate aspirin, clopidogrel, metoprolol, and atorvastatin. You want to initiate enoxaparin and reteplase. What is the enoxaparin dose for this patient?

   a. Loading dose of 30 mg IV once followed immediately by 1 mg/kg every 12 hours
   b. Loading dose of 30 mg IV once followed by 0.75 mg/kg every 12 hours
   c. 1 mg/kg daily
   d. 0.75 mg/kg every 12 hours

39. Which of the following is *not* a risk factor for intracranial hemorrhage in patients receiving fibrinolytic therapy in the treatment of ST-segment-elevation MI?

   a. HTN
   b. Body weight
   c. Age
   d. Time to presentation

40. R. M. is a 65-year-old man presenting to the emergency department (ED) with an ST-segment-elevation MI. It is decided to initiate thrombolytic therapy to induce reperfusion. The patient weighs 72 kg. What is the most effective dose of alteplase for this patient?

  a. 0.9 mg/kg, with a maximum of 90 mg
  b. 15 mg bolus; then 54 mg over 30 minutes; then 36 mg over 60 minutes
  c. 15 mg bolus; then 50 mg over 30 minutes; then 35 mg over 60 minutes
  d. 60 mg over 1 hour; then 20 mg per hour for 2 hours

Hyperlipidemia

41. M. R. is a 74-year-old man with a history of hypercholesterolemia treated with simvastatin. Two months ago he had a permanent pacemaker placed for sick sinus syndrome. He now presents with a 1-month history of fever, chills, and unexplained weight loss. On physical examination he has a new tricuspid regurgitation murmur. A transesophageal echocardiogram confirms your suspicion of endocarditis. Which of the following antibiotics increases the risk of rhabdomyolysis when given with simvastatin?

  a. Ceftriaxone
  b. Vancomycin
  c. Daptomycin
  d. Linezolid

42. Put the following regimens in order according to their low-density lipoprotein (LDL)-lowering ability.

  Atorvastatin, 10 mg daily (A)
  Cholestyramine, 8 g daily (C)
  Pravastatin, 20 mg daily (P)
  Gemfibrozil, 600 mg twice daily (G)

  a. A > P > C > G
  b. P > A > G > C
  c. A > P > G > C
  d. A > C > P > G

43. D. L. is a 76-year-old white man with a past medical history significant for DM type 2 and HTN. Chronic AFib was recently diagnosed with coronary artery disease (CAD) and hypercholesterolemia and he was initiated on gemfibrozil 600 mg twice daily and atorvastatin 40 mg daily. His other medications include glyburide, metoprolol, furosemide, levothyroxine, insulin, and aspirin. Two weeks later, he began to experience pain in his right calf, with pain and stiffness throughout his back, buttocks, and thigh. After another week, he was admitted to the hospital with similar heightened symptoms. On admission, his blood urea nitrogen was elevated, and the urinalysis showed orange, cloudy urine; protein, greater than 300; glucose, greater than 1,000; ketones, 2+; hemoglobin, 3+; red blood cell count, 6 to 10; and myoglobin, 1,367. Which of the following statements is *true*?

  a. The patient is experiencing rhabdomyolysis secondary to the drug interaction of atorvastatin and glyburide.
  b. Forced diuresis with urine alkalinization and discontinuation of gemfibrozil and atorvastatin are indicated for this patient.
  c. Atorvastatin is contraindicated in a patient with DM type 2 and HTN.
  d. If nicotinic acid, rather than gemfibrozil, had been used for hypercholesterolemia, this reaction would have been prevented.

Hypertension

44. N. H. is a 57-year-old man status post MI with a BP of 150/88 mmHg and a heart rate of 87 bpm. He is currently on aspirin, clopidogrel, atorvastatin, and lisinopril. Which agent would be the most appropriate addition for treatment of his HTN?

   a. Hydrochlorothiazide

   b. Metoprolol

   c. Clonidine

   d. Losartan

45. B. T. is a 56-year-old woman with long-standing HTN that is difficult to control. She is currently being treated with amlodipine 10 mg daily, lisinopril 40 mg daily, hydrochlorothiazide 25 mg daily, and clonidine 0.4 mg three times daily. She presented to the emergency room, and her initial BP was 200/110 mmHg. She states she had run out of one of her medications. Which one of her medications would most likely be implicated in causing hypertensive urgency?

   a. Amlodipine

   b. Lisinopril

   c. Hydrochlorothiazide

   d. Clonidine

46. C. P. is a 46-year-old white man admitted with worsening headache, and nausea and vomiting over 48 hours. The patient is status post single-lung transplant secondary to α_1-antitrypsin deficiency. His immunosuppression regimen includes cyclosporine, prednisone, and azathioprine. As a result of the cyclosporine, he has HTN and renal dysfunction (baseline serum creatinine, 1.9 mg/dL). His BP is controlled with clonidine 0.2 mg twice daily and metoprolol tartrate 25 mg twice daily. Two months ago, he was changed to metoprolol from amlodipine because of peripheral edema. The patient was in his usual state of health until approximately 1 week ago, when he experienced diarrhea, which has since resolved. On admission, his BP was 208/110 mmHg and his serum creatinine was 3.8 mg/dL. What is the most appropriate regimen to control this patient's BP?

   a. Change back to amlodipine 10 mg daily

   b. Initiate nitroprusside drip and give IV fluids

   c. Add captopril to the regimen and titrate to effect

   d. Give sublingual nifedipine

Heart Failure

47. R. W. is a 60-year-old woman with HF (left ventricular ejection fraction <30%) who has HTN with a BP of 152/90 mmHg. Her potassium is 4.0 mg/dL and serum creatinine is stable at 1.5 mg/dL. She is currently on digoxin and furosemide. Which regimen is most appropriate to initiate in this patient?

   a. Hydralazine 25 mg four times daily

   b. Metoprolol tartrate 12.5 mg twice daily

   c. Valsartan 20 mg twice daily

   d. Lisinopril 5 mg daily

48. A. V. is a 49-year-old woman with a history of HF presenting to the ED for the second time in a month with acutely decompensated HF. She has dyspnea at rest and 3+ edema in her lower extremities. Her serum creatinine is 1.8 mg/dL and BP is 90/60 mmHg. Her home regimen includes enalapril 20 mg twice daily, carvedilol 3.125 mg twice daily, and furosemide 40 mg PO daily. Which of the following is most appropriate for this patient?

a. Admit her to the hospital for IV furosemide therapy and hemodynamic monitoring.

b. Admit her to the hospital for diuresis with nesiritide.

c. Initiate an infusion of nesiritide in the ED and reassess in 4 hours.

d. Schedule intermittent outpatient infusions of nesiritide.

49. A patient with New York Heart Association class III HF was hospitalized 2 months ago for an exacerbation of his HF. The patient was discharged on lisinopril, furosemide, and digoxin. His lungs are clear and his vital signs are as follows: BP, 105/56 mmHg; heart rate, 84 bpm; and respiration rate, 18. Which regimen is most appropriate to initiate in this patient?

a. Atenolol 50 mg daily

b. Carvedilol 3.125 mg twice daily

c. Carvedilol 25 mg twice daily

d. Metoprolol tartrate 50 mg twice daily

50. Which β-blockers are recommended for use for patients with HF?

a. Metoprolol tartrate, pindolol, propranolol

b. Carvedilol, metoprolol succinate, bisoprolol

c. Metoprolol succinate, metoprolol tartrate, carvedilol

d. Metoprolol tartrate, carvedilol, bisoprolol

51. Y. J. is a 67-year-old African American man with HF who has been treated with lisinopril 20 mg daily, metoprolol succinate 25 mg daily, furosemide 40 mg twice daily, and spironolactone 12.5 mg daily. Despite his current therapy, he still complains of shortness of breath while conducting usual daily activities. What is the most appropriate change that should be made to his regimen?

a. Increase spironolactone

b. Start hydralazine

c. Initiate isosorbide dinitrate and hydralazine

d. Increase lisinopril

52. Which of the following statements is *true*?

a. Serum levels are used to guide the selection of the dose of digoxin.

b. Because spironolactone was found to have mortality benefit in the Randomized Aldactone Evaluation Study (RALES), the addition of spironolactone should be considered for all HF patients.

c. The benefit of long-term IV inotropic therapy may outweigh the increased mortality risk in refractory patients unable to be weaned from IV inotropic support.

d. Digoxin exhibits both symptomatic and mortality benefit in patients with HF.

Endocarditis

53. One month ago, a 37-year-old woman with sinus infection responded well to a 14-day course of amoxicillin/clavulanate 875/125 mg twice daily. She is scheduled for a root canal in 1 week. In the past, her dentist had prescribed one dose of clindamycin 600 mg, 1 hour prior to any dental work, for endocarditis prophylaxis because of her history of mitral valve prolapse. Realizing she has not received her prescription, the patient calls the dentist's office for an antibiotic. What prophylaxis is indicated for this patient?

a. Amoxicillin 2 g PO 1 hour before the procedure

b. Clindamycin 600 mg PO 1 hour before the procedure

c. Azithromycin 500 mg PO 1 hour before the procedure

d. No prophylaxis recommended in this patient

54. S. C. is a 59-year-old woman diagnosed with enterococcal endocarditis. She has no known drug allergies. Which of the following would exhibit standard therapy?

  a. Penicillin G, 5 million units IV every 4 hours for 4 to 6 weeks, plus gentamicin, 2.5 mg/kg IV every 8 hours for 4 to 6 weeks

  b. Ampicillin, 2 g IV every 4 hours for 4 to 6 weeks, plus gentamicin, 1 mg/kg IV every 8 hours for 4 to 6 weeks

  c. Ampicillin, 2 g IV every 4 hours for 4 to 6 weeks, plus gentamicin, 1 mg/kg IV every 8 hours for 3 to 5 days

  d. Vancomycin, 30 mg/kg per 24 hours in two equally divided doses for 4 to 6 weeks

ANSWERS   ● ● ●

1. **b.** 1,300 mg. To determine the loading dose of a one-compartment drug, three items are needed: (a) the drug's V_d (L/kg), (b) the desired steady-state concentration (Cpss [mg/L]), and (c) the patient's weight. Loading dose = V_d × Cpss. Kilograms and liters cancel, and you are left with the loading dose in milligrams.

2. **b.** 25%. The bioavailability of digoxin tablets is 75%. Therefore, when converting from PO to IV administration (bioavailability of 100%), there is a 25% increase in bioavailability. Without altering the dose of digoxin, this patient would most likely have an increase in digoxin level to approximately 2.4 ng/mL. This could lead to potential digoxin toxicity.

3. **c.** V_d and clearance. Half-life is a function of both clearance (Cl) and V_d. The elimination-rate constant (k_{el}) is determined by two independent factors: Cl and V_d. k_{el} = Cl/V_d. Half-life is determined by the equation 0.693/k_{el}. Therefore, as the apparent V_d and Cl change, the half-life of a drug may change.

4. **d.** Pharmacodynamics. Pharmacodynamics has been defined as the study of the biologic effects resulting from the interaction between drugs and biologic systems. Pharmacokinetic principles consider drug distribution, metabolism, clearance, and bioavailability, whereas pharmacodynamic principles take this one step further and relate these factors to pharmacologic response. Pharmacogenetics is the study of heredity on variations in drug response among individuals and populations. Pharmacogenetic studies have established that genetics play an important role in the dose–concentration–response relationships of medications, whereas pharmacology is simply the study of drugs.

5. **a.** Drug A is the most potent agent. This is based on the fact that at any given concentration of this agent, the effect is greater than that of the other drugs at similar concentrations. Drug B has the same maximal effect; however, it occurs at a higher concentration. Drug C is similar to drug B; however, it is less efficacious, because its maximal effect occurs at a concentration that is 50% lower than that of drug B.

6. **c.** Increases warfarin metabolism, decreases warfarin metabolism. Chronic ethanol consumption can lead to increased hepatic metabolism of many medications that are cleared through the liver. Increased hepatic metabolism is related to enhanced enzyme function. Therefore, chronic ethanol users typically need higher-than-usual doses of warfarin to achieve therapeutic INRs. Acute ingestion of large amounts of ethanol at a time may inhibit warfarin metabolism. This may lead to elevated INRs and increase the risk of hemorrhagic complications. Moderate ingestion of ethanol does not seem to affect the metabolism of warfarin.

7. **a.** Amiodarone. Amiodarone significantly increases the levels of digoxin. Amiodarone decreases the clearance of digoxin and inhibits p-glycoprotein. Amiodarone can increase digoxin levels by 50% to 70%. This interaction can occur in the first days of therapy and a 50% dosage reduction is required immediately. Metoprolol does not increase the levels of digoxin; however, it can have synergistic effects on lowering heart rate and should be monitored closely. Simvastatin and fenofibrate do not alter the levels of digoxin.

8. **c.** Sodium depletion is an important factor in the development of renal insufficiency associated with ACE inhibitors. Patients with hyponatremia, dehydration, and severe HF are most dependent on the maintenance of renal perfusion by angiotensin II–mediated vasoconstriction of the efferent arteriole. Prevention of hyponatremia by decreasing diuretics can reduce such risk. Numerous studies, including the Studies of Left Ventricular Dysfunction (SOLVD) treatment trial,

Veterans' Administration Heart Failure Trial (V-HeFT) II, and Cooperative North Scandinavian Enalapril Survival Study (CONSENSUS), have shown ACE inhibitors to reduce mortality in patients with ischemic and nonischemic cardiomyopathy and mild-to-moderate HF. ACE inhibitors are considered to be associated with a class benefit; however, not all ACE inhibitors carry the FDA indication for HF. The ACE inhibitors that are approved for the treatment of HF include captopril, enalapril, lisinopril, quinapril, fosinopril, and ramipril. In 1998, the Assessment of Treatment with Lisinopril and Survival (ATLAS) trial showed that high doses of lisinopril were superior to low doses in decreasing risk of death or hospitalization. Therefore, an effort to use target doses used in clinical trials is important (e.g., captopril 50 mg thrice daily, enalapril 10 mg twice daily, and lisinopril 20 mg daily). Potassium retention of ACE inhibitors is caused by a reduction in the feedback of angiotensin II to stimulate aldosterone release. Caution is necessary when initiating a potassium supplement in a patient on ACE inhibitor therapy.

 9. **c.** (1) ii; (2) iii; (3) i; (4) iv. Agents exhibiting α-blockade include labetalol and carvedilol. Agents with ISA are pindolol, penbutolol, carteolol, and acebutolol. Agents with membrane-stabilizing activity are propranolol, labetalol, and acebutolol. β_1-Selective agents include bisoprolol, betaxolol, atenolol, acebutolol, and metoprolol.

10. **a.** Diltiazem and verapamil decrease conduction velocity within the AV node and increase refractory period of nodal tissue. This then causes slowing of ventricular rate.

11. **d.** Nimodipine. Nimodipine is the only agent indicated for patients with subarachnoid hemorrhage. Nimodipine decreases the influx of extracellular calcium, thus preventing vasospasm.

12. **a.** Ethacrynic acid. Ethacrynic acid is the only loop diuretic that is not a sulfonamide. It is used only in patients allergic to other either loop or thiazide diuretics. Disadvantages of ethacrynic acid include gastrointestinal intolerance and a narrower dose–response curve.

13. **b.** False. Conivaptan is a dual vasopressin antagonist indicated for the treatment of euvolemic and hypervolemic hyponatremia. Its predominant pharmacodynamic effect is through the V_2 antagonism of vasopressin in the renal collecting ducts that results in excretion of free water. Because of the limited number of HF patients with hypervolemic hyponatremia treated with conivaptan, safety in HF patients has not been established; therefore, its use in HF patients may be considered only when the clinical benefit outweighs the risk of adverse effects.

14. **a.** Inhibition of the Na^+/K^+-adenosine triphosphatase. Digoxin inhibits the Na^+/K^+-adenosine triphosphatase pump on the myocardial cell surface. This inhibits the ability of the cell to exchange potassium for sodium and thus leads to an increase in intracellular sodium. This increase in intracellular sodium leads to exchange of sodium for calcium, increasing intracellular calcium concentrations. Increased intracellular calcium enhances contraction coupling.

15. **b.** Discontinue the digoxin and administer digoxin-specific antibodies. Digoxin-immune Fab is indicated for patients with life-threatening ventricular arrhythmias relating to digoxin toxicity. It is also indicated in patients with progressive bradyarrhythmias, such as severe sinus bradycardia or second- or third-degree heart block not responsive to atropine. It should not be used for milder forms of digoxin toxicity. Also, in the setting of hyperkalemia and digitalis intoxication, digoxin-immune Fab fragment is indicated. Digoxin-immune Fab fragment is ovine derived; there is a potential for hypersensitivity reactions, and there are no data available in regard to readministration.

16. **c.** Milrinone. Milrinone is a phosphodiesterase inhibitor classified as inodilator. Thus, milrinone produces positive inotropic effects and vasodilation. Milrinone inhibits the phosphodiesterase III enzyme, leading to an increase in intracellular cAMP, thus causing increased intracellular levels of calcium. In addition, milrinone will decrease pulmonary pressures and left ventricular (LV) end-diastolic pressures more predictably than the other agents listed. These combined effects lead to minimal increases in myocardial O_2 consumption. Also, milrinone may be useful in this patient secondary to chronic metoprolol therapy.

17. **c.** IV vitamin K works faster to lower the INR than oral vitamin K at similar doses. The onset of action of IV vitamin K is 1–2 hours compared to 6–10 hours for oral vitamin K. As a result, INR values return to normal quicker with IV vitamin K. The overall reduction in INR is dose dependent and not route dependent when comparing IV and oral formulations. Subcutaneous vitamin K has variable absorption which can lead to variations in time to onset as well as INR lowering effect.

18. **b.** Fondaparinux. Fondaparinux, a pentasaccharide, selectively inhibits activated Xa through its binding to antithrombin. Enoxaparin and UFH bind to both thrombin (IIa) and activated Xa, whereas bivalirudin binds directly to thrombin. UFH binds to thrombin and activated factor Xa in a 1:1 ratio, whereas LMWHs vary in their binding ratios.

19. **c.** Warfarin, with a target goal international normalized ratio (INR) of 2.5. This patient is at high risk for a thromboembolic event. Recommendations for antithrombotic therapy include risk stratification. Risks are stratified into high, moderate, and low. High-risk patients include patients with prior stroke or transient ischemic attack or systemic embolus, history of HTN, poor LV systolic function, age older than 75 years, rheumatic mitral valve disease, and a prosthetic heart valve. Moderate risk factors include age between 65 and 75 years, DM, and CAD with preserved LV systolic function. Low-risk patients are those younger than 65 years old with no clinical or transthoracic echocardiogram evidence of cardiovascular disease.

20. **c.** Warfarin with a target INR of 2.5 for 3 weeks before cardioversion and continued for 4 weeks after cardioversion. Recommendations from the Sixth ACCP Consensus Conference on Antithrombotic Therapy state that patients undergoing elective cardioversion for AFib should be initiated on oral anticoagulant therapy for 3 weeks before and at least 4 weeks after elective direct current cardioversion. The grade of evidence is 1C+. Also, an alternative approach would be to initiate anticoagulation, have the patients undergo a transesophageal echocardiography, and have the cardioversion performed if no thrombi are seen. Warfarin should be continued for at least 4 weeks, as long as the patient maintains normal sinus rhythm. This is a grade 1C recommendation.

21. **a.** Antithrombin. Heparin must first bind to antithrombin to exert its anticoagulant effect. This complex accelerates antithrombin effect. Heparin potentiates antithrombin's effect by binding to a glucosamine unit within a pentasaccharide sequence.

22. **b.** 50 mg. Every 1 mg of protamine will antagonize approximately 100 units of heparin. Because this patient just received the bolus, she would require 50 mg of protamine. If she had received the dose 30 to 60 minutes ago, then a dose of 0.50 to 0.75 mg of protamine per 100 units of heparin would be required. If she had been on a continuous infusion of heparin, then the dosing would be dependent on the time and dose of the last bolus of heparin and the rate of infusion. In this scenario, most patients require approximately 25 to 50 mg of protamine.

23. a. 90% to 100%. There have been several reports of patients who have heparin-induced thrombocytopenia being treated with LMWH. However, the cross-reactivity in vitro approaches 100%. The use of LMWH should be considered a contraindication unless there is a documented negative test for antibodies against LMWH.

24. c. Argatroban, 2 µg/kg/min. Argatroban is hepatically cleared and, therefore, does not require dosing adjustment for patients with renal dysfunction and may be a safer alternative for anticoagulation. Lepirudin is reasonable as well; however, patients with significant renal dysfunction require appropriate dosing adjustments. Continuous infusion should not be used in patients with a creatinine clearance <15 mL/min because of accumulation of drug. LMWHs have a high likelihood for in vitro and in vivo cross-reactivity of 80% to 100%, and there is a potential for an increase in thrombotic complications.

25. b. 100 mg. The Ticagrelor versus Clopidogrel in Patients with Acute Coronary Syndromes (PLATO) trial evaluated antiplatelet strategies in addition to aspirin post-ACS. The trial did not mandate a specific aspirin maintenance dose which was left to the discretion of the provider. After trial completion, a subset analysis was performed which favored ticagrelor use with low maintenance dose aspirin (<100 mg) as higher doses resulted in decreased ticagrelor effectiveness. The package insert for ticagrelor recommends the maintenance dose of aspirin to be 75–100 mg daily if being used concomitantly with ticagrelor. An initial 325 mg dose of aspirin should still be given with ticagrelor in the ACS setting.

26. d. The number of days to discontinue therapy prior to CABG. The recommended number of days prior to CABG surgery to stop clopidogrel or ticagrelor is 5. Patients in both the Ticagrelor versus Clopidogrel in Patients with Acute Coronary Syndromes (PLATO) trial and the Effects of Clopidogrel in Addition to Aspirin in Patients with Acute Coronary Syndromes without ST-Segment Elevation (CURE) trial had increased bleeding if the agents were not stopped at least 5 days prior to surgery. Although the competitive antagonist property of ticagrelor at the $P2Y_{12}$ receptor and its short half-life (~7 hours) would lead clinicians to believe that ticagrelor could be stopped earlier than 5 days prior to surgery, that has not proven to be true.

27. c. In the Ticagrelor versus Clopidogrel in Patients with Acute Coronary Syndromes (PLATO) trial, patients were more likely to experience dyspnea in the ticagrelor arm versus the clopidogrel arm (14% vs. 8 %). Also, more patients had to discontinue ticagrelor than clopidogrel because of dyspnea (0.9% vs. 0.1%). The mechanism for increased dyspnea is hypothesized to be triggered by adenosine. Ticagrelor inhibits the clearance of adenosine thereby increasing its concentration in the circulation. Although, more dyspnea results from ticagrelor use, there were no differences in forced expiratory volume in 1 second (FEV1) between ticagrelor and clopidogrel.

28. c. Neutropenia. Ticlopidine causes neutropenia in 2.4% of patients who are initiated on therapy. Nearly 1% of patients develop severe neutropenia. Therefore, a complete blood count is required every 2 weeks during initiation of therapy for the first 3 months of therapy. Both agents can cause diarrhea and rash. Structurally, these two drugs are so similar that allergic cross-reactivity is expected. Thrombotic thrombocytopenic purpura has been reported with both agents. There have been >100 cases of thrombotic thrombocytopenic purpura reported with the use of ticlopidine and clopidogrel.

29. c. Adenosine diphosphate (ADP) inhibitor. ADP is released from red blood cells, activated platelets, and damaged endothelial cells, leading to platelet adhesion and aggregation. However, the precise mechanism of its action has not been completely identified. ADP blockade decreases the expression of the glycoprotein IIb/IIIa receptor. Platelet inhibition occurs at maximal effect within 3 to 5 days and produces approximately 40% to 50% platelet inhibition. The onset and degree of platelet inhibition can be expedited with use of loading doses (300 to 600 mg).

30. b. Abciximab. All glycoprotein IIb/IIIa inhibitors may cause thrombocytopenia. However, abciximab has the highest rate of all, based on the clinical trials.

31. c. Abciximab. Abciximab has a serum half-life of 10 to 30 minutes; however, because of its high binding affinity to the glycoprotein IIb/IIIa receptor, it maintains its activity for many hours after discontinuation of therapy, and abciximab can be detected in the serum for longer than 2 weeks. The short-acting inhibitors have half-lives of approximately 2 hours, depending on renal function; however, because of their competitive inhibiting nature, once the infusion is discontinued, their effects wane relatively quickly.

32. c. NYHA class IV heart failure. The Antiarrhythmic Trial with Dronedarone in Moderate-to-Severe Congestive Heart Failure Evaluating Morbidity Decrease (ANDROMEDA) was a mortality trial comparing dronedarone to placebo in patients with moderate to severe heart failure for rhythm control. The trial was prematurely terminated as a significantly higher mortality rate was seen in the dronedarone arm versus placebo (8.1% vs. 3.8%). The risk of death was highest in patients with severely depressed left ventricular systolic function. The package insert for dronedarone states the drug is contraindicted in patients with NYHA Class IV heart failure or symptomatic heart failure with recent decompensation requiring hospitalization because it doubles the risk of death.

33. a. Dofetalide. Structural heart failure limits the use of antiarrythmic therapies for rhythm control in atrial fibrillation due to mortality concerns. Dofetalide has not shown to increase mortality in patients with atrial fibrillation who also have heart failure unlike dronedarone, flecanide, and quinidine. The agent of choice in this situation; however, would likely be amiodarone unless the patient has other contraindications for amiodarone therapy.

34. b. Amiodarone. Although amiodarone does not carry an FDA indication for the treatment of AFib, it can convert to and maintain normal sinus rhythm. The other agents listed are only used for rate control when used for AFib.

35. b. Amiodarone. The most recent advanced cardiac life support guidelines recommend that amiodarone be the first-line agent in patients with pulseless VT/VF. This recommendation is based on the Amiodarone for Resuscitation after Out-of-Hospital Cardiac Arrest due to Ventricular Fibrillation (ARREST) trial, which showed that amiodarone increased the likelihood of admission to the hospital after an out-of-hospital arrest. This is further supported by the recently presented Amiodarone versus Lidocaine in Pre-Hospital Refractory Ventricular Fibrillation Evaluation (ALIVE) trial. Lidocaine is now considered Class Indeterminate based on the lack of controlled trials supporting its use in pulseless VT/VF. Procainamide administration is prolonged and not suitable for rapid administration. Bretylium is no longer available secondary to lack of raw materials.

36. c. Loading dose of 180 µg/kg and a maintenance dose of 1 µg/kg/min. Based on product information, eptifibatide loading dose should not be changed and the maintenance infusion should be initiated at 1 µg/kg/min. Eptifibatide is contraindicated in patients on dialysis and there is limited experience using this agent in this patient population. Tirofiban is not contraindicated in patients on dialysis; however, there are limited data to support its use in dialysis patients.

37. b. Enoxaparin 1 mg/kg daily. Enoxaparin is approved for both ST-segment-elevation and non-ST-segment-elevation MI. In patients with a creatinine clearance >30 mL/min then the standard dose of 1 mg/kg every 12 hours is appropriate. However, when the creatinine clearance is <30 mL/min then the dose should be reduced to 1 mg/kg once daily. Fondaparinux is contraindicated in patients with a creatinine clearance <30 mL/min.

38. d. Loading dose of 30 mg IV once followed by 0.75 mg/kg every 12 hours. Enoxaparin was recently approved for the treatment of ST-segment-elevation MI with fibrinolysis based on the ExTRACT-TIMI 25 trial. In the older patients, lower enoxaparin doses were used to minimize bleeding. There was a lower risk of the primary endpoint in those that received enoxaparin versus those receiving UFH. There was no difference in intracranial hemorrhage; however, there was a significantly higher rate of major bleeding with enoxaparin (2.1% versus 1.4%).

39. d. Time to presentation. Time to presentation is not a risk factor for intracranial hemorrhage in patients receiving thrombolytic therapy. In clinical trials, the risks for intracranial hemorrhage included age older than 65 years, low body weight (<70 kg), HTN on hospital admission, and the use of alteplase. Also, the levels of concomitant anticoagulation can also increase the risk of intracranial hemorrhage.

40. c. 15 mg bolus; then 50 mg over 30 minutes; then 35 mg over 60 minutes. Based on the first GUSTO trial, the most effective dosing for acute ST-segment-elevation MI is front-loaded tissue plasminogen activator. The maximum dose should be 100 mg and, therefore, Answer b may increase the risk of major bleeding, specifically intracranial hemorrhage. Answer d is standard dosing of recombinant tissue-type plasminogen activator and was found inferior to front loading. Finally, Answer a is the recommended dosing for acute ischemic stroke.

41. c. Daptomycin. Daptomycin may cause elevations in creatine phosphokinase (CPK) levels. The product literature for daptomycin recommends temporary discontinuation of medications that can raise CPK levels when a patient is receiving this antibiotic. Even though this adverse reaction is rare, CPK levels should be monitored weekly in patients receiving daptomycin alone and more frequently if statin therapy is continued.

42. a. A > P > C > G. HMG-CoA reductase inhibitors decrease LDL by 18% to 55%. Atorvastatin is the most potent agent statin of the group. Bile-acid sequestrants decreased LDL by 15% to 30%. Fibrates decrease LDL by 5% to 20%.

43. b. Forced diuresis with urine alkalinization and discontinuation of gemfibrozil and atorvastatin are indicated for this patient. Rhabdomyolysis secondary to the interaction of atorvastatin and gemfibrozil is responsible for this clinical picture. Rhabdomyolysis is defined as the disintegration of muscle, associated with the excretion of myoglobin in the urine. Clinical signs and symptoms include myalgias, elevated creatine kinase, elevated urine and serum myoglobin, and dark urine. Complications of rhabdomyolysis are numerous and may include renal failure, disseminated intravascular coagulation, metabolic acidosis, and cardiomyopathy. HMG-CoA (3-hydroxy-3-methyl-glutaryl-CoA) reductase inhibitors (statins) can be considered direct myotoxins and may induce rhabdomyolysis when used alone. However, the risk of toxicity increases when statins are used in combination with fibric acid derivatives (gemfibrozil or fenofibrate), nicotinic acid, cyclosporine, itraconazole, or erythromycin, to name a few. Treatment of the underlying cause, in this case discontinuation of the offending agents, is necessary. In addition, renal failure caused by products of tissue degradation must be combated with urinary alkalinization and maintenance of a high urine volume.

44. **b.** Metoprolol. The American College of Cardiology (ACC) and American Heart Association (AHA) recommend the use of β-blockers in patients after surviving an MI to decrease mortality, sudden death, and reinfarction. Therefore, if this patient is not already on a β-blocker, one would be indicated, not only for HTN but also for secondary prevention.

45. **d.** Clonidine. Abrupt withdrawal of an α2-agonist is the most likely cause of severe rebound HTN. Typically, this is seen within 24 to 48 hours of discontinuation of clonidine and typically occurs in patients taking large doses for longer than 3 months. The best treatment for this is to restart clonidine. β-Blockers could make the situation worse by causing unopposed α1-stimulation.

46. **b.** Initiate nitroprusside drip and give IV fluids. Hypertensive emergencies are defined by the presence of end-organ damage in the face of high BP. This patient was dehydrated from diarrhea and had uncontrolled BP because of the medication change that occurred. Use of nitroprusside would be most appropriate in this patient because of the emergent situation of the renal insufficiency and possible cerebrovascular involvement exhibited by the headache. Typically, parenteral antihypertensive agents are initiated for hypertensive emergencies. In addition, it is necessary to correct the underlying cause of the hypertensive episode, if it can be identified; therefore, rehydration in this patient is prudent. Nitroprusside is the drug of choice because it has a quick onset of action yet is easily titratable. Sublingual nifedipine is no longer advocated because of the precipitous drop in BP and the subsequent adverse effects.

47. **d.** Lisinopril 5 mg daily. Because the patient is not already receiving ACE inhibitor therapy, an ACE inhibitor is indicated in patients with HF and a reduced ejection fraction (less than 35% to 45%) to decrease morbidity and mortality, as shown in the SOLVD, V-HeFT, and CONSENSUS trials. The patient has no contraindications to such therapy. If the patient's renal function were changing, thereby making an ACE inhibitor inappropriate, then hydralazine plus a nitrate would be indicated, because V-HeFT I showed mortality benefit compared with placebo and an α-blocker. An angiotensin receptor blocker (ARB), like valsartan, would be indicated if the patient were intolerant to ACE inhibitors in the past. Both ACE inhibitors and ARB should be initiated at low doses, and titrated (as tolerated) to doses proven in clinical trials to reduce cardiovascular events.

48. **a.** Admit her to the hospital for IV furosemide therapy and hemodynamic monitoring. Nesiritide is contraindicated for use in patients with systolic BP <90 mmHg. However, based on meta-analyses that raised questions of increased renal dysfunction and mortality associated with nesiritide, the FDA convened a panel to assess available data and provide recommendations regarding appropriate use of nesiritide. These recommendations state that nesiritide should be limited to hospitalized patients with decompensated HF with dyspnea at rest and it should not be used to replace diuretics. Furthermore, because of insufficient evidence, nesiritide should not be used for intermittent outpatient infusions, for scheduled repetitive use, to improve renal function, or to enhance diuresis. A large-scale clinical trial to assess outcomes and further assess the risks of nesiritide versus standard therapy is currently being conducted.

49. **b.** Carvedilol 3.125 mg twice daily. All patients with stable, class II or III HF should be initiated on a β-blocker, unless a contraindication (bronchospastic disease, symptomatic bradycardia, or advanced heart block) or intolerance is exhibited. Initiation of β-blocker therapy is recommended in stable patients with mild-to-moderate HF and a low ejection fraction (less than 35% to 40%). The mortality benefit of β-blocker use was seen when added to a preexisting regimen of an ACE inhibitor and diuretic, with or without digoxin. It should be noted that β-blockers must be initiated at very low doses and only gradually increased if low doses have been well tolerated.

50. **b.** Carvedilol, metoprolol succinate, bisoprolol. Overwhelming mortality benefit in patients with chronic HF has been proven in clinical trials for carvedilol, metoprolol succinate, and bisoprolol when added to standard HF therapy. These agents are specifically recommended in the ACC/AHA guidelines for the management of chronic heart failure. Despite survival benefit with each of these β-blockers, a class effect with all β-blockers should not be assumed as demonstrated by the Carvedilol or Metoprolol European Trial (COMET). The COMET compared carvedilol with metoprolol tartrate in HF patients and concluded that carvedilol exhibited superior mortality benefit. β-Blockers with ISA should not be used on patients with HF. Pindolol and others with ISA (such as penbutolol, carteolol, and acebutolol) are partial β-agonists and can maintain normal sympathetic tone. This activity prevents the benefits seen with the reduced heart rate, cardiac output, and peripheral blood flow caused by other β-blockers.

51. **c.** Initiate isosorbide dinitrate and hydralazine. The ACC/AHA guidelines recommend the initiation of isosorbide dinitrate and hydralazine as a reasonable addition to standard therapy in blacks with New York Heart Association class III/IV HF. The A-HeFT trial evaluated a proprietary drug combination (hydralazine 37.5 mg and isosorbide dinitrate 20 mg per tablet) in African Americans with HF along with standard treatment; because of significant mortality benefit, the study was prematurely discontinued.

52. **c.** The benefit of long term IV inotropic therapy may outweigh the increased mortality risk in refractory patients unable to be weaned from IV inotropic support. Because long-term IV positive inotropic therapy may cause an increased risk of death, such therapy is not regularly recommended. This risk, however, may be outweighed in patients who cannot be weaned from continuous support. Such patients with refractory HF may experience an improved quality of life because of the relative clinical stability afforded by the inotrope; therefore, IV positive inotropic therapy may be considered as a palliative measure in end-stage HF. The DIG (Digitalis Investigation Group) trial showed that digoxin's benefit in HF was the alleviation of symptoms and improvement in clinical status. These findings were associated with a decreased morbidity (fewer hospitalizations) but not mortality. Because digoxin has negligible effect on survival, it is recommended that digoxin be used in conjunction with diuretics, ACE inhibitors, and β-blockers to decrease the clinical symptoms of HF. Furthermore, little evidence supports the practice of dosing digoxin according to serum levels. This is because of the lack of data exhibiting a relationship between digoxin serum concentrations and therapeutic effect. In the RALES trial, spironolactone was shown to be associated with reduced mortality and morbidity. However, the patients who were included in this trial were patients with class IV HF. Therefore, it would only be prudent to consider spironolactone in patients with recent or current severe HF symptoms. Efficacy and safety of spironolactone's use in patients with mild-to-moderate HF is yet to be determined.

53. **d.** No prophylaxis is recommended in this patient. The recommendations according to the 2007 Guidelines for Prevention of Infective Endocarditis no longer recommend prophylactic antibiotics prior to dental procedures for people with mitral valve prolapse, rheumatic heart disease, bicuspid valve disease, calcified aortic stenosis, or congenital heart conditions such as ventricular septal defect, atrial septal defect, and hypertrophic cardiomyopathy.

54. **b.** Ampicillin, 2 g IV every 4 hours for 4 to 6 weeks, plus gentamicin, 1 mg/kg IV every 8 hours for 4 to 6 weeks. Treatment of enterococcal endocarditis is complicated because of the high levels of resistance to penicillin, extended-spectrum penicillins, and vancomycin. However, penicillin, ampicillin, or vancomycin in combination with an aminoglycoside causes synergistic bactericidal effect on these organisms. Treatment with an aminoglycoside for the full 4 to 6 weeks at a synergistic dose (1 mg/kg IV every 8 hours) in addition to the penicillin agent or vancomycin is required.

SUGGESTED READINGS

Anderson JL, Adams CD, Antman EM, et al. ACC/AHA 2007 guidelines for the management of patients with unstable angina/non–ST-elevation myocardial infarction: a report of the American College of Cardiology/American Heart Association Task Force on Practice Guidelines (Writing Committee to Revise the 2002 Guidelines for the Management of Patients with Unstable Angina/Non–ST-Elevation Myocardial Infarction): developed in collaboration with the American College of Emergency Physicians, American College of Physicians, Society for Academic Emergency Medicine, Society for Cardiovascular Angiography and Interventions, and Society of Thoracic Surgeons. *J Am Coll Cardiol.* 2007;50:e1–e157.

Antman EM, Hand M, Armstrong PW, et al. 2007 Focused update of the ACC/AHA 2004 Guidelines for the Management of Patients with ST-Elevation Myocardial Infarction: a report of the American College of Cardiology/American Heart Association Task Force on Practice Guidelines (Writing Group to Review New Evidence and Update the ACC/AHA 2004 Guidelines for the Management of Patients with ST-Elevation Myocardial Infarction). *Circulation.* 2008;117:296–329.

Expert Panel of Detection, Evaluation, and Treatment of High Blood Cholesterol in Adults. Executive summary of the third report of the National Cholesterol Education Program (NCEP) Expert Panel on Detection, Evaluation, and Treatment of High Blood Cholesterol in Adults (Adult Treatment Panel III). *JAMA.* 2001;285:2486–2497.

Hunt SA, Abraham WT, Chin MH, et al. ACC/AHA 2005 guideline update for the diagnosis and management of chronic heart failure in the adult: a report of the American College of Cardiology/American Heart Association Task Force on Practice Guidelines (Writing Committee to Update the 2001 Guidelines for the Evaluation and Management of Heart Failure). *Circulation.* 2005;112(12):e154–e235. Available at: http://www.acc.org/clinical/guidelines/failure//index.pdf

The sixth report of the National Committee on detection, evaluation, and treatment of high blood pressure (JNC-VI). *Arch Intern Med.* 1997;157:2413–2446.

Wilson W, Taubert KA, Gewitz M, et al. Prevention of infective endocarditis: guidelines from the American Heart Association: a guideline from the American Heart Association Rheumatic Fever, Endocarditis, and Kawasaki Disease Committee, Council on Cardiovascular Disease in the Young, and the Council on Clinical Cardiology, Council on Cardiovascular Surgery and Anesthesia, and the Quality of Care and Outcomes Research Interdisciplinary Working Group. Published online on April 19, 2007 (DOI: 10.1161/CIRCULATIONAHA.106.183095). *Circulation.* 2007;116:1736–1754. Available at: http://circ.ahajournals.org/cgi/content/full/116/15/1736

chapter 6

Aorta

Craig R. Asher • Gian M. Novaro

QUESTIONS ● ● ●

Case 1 (Questions 1 to 3)

A 78-year-old woman is referred to cardiology clinic for management of aortic regurgitation. The patient has no cardiac risk factors except mild hypertension (HTN) on monotherapy and has not previously undergone cardiac testing. A review of systems is notable for recent onset of headaches and myalgias.

Physical Examination

Blood pressure (BP)—138/78 mmHg in both arms; pulse—62 bpm.

Funduscopic examination reveals no changes consistent with hypertensive retinopathy. The heart examination is notable for a normal S_1 and increased intensity S_2 (A_2). An S_4 gallop, II/VI diastolic decrescendo murmur heard best at the right sternal border, and III/VI early-peaking systolic ejection murmur heard at the left sternal border are present. There is no systolic ejection click. The carotid pulse is of normal intensity and contour and the pulses in the upper and lower extremities are strong and equal.

Electrocardiogram (ECG) reveals sinus rhythm with nonspecific ST changes.

1. What is the most likely explanation for the patient's heart murmur?

   a. Bicuspid aortic valve with severe aortic regurgitation
   b. Bicuspid aortic valve with severe aortic stenosis and moderate aortic regurgitation
   c. Degenerative severe aortic valve stenosis and moderate aortic regurgitation
   d. Aortic dilatation with moderate aortic regurgitation and mild aortic stenosis

A transthoracic echocardiogram (TTE) is performed showing normal left ventricular (LV) size and function with a trileaflet aortic valve. Aortic measurements are as follows: sinus of Valsalva—4.0 cm; sinotubular junction—4.4 cm; mid-ascending aorta—4.5 cm with moderate effacement of the sinotubular junction. Peak and mean aortic gradients are 22/13 mmHg with moderate (2+) aortic regurgitation. A small circumferential pericardial effusion is present. Laboratory tests reveal an erythrocyte sedimentation rate of 74.

2. What additional test would be most helpful in determining the etiology of the patient's aortic dilatation and aortic regurgitation?

   a. Coronary angiogram and aortography
   b. Magnetic resonance angiography (MRA) of the great vessels

   c. Computed tomographic angiography (CTA) of the ascending aorta
   d. Transesophageal echocardiography (TEE)

3. What is the most likely diagnosis to explain the patient's aortic dilatation and aortic regurgitation? See Figure 6.1.

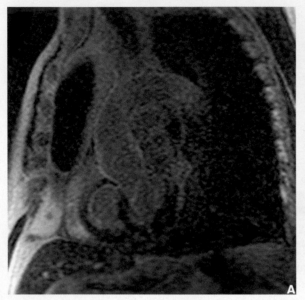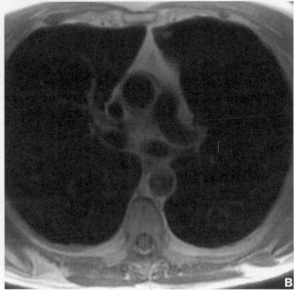

Figure 6.1

   a. Takayasu arteritis
   b. Degenerative aortic disease
   c. Connective tissue disorder
   d. Giant cell arteritis

Case 2 (Questions 4 to 6)

An 18-year-old woman presents for her annual physical examination. She had a brother with Marfan syndrome who was 24 years old when he died suddenly. She is active and asymptomatic.

Physical Examination

   5 feet 7 inches (170 cm) and 150 pounds (68 kg).

   Arm span-to-height ratio = 1.07.

   Head and neck examination is notable for a high-arched palate and a slit-lamp examination shows ectopia lentis. Musculoskeletal examination is notable for a pectus carinatum and positive wrist and thumb sign. Cardiac examination is notable for a mitral valve click and a soft murmur of mitral regurgitation.

4. What additional testing is needed to determine whether this young woman has Marfan syndrome?

   a. TTE
   b. Genetic testing
   c. CT angiogram of the aorta
   d. No additional testing

A TTE is performed that shows mitral valve prolapse with mild (1+) mitral regurgitation. The aortic root is dilated at 5.0 cm with effacement of the sinotubular junction and a mid-ascending aortic measurement of 3.6 cm. The aortic valve is trileaflet with no aortic regurgitation.

5. What is the most important recommendation to be made to this patient?

   a. Repeat the TTE in 6 months

   b. Initiate a β-blocker

   c. Avoid strenuous exertion, contact sports, and pregnancy

   d. Elective aortic replacement

The patient wishes to schedule surgery but prefers to wait 2 months until the end of the school year. Her father who is an internal medicine physician has read about the potential benefit of angiotensin receptor blockers (ARBs) for patients with aneurysms and asks your advice regarding treatment.

6. What is the postulated mechanism of action whereby ARBs reduce progression of aortic disease in Marfan syndrome?

   a. Reduction of BP through angiotensin II type 1 receptor blockade

   b. Complete blockade of the renin–angiotensin–aldosterone system

   c. Reduction in activity of transforming growth factor (TGF)-β

   d. Increase production of matrix metalloproteinases (MMPs)

Case 3 (Questions 7 and 8)

A 67-year-old man with long-standing HTN presents to the emergency room (ER) with sudden-onset chest pain described as ripping in quality, subsiding since its onset. He underwent a cardiac catheterization 6 months previously that showed a 40% lesion in the mid-left anterior descending coronary artery. His medications include aspirin, gemfibrozil, and nifedipine.

Physical Examination

   He appears diaphoretic. HR—110 bpm; BP—106/54 mmHg (right arm); 72/35 mmHg (left arm). Jugular venous pressure—12 cm H_2O. Heart sounds are soft and there is no audible systolic or diastolic murmur. Left radial and brachial pulses are weak.

   ECG on presentation shows ST elevations in the inferior leads and low voltage.

   Chest X-ray (CXR) shows cardiomegaly with a globular-shaped heart and interstitial edema.

7. Which of the following is the first diagnostic test that should be performed?

   a. Cardiac enzymes

   b. MRA of the aorta

   c. TTE

   d. Cardiac catheterization

A TTE was performed showing a pericardial effusion and signs of cardiac tamponade. A CT angiogram is also performed and shown in Figure 6.2.

8. What intervention should be performed next for the management of this patient?

   a. Cardiac catheterization

   b. Emergent aortic surgery

   c. Swan-Ganz catheterization

   d. Pericardiocentesis

Case 4 (Questions 9 and 10)

A 36-year-old man with a bicuspid aortic valve develops sudden onset of headache, mental status changes, and unequal pupils. He is rushed to an ER and a head CT scan is done that shows an intracranial bleed. BP on presentation is 158/78 mmHg.

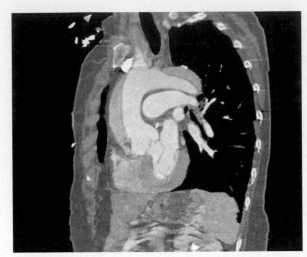

Figure 6.2

Except for a history of HTN, he has no known medical problems and no history of drug abuse. A visit to his physician's office 1 week earlier revealed a BP of 120/75 mmHg on metoprolol and ramipril.

9. What is the most likely reason for the patient's intracranial bleed?

   a. Hypertensive crisis

   b. Aortic dissection

   c. Cerebral aneurysm rupture

   d. Mycotic aneurysm associated with endocarditis

10. What other structural abnormality is most commonly associated with coarctation of the aorta?

   a. Atrial septal defect

   b. Ventricular septal defect

   c. Pulmonary stenosis

   d. Mitral valve prolapse

Case 5 (Questions 11 and 12)

A 74-year-old man presents to the ER with upper back pain ongoing for 3 hours. The pain is described as sharp and severe occurring at rest. He has no associated symptoms of shortness of breath, chest pain, or presyncope. His past medical history is notable for a coronary artery bypass graft (CABG) 2 years previously, HTN, and ongoing tobacco use. At the time of his CABG, he was noted to have a 4.4-cm ascending aortic aneurysm that was not repaired. His medications include aspirin, an angiotensin-converting enzyme inhibitor, and a β-blocker.

Physical Examination

   BP—180/110 mmHg.

   Pulse rate—90 bpm.

   Lung and cardiac examinations are unremarkable and no cardiac murmur is heard. The abdomen is mildly tender with no bruit. Pulses are equal but diminished in the lower extremities.

   ECG shows sinus rhythm with nonspecific ST changes and an old inferior myocardial infarction (MI).

   Laboratory tests including cardiac enzymes, liver function tests, amylase, and lipase are normal.

11. What is the most appropriate diagnostic procedure to perform next?

   a. TTE

   b. TEE

   c. CTA of the chest and abdomen

   d. Aortography

A CT scan demonstrates an ascending aortic aneurysm of 4.8 cm and a descending thoracic aortic aneurysm of 6.0 cm but no evidence of dissection. There is no abdominal aortic aneurysm (AAA). The patient continues to have ongoing pain despite high doses of β-blockers, sodium nitroprusside, and opioid analgesics.

   ECG and cardiac enzymes remain normal.

   D-dimer level is >500 ng/mL.

12. What is the most appropriate next decision for management?

   a. Cardiac catheterization

   b. MRA of the chest/aorta

   c. TEE

   d. Intensify medical therapy

Case 6 (Question 13)

A 62-year-old man presents for a routine annual examination. He has a history of HTN that is managed with monotherapy. He is active and has no symptoms.

Physical Examination

BP—162/88 mmHg in both arms. Pulse rate—70 bpm. Heart and lung examination is unremarkable. Abdominal examination reveals a pulsatile mass.

ECG shows sinus rhythm and a complete right bundle branch block.

Abdominal ultrasound shows an infrarenal AAA of 4.2 cm.

13. What is the most appropriate management step?

   a. Initiate a β-blocker and repeat ultrasound in 6 months

   b. Initiate a β-blocker and repeat ultrasound in 3 months

   c. No medical therapy and repeat ultrasound in 1 year

   d. No medical therapy and repeat ultrasound in 2 years

Case 7 (Questions 14 and 15)

A 76-year-old man presents to the ER with severe sharp chest pain that began 2 hours previously. He has a history of HTN and had CABG 3 years ago after an MI. He continues to smoke. The CABG was performed off-pump because of severe atheroma in the ascending aorta seen by intraoperative TEE. The patient's pain has not subsided with the initiation of IV heparin, nitroglycerin, and β-blockers. The pain is different in character from the pain before his MI.

Physical Examination

BP—160/94 mmHg.

Pulse—76 bpm.

Heart and lung sounds are normal. Pulses are diminished in the lower extremities.

ECG shows a left bundle branch block.

Cardiac enzymes are normal × 1.

Despite severe atheroma in the aorta, the physician taking care of the patient is not convinced that he does not have an acute coronary syndrome and performs a cardiac catheterization. It shows that the grafts are patent and there is no culprit lesion in the native vessels. He then decides to perform aortography and a focal out-pouching is seen in the aortic wall in the distal ascending aorta (Fig. 6.3A). Contrast dye collects slowly in this region. The patient's chest pain is intensifying. A TEE is also performed (Fig. 6.3B).

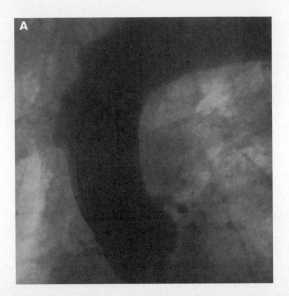

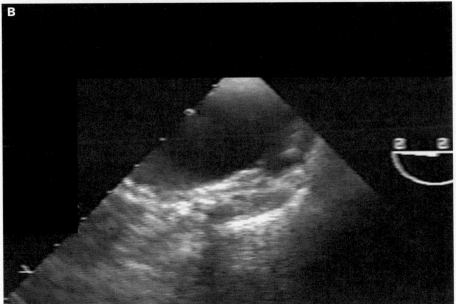

Figure 6.3

14. What is the correct diagnosis?

    a. Aortic dissection
    b. Aortic aneurysm
    c. Intramural hematoma
    d. Penetrating aortic ulcer

15. What is the most appropriate next management step to take?

    a. Medical management with β-blockers and afterload reduction
    b. Transfer to the operating room immediately for replacement of the ascending aorta

c. Medical management and obtain a CT chest/aorta

d. Medical management and obtain an MRA of the aorta

Case 8 (Questions 16 and 17)

A 45-year-old woman presents with discomfort in her left leg with walking, dizziness, headaches, and a cold right hand. She has no chest pain or shortness of breath. There is no significant past medical history and she does not smoke.

Physical Examination

BP—170/82 mmHg (left arm) and 140/68 mmHg (right arm). Lung sounds are clear. Cardiac examination is notable for a normal S_1 and S_2 and II/VI diastolic decrescendo murmur at the left sternal border. The right brachial pulse is diminished and lower extremity pulses are diminished. A bruit is heard over the left carotid artery and right subclavian artery.

16. What test would be most useful for diagnosing the patient's condition?

a. TEE

b. Carotid duplex ultrasound

c. Magnetic resonance imaging (MRI) of the head

d. Angiography

17. What is the most likely diagnosis?

a. Behçet disease

b. Relapsing polychondritis

c. Giant cell arteritis

d. Takayasu arteritis

Case 9 (Questions 18 to 21)

A 21-year-old woman with Turner syndrome has a history of surgical repair for periductal coarctation of the aorta at age 4 years. Her presentation was for HTN and heart failure, both of which resolved after the procedure. She was lost to follow-up after childhood and recently reestablished with a cardiologist. She has been experiencing dyspnea and claudication in the past year.

Physical Examination

BP—188/94 mmHg (left arm); 192/100 mmHg (right arm); 100/60 mmHg (right leg).

Pulses are notable for normal upper extremity and reduced lower extremity pulses with a brachial–femoral delay. Cardiac examination is notable for normal S_1 and paradoxically split S_2 with an ejection click and S_4 gallop. A continuous murmur III/VI in intensity is heard under the left scapula.

18. Which of the following statements is correct regarding the echocardiographic image from this patient obtained from the suprasternal notch (Fig. 6.4)?

a. Pressure gradients are usually underestimated using the simplified Bernoulli equation

b. Pressure gradients are usually accurate using the simplified Bernoulli equation

c. Pressure gradients shown are not consistent with severe coarctation

d. Presence of systolic and diastolic flow is consistent with severe coarctation

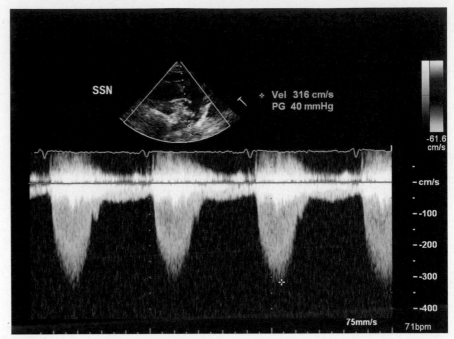

Figure 6.4

19. Which of the following statements is correct regarding the echocardiographic image from this patient obtained from the abdominal aorta (Fig. 6.5)?

    a. The hallmark of coarctation is the presence of low systolic velocities

    b. The presence of coarctation cannot be determined without knowing the timing of the pulse delay relative to aortic ejection

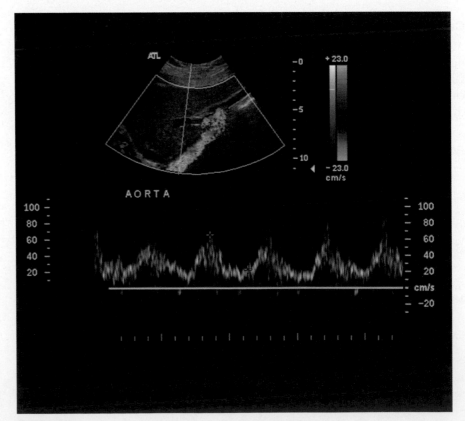

Figure 6.5

c. The hallmark of coarctation is the presence of persistent antegrade flow in diastole

d. The presence of coarctation cannot be determined without additional Doppler images proximal to the coarctation site

20. Which of the following recommendations is most appropriate regarding reintervention in this patient (Fig. 6.6)?

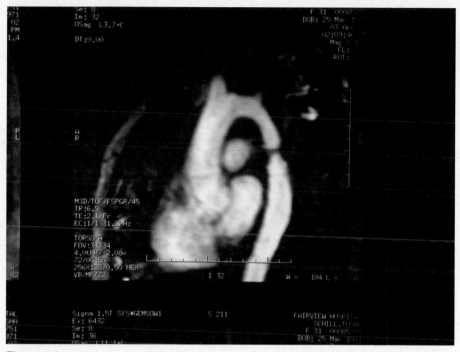

Figure 6.6

a. Surgery is generally recommended

b. No intervention should be performed until maximal medical therapy is attempted

c. Balloon angioplasty with or without stents is generally recommended

d. There is no consensus and either surgery or balloon aortoplasty (with or without stenting) are equal options

21. Which of the following is an indication for aortic coarctation intervention?

a. Symptomatic patient with dyspnea at rest, regardless of the coarctation gradient

b. Asymptomatic patient with normal BP at rest and with exercise and a peak-to-peak gradient across the coarctation site of 19 mmHg

c. Asymptomatic patient with a peak-to-peak gradient across the coarctation site of 15 mmHg with extensive collaterals

d. Symptomatic patient with a bicuspid aortic valve and severe aortic regurgitation undergoing aortic valve replacement and a peak-to-peak gradient across the coarctation of 15 mmHg

Case 10 (Question 22)

A 30-year-old man is referred to cardiology clinic for evaluation of a heart murmur. He had an uneventful childhood except that on four separate occasions he fractured his arms or legs requiring multiple surgical repairs. He has no family history of heart disease or congenital abnormalities.

Physical Examination

Normal stature. Vital signs are normal. Arm span-to-height ratio is normal.

No pectus deformity, scoliosis, wrist sign. Cardiac examination is notable for a decreased S_1 and normal S_2 intensity with a III/VI diastolic decrescendo murmur and no gallops. Pulses are normal and the extremities are hypermobile. No abnormality of the skin is present.

TTE shows a dilated sinus of Valsalva of 4.7 cm with severe aortic regurgitation. Left ventricular ejection fraction (LVEF) = 65% with LV dimensions of (diastole 6.4 cm; systole 5.1 cm).

22. What is the most likely diagnosis for this patient?

   a. Ehlers-Danlos syndrome

   b. Marfan syndrome

   c. Osteogenesis imperfecta

   d. Homocystinuria

Case 11 (Questions 23 and 24)

A 65-year-old man presents to the ER with severe, tearing lower back pain that started while he was shoveling snow. He has a history of poorly controlled HTN and coronary artery disease with a stent to the left anterior descending coronary artery 4 months previously. Other medical problems include severe O_2-dependent chronic obstructive pulmonary disease.

Physical Examination

BP—190/110 mmHg.

Pulse—90 bpm.

Cardiac examination is notable for a normal S_1 and S_2 with an S_4 gallop and II/VI early-peaking systolic ejection murmur at the left sternal border.

ECG shows sinus rhythm and no ST changes.

An initial set of cardiac enzymes is normal.

23. What is the most appropriate initial medical therapy?

   a. Intravenous metoprolol

   b. Intravenous diltiazem

   c. Intravenous enalapril

   d. Intravenous nitroprusside

A CT angiogram is performed (Fig. 6.7).

24. Which of the following statements regarding the appearance of this form of acute aortic syndrome is most accurate?

   a. There is low attenuation of the aortic wall

   b. It is not continuous

   c. Intimal calcium is nondisplaced

   d. It is circumferential or crescentic

Case 12 (Questions 25 to 28)

A 44-year-old man is admitted to the hospital because of a left hemisphere stroke with right arm and leg weakness. He has no history of HTN or smoking, although his total cholesterol level is 334. ECG shows sinus rhythm. Carotid duplex ultrasound shows less than 20% obstruction bilaterally. Head CT demonstrates a recent stroke in

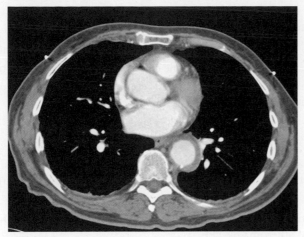

Figure 6.7

the left cortex in the region of the middle cerebral artery. A TTE shows normal valves, chamber sizes, and LV function.

25. Which test is most likely to reveal the etiology of the patient's stroke?

    a. TTE with bubble study

    b. 30-Day event recorder

    c. MRA of the head and neck

    d. TEE

26. Which of the following medical regimens is most appropriate for a patient with a cardioembolic stroke and the following finding seen on TEE (Fig. 6.8)?

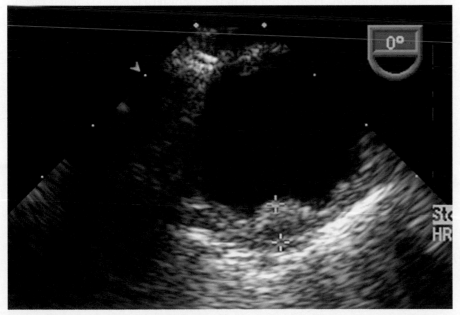

Figure 6.8

    a. Statin and aspirin

    b. Statin and warfarin

    c. Aspirin and dipyridamole

    d. Statin, antiplatelet agent, and warfarin

27. Which of the following atheromatous plaques is least likely to be associated with a cardioembolic event?

   a. 3-mm plaque with severe calcification and no mobile components

   b. 4-mm plaque with small mobile components and no calcification

   c. 5-mm plaque with multiple mobile components, no calcification, and a small ulceration

   d. 2-mm plaque with calcification, a small mobile component, and large ulceration

28. Which statement is correct regarding performing CABG in a similar patient with aortic arch atheroma and focal areas of atheroma in the ascending aorta?

   a. Palpation of the aorta by the surgeon for calcified plaque correlates with findings of atheroma by TEE.

   b. Alternative sites for cross-clamping or cannulation may reduce stroke risk.

   c. Aortic arch endarterectomy is recommended.

   d. Replacement of the ascending aorta is recommended because of increased likelihood of stroke.

Case 13 (Question 29)

A 21-year-old man is referred to a cardiology clinic for exertional dyspnea. As a child he was evaluated for a heart murmur by a pediatric cardiologist.

Physical Examination

   BP—140/84 mmHg (left arm); 120/68 (right arm).

   Cardiac examination is notable for a normal S_1 and increased intensity S_2/A_2, absence of an ejection click, and III/VI systolic ejection murmur heard best in the first right intercostal space radiating to the neck and increases with expiration. There is a thrill in the suprasternal notch. The left carotid and brachial pulses are diminished relative to the right carotid and brachial pulses.

29. What diagnosis best explains the patient's disorder?

   a. Patent ductus arteriosus

   b. Coarctation of the aorta

   c. Supravalvular pulmonary stenosis

   d. Williams syndrome

Case 14 (Questions 30 to 32)

A 30-year-old man with a history of congenital heart disease is referred to you because of symptoms of dysphagia and an abnormal CXR. As a child he was told that his CXR was abnormal because of an "aortic anomaly" and that it was benign.

Physical Examination

   Vital signs are normal.

   Cardiac examination is notable for normal intensity S_1 and S_2 heart sounds. An ejection click is heard in the right upper sternal border (RUSB) though no murmur is audible. Upper and lower extremity pulses are equal.

30. The CXR (Fig. 6.9) shows what abnormality?

   a. Bovine aortic arch

   b. Cervical aortic arch

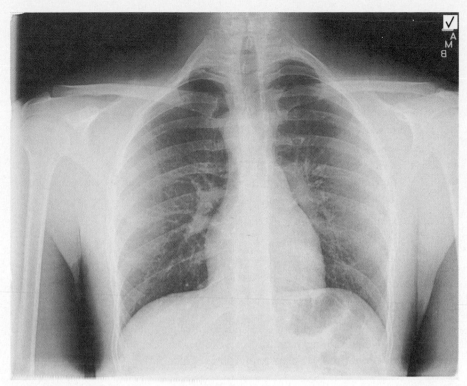

Figure 6.9

    c. Right-sided aortic arch

    d. Aberrant right subclavian artery

31. What is the most common congenital defect associated with the aortic anomaly seen in Question 30?

    a. Tetralogy of Fallot

    b. Truncus arteriosus

    c. Atrial septal defect

    d. Transposition of the great vessels

32. The patient's dysphagia is likely caused by what abnormality associated with his aortic anomaly?

    a. Aberrant left subclavian artery and diverticulum of Kommerell

    b. Coarctation of the aorta

    c. Isolated aberrant right subclavian artery

    d. Interrupted aortic arch

Case 15 (Questions 33 and 34)

A 30-year-old man presents for follow-up after undergoing a surgical coarctation repair at age 9. He has no records and is uncertain of the type of repair. He has not had any testing done in the past 10 years. He has used antibiotic prophylaxis for dental procedures. He takes no other medications. He feels well, is active, and has no complaints.

Physical Examination

    BP—138/72 mmHg (right arm); 126/70 mmHg (left arm); pulse—80 bpm, regular.

    Heart sounds are of normal intensity. An aortic ejection click is present in the RUSB. There is a brief, short duration systolic ejection murmur in the RUSB without a diastolic murmur. Upper and lower extremity pulses are equal and there is no radial or brachial to femoral delay.

33. Which test would be least appropriate for this patient?

    a. TTE

    b. CTA of the chest/aorta

    c. Exercise treadmill stress test

    d. 24-Hour Holter monitoring

34. How often should the coarctation repair site be evaluated by chest imaging in this patient (CTA or MRA)?

    a. Generally every 5 years

    b. Generally every 10 years

    c. Generally every 2 years

    d. Not recommended unless there is specific concern

Case 16 (Questions 35 and 36)

A 38-year-old man is referred for a cardiac surgical evaluation for bicuspid aortic regurgitation. He has a long-standing aortic valve disorder for 10 years. He is fully active with no limitations. He plays tennis on a regular basis.

Physical Examination

BP—120/40 mmHg; pulse—68 bpm. Cardiac examination is notable for a reduced intensity S_1 and increased intensity S_2/A_2. Three murmurs are present, a mid-peaking crescendo/decrescendo systolic ejection murmur beginning after an ejection click, a long-duration high-pitched diastolic decrescendo murmur along the left sternal border and a low-pitched mid-diastolic rumble heard at the apex.

Stress echocardiography is performed and shows a bicuspid aortic valve with right–left fusion. There is calcification of the raphe between the conjoined leaflets. Peak/mean gradients = 30/15 mmHg. Holodiastolic flow reversal is present in the descending aorta. The aortic root measures 4.0 cm and the mid-ascending aorta is 3.9 cm with no sinotubular junction effacement. LV cavity measurements are as follows: LVIDd—5.8 cm; LVIDs—3.9 cm; LVEF—58%. There is reduction in LV cavity size with 13 metabolic equivalents of exercise and no symptoms.

35. What is the most appropriate surgical recommendation?

    a. Elective aortic valve surgery and ascending aortic grafting

    b. Elective aortic valve surgery without ascending aortic grafting

    c. Medical therapy/observation and add a β-blocker

    d. Observation only

Six months later the patient has developed dyspnea with moderate exertion and a significant reduction in exercise tolerance. Repeat echocardiogram shows similar LV cavity dimensions and LVEF calculated at 57%. Aortic root dimension is 4.0 cm and the mid-ascending aorta is 4.6 cm.

36. What is the appropriate recommendation at this time?

    a. Aortic valve replacement

    b. Aortic valve repair

    c. Aortic valve replacement and aortic graft

    d. Stress echocardiogram to confirm change in exercise tolerance

Case 17 (Questions 37 to 40)

A 66-year-old man is seen by his internist for an annual evaluation. Past medical history is notable for HTN and tobacco use. His BP is 136/80 mmHg on monotherapy. Cardiac and abdominal examinations are unremarkable.

He has a friend who was detected to have an AAA on routine screening and asks his physician whether it is indicated for him to be screened.

37. Which of the following statements regarding AAA screening is correct?

   a. Consensus guidelines recommend routine screening of all women >60 years of age or older

   b. Screening men >65 years old is associated with a reduction in aneurysm-related deaths compared with unscreened males of similar ages

   c. Sensitivity and specificity of ultrasound screening in appropriate patients in accredited laboratories are >70%, respectively

   d. After a negative screening examination in a man aged 65 years or older, a repeat examination should be performed 5 years later

A screening abdominal ultrasound is performed in this patient and shows an infrarenal AAA of 5.5 cm. The patient is advised to undergo repair though wishes to consider the option of an endovascular stent graft (EVAR) rather than an open repair.

38. Which of the following statements is true regarding recommendations for AAA repair?

   a. Repair is indicated for any AAA > 5.0 cm

   b. Size cutoffs for AAA repair should be based on age, weight, and height

   c. Inflammatory or infectious aneurysms should be repaired at any size

   d. Women should undergo repair only for AAA > 5.5 cm

39. Which statement regarding EVAR is correct?

   a. Open repair and EVAR are associated with similar 30-day mortality

   b. Open repair and EVAR are associated with similar long-term mortality

   c. EVAR is associated with decreased late complications compared with open repair

   d. EVAR is associated with less repeat interventions compared with open repair

40. Which of the following statements regarding endoleaks is correct?

   a. They occur with a similar prevalence with EVAR and open procedures

   b. Endoleaks may occur as a result of retrograde flow of small arterial branches back into the aneurysm sac

   c. They are rare and generally do not lead to repeat procedures

   d. Type IV endoleaks (leakage through graft material) are the most common

Case 18 (Questions 41 and 42)

A 38-year-old woman is admitted to the internal medicine service for chest pain. She is experiencing sharp chest pain unrelated to exertion and dyspnea for 2 days. Her family history is unknown since she was adopted. Past medical history is not well defined but notable for an uncharacterized connective tissue disorder. She was told at a younger age to avoid pregnancy.

Admission ECG and cardiac enzymes are negative. She is unable to exercise because of her symptoms and therefore is sent for an adenosine nuclear stress test. The test shows mild anteroseptal ischemia with no ECG changes.

The cardiology service is consulted for a cardiac catheterization.

Physical Examination

She is thin and in mild distress. Vital signs are normal. General examination and skin examination are notable for a translucent appearance to the skin, joint hypermobility, hyperextensible skin, and bruises. There are no findings suggestive of Marfan syndrome. Cardiac examination reveals a normal S_1 and S_2 and a soft diastolic decrescendo murmur at the right sternal border.

41. What do you recommend?

    a. Coronary angiography

    b. No further testing

    c. Cardiac MRI to assess for coronary anomalies

    d. CTA of the chest and aorta

42. What should be done to more definitively characterize the patient's condition?

    a. Diagnosis based on clinical criteria

    b. DNA sequencing

    c. Blood analysis for chromosomal abnormalities

    d. Clinical laboratory markers of inflammation

Case 19 (Questions 43 to 45)

A 24-year-old man is referred to cardiology clinic for consultation regarding an aortic aneurysm. He has a family history of ascending aortic aneurysms. Echocardiography showed a trileaflet aortic valve and mid-ascending aortic aneurysm of 4.4 cm that is confirmed by CTA.

Physical Examination

    BP—120/64 mmHg; pulse—70 bpm. Head and neck examination is notable for widely set eyes. The oropharynx is shown (Fig. 6.10). Cardiac and skin examinations are normal.

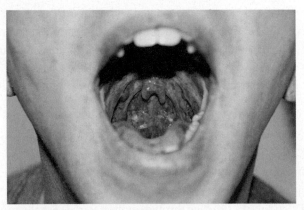

Figure 6.10

43. What is the patient's diagnosis?

    a. Cogan syndrome

    b. Loeys-Dietz syndrome

    c. Ormond disease

    d. Behçet disease

44. What is the gene defect associated with this condition?

    a. COL3A1

    b. TGFBR1 or TGFBR2

    c. ACTA2

    d. FBN1

45. What further recommendation is correct regarding management of this patient?

    a. Start a β-blocker

    b. Start an ARB

    c. Recommend aortic repair

    d. Observation only

Case 20 (Question 46)

A 40-year-old man is transferred via air ambulance to a level 1 trauma center after a motor vehicle accident (MVA). He had a head-to-head collision with another car traveling at a high speed and was propelled forward but was partially restrained by his seat belt and deployed air bags.

Physical Examination

BP—162/62 mmHg (right arm); HR—110 bpm. General condition notable for intubated, sedated man with a cervical collar. Cardiac examination is notable for normal heart sounds and a soft systolic murmur. Lower extremities are mottled and pulseless.

ECG shows sinus tachycardia with no ST changes.

CXR shows no broken ribs bilaterally, a widened mediastinum, and left pleural effusion.

46. Which of the following diagnoses are most likely for this patient?

    a. Complete aortic transection

    b. Ascending aortic dissection and cardiac tamponade

    c. Descending aortic partial transection with pseudoaneurysm

    d. Descending aortic intramural hematoma/dissection

Case 20 (Questions 47 and 48)

A 79-year-old man with HTN underwent a routine CXR and is found to have a thoracic aneurysm. He is asymptomatic with well-controlled BP on a β-blocker. A CT angiogram of the chest is performed showing a descending thoracic aortic aneurysm of 5.4 cm distal to the left subclavian artery with a chronic dissection. The aneurysmal segment does not extend into the abdomen. The ascending aorta is 4.5 cm in the mid-portion and 4.0 cm in the mid-arch. The patient has no other comorbid conditions.

47. What recommendation is most appropriate for this patient based on current guidelines?

    a. Open repair is recommended

    b. TEVAR (thoracic endovascular aortic repair) is recommended

    c. Medical therapy is recommended

    d. An elephant trunk procedure is recommended

48. Which statement is correct comparing TEVAR with open repair for thoracic aortic aneurysms?

    a. TEVAR is associated with higher rates of hospital mortality

    b. TEVAR is associated with higher risks of paraplegia

    c. TEVAR is associated with a 30-day risk of endoleaks of 10%

    d. TEVAR is associated with lower long-term mortality in randomized trials

Case 21 (Questions 49 and 50)

A 45-year-old woman with a history of fibromuscular dysplasia presents to the ER with an acute ST-elevation inferior MI. She is taken immediately to the cardiac catheterization laboratory for primary percutaneous intervention of the right coronary artery (RCA). The first injection of the RCA shows a dissection extending from the ostium to the posterior descending artery. A subsequent aortogram after stenting of the RCA is performed (Fig. 6.11).

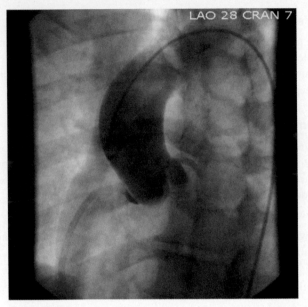

Figure 6.11

49. What does the aortogram show?

   a. Aortic root aneurysm

   b. Aortic root pseudoaneurysm

   c. Anomalous RCA from the left cusp

   d. Aortic root localized dissection

50. What further evaluation or management do you recommend for this patient?

   a. Observation and medical therapy

   b. Open heart surgery

   c. Intravascular ultrasound of the RCA

   d. TEE

ANSWERS

1. **d.** Aortic dilatation with moderate aortic regurgitation and mild aortic stenosis. A bicuspid aortic valve is not likely in a 78-year-old with an initial presentation of aortic valve disease. An aortic ejection click is often present in patients with bicuspid aortic valve disease when the valve is still pliable and is not heard in this patient. Furthermore, the examination is not consistent with severe aortic regurgitation because the diastolic BP is normal (not reduced), the S_1 sound is normal in intensity (not reduced as a result of premature closure of the mitral valve), and the carotid pulsations are normal (not bisferiens). The examination is not consistent with severe aortic stenosis because the murmur is early peaking and S_2 (A_2) is audible and not reduced in intensity. The intensity of a systolic ejection murmur is related in part to the stroke volume and not a good single indicator of severity of stenosis. Therefore, the most likely explanation for the heart murmur is aortic dilatation with nonsevere aortic regurgitation and stenosis. Of note, aortic regurgitant murmurs originating from aortic abnormalities are generally heard best along the right sternal border and those originating from valvular disease heard best along the left sternal border.

2. **b.** Magnetic resonance angiography (MRA) of the great vessels. The presence of a pericardial effusion and an elevated erythrocyte sedimentation rate in a patient with aortic dilatation suggests an inflammatory etiology. Etiologies of aortic aneurysms are listed in Table 6.1. Inflammatory aortitis includes systemic diseases and primary large-vessel vasculitis. Numerous systemic diseases may involve the aorta, including systemic lupus erythematosus, rheumatoid and psoriatic arthritis, inflammatory bowel disease, ankylosing spondylitis, systemic sclerosis, relapsing polychondritis, Behçet syndrome, and Reiter syndrome. Primary vascular disorders include Takayasu and giant cell arteritis. MRA of the aorta may distinguish characteristic thickening and tissue edema that are diagnostic of aortitis.

3. **d.** Giant cell arteritis. The presence of systemic symptoms including headaches and myalgias with an elevated sedimentation rate in an elderly woman is suggestive of temporal arteritis. Temporal arteritis affects women twice as often as it does men and is most commonly seen after age 55 years. Temporal artery tenderness may be present with the potential for blindness to occur. Biopsy of the temporal arteries is diagnostic. Associated giant cell arteritis with involvement of the

TABLE 6-1	Etiologies of Aortic Aneurysms

- Degenerative (HTN, arteriosclerosis, age related)
- Systemic connective tissue disorders
- Trauma (deceleration injury, dissection)
- Infectious diseases (syphilitic, mycotic)
- Primary vasculitis (Takayasu and giant cell aortitis, postoperative aortitis)
- Genetic (Marfan syndrome, Loeys-Dietz syndrome, Ehlers-Danlos type IV, familial thoracic aneurysm and dissection syndrome/FTAAD, Turner and Noonan syndrome)
- Congenital (unicuspid, bicuspid aortic valve, coarctation)
- Miscellaneous conditions (pregnancy, polycystic kidney disease, idiopathic, cocaine, steroids)

HTN, hypertension; FTAAD, familial thoracic aortic aneurysm disease.

aorta and branch vessels with aneurysm formation may occur. Diagnostic criteria are sensitive and specific for giant cell arteritis if at least three of the following findings are present: (a) >50 years of age, (b) recent onset of localized headaches, (c) temporal artery tenderness or pulse attenuation, (d) erythrocyte sedimentation rate >50 mm/h, and (e) arterial biopsy showing necrotizing vasculitis.

The MRA of this patient shows features of vessel thickening of the ascending aorta and arch with "edema"-weighted characteristics and mural enhancement suggestive of an inflammatory aortitis and consistent with giant cell aortitis. Corticosteroids therapy can be used to reduce inflammation seen with aortitis with guidance from serial MRA imaging. Cardiac MRI. Sagittal delayed enhancement (phase-sensitive inversion recovery) image (**A**) and axial black-blood (double IR) (**B**) images demonstrating diffuse mural enhancement (**A**) and thickening of the ascending aorta and arch (**B**) consistent with an inflammatory arteritis. This patient has giant cell arteritis of the aorta (see Figure 6.1).

4. **d.** No additional testing. The revised Ghent criteria are based primarily on clinical criteria although genetic testing for the FBN1 mutation can aid in diagnosis. There are criteria for individuals with and without a family history of Marfan syndrome (see Table 6.2). The patient presented has ectopia lentis and a family history of Marfan syndrome. Therefore, no additional information is required to make a diagnosis. She does additionally have systemic criteria that are consistent with the diagnosis, including pectus carinatum, wrist and thumb sign, high-arched palate, and mitral valve prolapse. An increased arm span-to-height ratio is no longer considered a diagnostic criterion for Marfan syndrome.

5. **d.** Elective aortic replacement. The timing of surgery for patients with ascending aortic aneurysms caused by Marfan syndrome is addressed in the 2010 guidelines for thoracic aortic diseases. Surgery is recommended for asymptomatic patients with Marfan syndrome or other genetic etiologies for thoracic ascending aortic aneurysms between 4.0 and 5.0 cm (class I) or when the ratio of the maximal ascending aortic or aortic root area ($\pi \times radius^2$) in cm^2 divided by the patient's height in meters exceeds 10 (class IIa). In this patient, the calculation

TABLE 6-2	Revised 2010 Ghent Criteria for Marfan Syndrome

In the absence of family history or findings consistent with other syndromes—the following criteria are sufficient for the diagnosis of Marfan syndrome:

1. Aortic root dilatation or dissection and ectopia lentis
2. Aortic root dilatation or dissection and FBN1 mutation
3. Aortic root dilatation or dissection and systemic score ≥7 points
4. Ectopia lentis and FBN1 mutation

In the presence of family history—any of the following criteria are sufficient for the diagnosis of Marfan syndrome:

1. Ectopia lentis
2. Systemic score ≥7 points
3. Aortic root dilatation

Systemic score:

3 points = wrist and thumb sign

2 points = pectus carinatum deformity, hindfoot deformity, spontaneous pneumothorax, dural ectasia, protucio acetabulae

1 point = wrist or thumb sign, pectus excavatum or chest asymmetry, plain flat foot, scoliosis or thoracolumbar kyphosis, reduced elbow extension, three of five facial features, skin striae, severe myopia, mitral valve prolapse

TABLE 6-3   Timing of Surgery for Thoracic Aortic Aneurysms

Aortic Root or Ascending Aorta	Size
Degenerative etiology	≥5.5 cm or >0.5 cm growth/yr
Chronic aortic dissection	≥5.5 cm
Genetic etiology[a]	4.0–5.0 cm, >10:1 ratio[b] or >0.5 cm growth/yr
Bicuspid aortic valve	4.0–5.0 cm, >10:1 ratio[b] or >0.5 cm growth/yr
	>5.5 cm[c]
	>5.0 cm[c] (and ≥ 0.5 cm growth/yr or FH dissection
Loeys-Dietz syndrome	≥4.4 cm
Marfan syndrome (anticipating pregnancy)	>4.0 cm
Aortic valve repair or replacement (bicuspid valve or genetic etiology)	>4.5 cm
Aortic Arch	
Low risk	>5.5 cm
Descending Aorta	
Low risk	>5.5 cm
High risk (limited endovascular options)	>6.0 cm
Abdominal Aorta	
All patients	>5.5 cm
Women and smaller men	>5.0 cm

[a]See Table 6.1 for genetic etiologies.
[b]Ratio of maximal aortic root or ascending aortic area (πr^2) in cm² divided by the patient's height in meters.
[c]2014 American Heart Association/American College of Cardiology Guideline for the Management of Patients with Valvular Heart Disease
FH = family history

would be as follows: ($\pi \times 2.5^2 = 3.14 \times 6.25 = 19.6$ cm²/1.70 m = 11.5), well above the 10:1 ratio. For women anticipating pregnancy, elective surgery should be performed when the ascending aortic dimension is >4.0 cm. Additional factors of importance include rate of change of aortic size >0.5 cm/year, presence and severity of aortic regurgitation, family history of dissection or sudden cardiac death, and the extent of aortic involvement. See Table 6.3 for timing of surgery in aortic diseases. An open-label study of adult patients with aortic dilatation and Marfan syndrome who were randomized to propranolol or no treatment showed less aortic dilatation and aortic complications among patients on propranolol. Therefore, β-blockers should be advised for this patient although this is not the most important recommendation.

6.   c. Reduction in activity of transforming growth factor (TGF)-β. The ARB losartan has been associated with a reduction in the rate of aortic dilatation and aneurysm growth in both experimental mouse studies and recently an open-label randomized trial of Marfan syndrome patients (COMPARE trial). A larger prospective randomized trial comparing atenolol versus losartan sponsored by the NIH is in progress. The postulated mechanism of action is independent of BP lowering. Because of defective production in fibrillin due to the FBN1 mutation, there is overexpression of TGF-β activity. TGF-β activity leads to an increase in destructive MMPs, which cause aortic wall weakening. Losartan appears to block the overproduction of TGF-β and MMPs so that aortic wall integrity is maintained.

7.   c. TTE. A TTE should be performed immediately in this patient since the clinical findings are highly suggestive of a proximal ascending aortic dissection (character of chest pain, differential BPs, and weak pulses) and cardiac tamponade (tachycardia, elevated jugular venous pressure, soft heart sounds, and globular-shaped heart on CXR with interstitial edema). Cardiac enzymes may determine the presence of myocardial injury but not reveal the cause. An acute inferior MI is likely due to the aortic dissection involving the origin of the RCA and not due to occlusive coronary artery disease.

The advantages and disadvantages of CTA, MRA, and TEE for the diagnosis of aortic dissection have been reviewed in detail. Each of these tests has high diagnostic accuracy for diagnosing aortic dissection. The test of choice for a given patient should be determined based on the relative expertise of each institution, the rapid availability of the test and its interpretation, and the specific individual circumstances of a patient. Given the likelihood of an aortic dissection and the possibility of cardiac tamponade in this patient, a TTE or a TEE is best suited for this patient. A limited TTE could assess whether a pericardial effusion and cardiac tamponade are present followed by either a TEE or CTA of the aorta to confirm and determine the location and extent of dissection.

8.   b. Emergent aortic surgery. A proximal aortic dissection with hypotension or cardiac tamponade should be treated by emergent aortic surgery. A rapid confirmatory test can be performed on the way to or in the operating room. Small retrospective reviews have raised concerns regarding pericardiocentesis in patients with cardiac tamponade and aortic dissection. Rapid decompensation and death can occur in some patients due to propagation of dissection and increased bleeding into the pericardium. Most importantly, the presence of cardiac tamponade with aortic dissection should mandate immediate surgery. Pericardiocentesis can be performed if the patient is deteriorating rapidly and surgical assistance is not readily available or if the patient is in pulseless electrical activity.

Controversy also exists regarding cardiac catheterization for patients with proximal aortic dissection. Proponents of cardiac catheterization argue that patients with severe obstructive coronary disease require grafting at the time of surgery and that failure to do so will increase the risk of perioperative and postoperative cardiac events. Those who favor not performing cardiac catheterization argue that any delay may increase the risk of death and that an invasive procedure will add further risk of dissection, tamponade, or rupture. One study comparing outcomes of patients undergoing surgery for aortic dissection found that those not undergoing cardiac catheterization had similar mortality than those undergoing the procedure. The 2010 guidelines for thoracic aortic diseases recommend that coronary angiography should be considered if the patient is over 40 years of age, stable, and has either known CAD, significant risk factors for CAD, or an ischemic presentation. Computed tomographic angiography of the chest. Sagittal oblique reconstruction shows an ascending aortic and aortic arch aneurysm with a dual lumen consistent with a type A aortic dissection (see Figure 6.2).

9.   c. Cerebral aneurysm rupture. The history of HTN requiring treatment in a young man with a bicuspid aortic valve suggests the likelihood of an aortic coarctation. Given his recent well-controlled BP, aortic dissection, hypertensive crisis, and endocarditis are unlikely. A known association between aortic coarctation and cerebral aneurysms involving the circle of Willis is well established. Testing for this abnormality with MRA or CTA of the brain should be performed for coarctation patients when any neurologic symptoms are present. However, at least a 1 time scan of the brain for intracranial aneurysms is recommended for all patients with coarctation accordingly to the 2008 guidelines for management of congenital heart disease.

10. **b.** Ventricular septal defect. Several cardiac structural lesions are associated with coarctation of the aorta. The most common is a bicuspid aortic valve occurring in up to 85% of patients. Valvular, subvalvular, or supravalvular stenosis may occur. Aortic ectasia or aneurysm involving the ascending thoracic aorta and arch is often present. Other associated structural abnormalities include patent ductus arteriosus, perimembranous ventricular septal defect, and mitral stenosis (parachute mitral valve) as part of the Shone complex of left heart obstructive lesions.

11. **c.** CTA of the chest and abdomen. The patient's history is most suggestive of a thoracic aortic aneurysm or AAA or dissection. He is known to have thoracic aortic dilatation and atherosclerosis, and presents hypertensive with back pain and diminished pulses. Although TEE may be accurate for diagnosis of aortic dissection above the diaphragm, a CT scan may extend imaging to the entire aorta including the abdominal aorta and provide information regarding the involvement of branch vessels. Therefore, CT imaging would be preferable. Aortography is invasive and could cause further injury to the aorta. However, it could provide useful information along with angiography regarding the patency of the patient's bypass grafts and native circulation.

12. **b.** MRA of the chest/aorta. The patient is experiencing ongoing pain refractory to medical therapy and the clinical history remains suggestive of an acute aortic syndrome. The types of acute aortic syndromes are listed in Table 6.4. Although CT imaging is highly accurate in diagnosing aortic dissection, there are false-negative readings. In the International Registry of Aortic Dissection (IRAD) registry, many patients with suspected aortic dissection required more than one imaging test. Therefore, additional imaging should be performed in this patient especially since an alternative diagnosis for the patient's symptoms is not available. An acute coronary syndrome is not likely in view of recent CABG and unremarkable ECG and cardiac enzymes. Biomarkers are emerging as a diagnostic aide in diagnosing acute aortic syndromes. A D-dimer level <500 ng/mL and a low C-reactive protein make aortic dissection unlikely.

13. **a.** Initiate a β-blocker and repeat ultrasound in 6 months. To determine the stability of an AAA between 4.0 and 4.9 cm (4.2 cm in this patient), it is generally recommended to do an initial follow-up ultrasound in 6 months. However, most patients with AAA size = 4.5 cm should be referred to a vascular surgeon for subsequent follow-up and risk assessment for surgical consideration and have a

TABLE 6-4	Types of Aortic Syndromes

- Classic dissection (intimal tear with double lumen)
- Intramural hematoma (no intimal tear)
- Limited dissection (rare without hematoma, most often in Marfan syndrome)
- Penetrating aortic ulcer (associated localized hematoma or saccular aneurysm)
- Iatrogenic (catheter or trauma related)
- Symptomatic aneurysm

baseline CT of the aorta to assess for anatomic feasibility for endovascular repair. β-Blockers have been shown to delay the rate of AAA enlargement and would be indicated for this patient with suboptimal control of BP.

14. **d.** Penetrating aortic ulcer. A penetrating aortic ulcer occurs when aortic atheroma ruptures into the aortic media through the internal elastic lamina. Subsequently, an aneurysm, pseudoaneurysm, localized dissection, hematoma, or aortic rupture may develop. Penetrating ulcers can be diagnosed by aortography, CTA, MRA, or TEE. They more typically occur in the descending aorta. Typical findings include a focal outpouching or ulcer crater in the region of severe, calcified atheroma. Localized flow may be seen by contrast opacification or color Doppler. The aortogram in this patient shows multiple penetrating aortic ulcers, seen as outpouching on the greater curvature of the ascending aortic wall. Contrast aortogram (**A**) shows several outpouchings on the greater curvature of the ascending aorta consistent with penetrating ulcers. Transesophageal echocardiogram (**B**) showing a break in the lesser curvature of the aorta in the same patient in the region of diffuse calcific atheroma also consistent with a penetrating aortic ulcer (see Figure 6.3).

15. **b.** Transfer to the operating room immediately for replacement of the ascending aorta. The patient has an acute aortic syndrome with a symptomatic penetrating ulcer in the ascending aorta. Immediate surgery is indicated to prevent the possibility of aortic rupture. Further confirmatory imaging is not required.

16. **d.** Angiography. The patient presents with pulse deficits, bruits, and symptoms consistent with arterial insufficiency in multiple distributions, including the upper and lower extremities. Angiography (either CTA/MRA or invasive) of the arterial system would define the site and extent of arterial disease. The appearance of the lesions may also help with determining the etiology of the vascular disease (i.e., atherosclerotic versus vasculitic).

17. **d.** Takayasu arteritis. Takayasu arteritis ("pulseless disease") is an inflammatory disease of large sized arteries. Both stenotic lesions and aneurysms may be present with involvement of proximal segments of the aortic arch vessels. Aortic regurgitation is not uncommon due to involvement of the aortic root and aortic valve with inflammatory disease. Although most commonly described in Japanese patients, it has been described throughout the world.

    A diagnostic classification proposed by the American College of Rheumatology requires three of six criteria: (a) age at onset younger than 40 years, (b) intermittent claudication, (c) diminished brachial artery pulse, (d) >10 mmHg difference in systolic BP between arms, (e) bruit of the subclavian arteries or the aorta, or (f) angiographic narrowing or occlusion of the aorta or branches.

18. **d.** Presence of systolic and diastolic flow is consistent with severe coarctation. The peak Doppler pressure gradient as obtained from the simplified Bernoulli often overestimates the gradient obtained across the coarctation as measured by invasive hemodynamics. Since the pre-coarctation velocity is often increased due to abnormality of aortic valve, it must be accounted for in the Bernoulli equation. This requires using the modified Bernoulli equation, where pressure = 4 $(V_2^2 - V_1^2)$, in which V_2 is the peak Doppler velocity across the coarctation and V_1 is the pre-coarctation velocity. The typical sawtooth pattern of aortic coarctation is shown in this example with an elevated systolic velocity and a lower velocity forward flow in diastole. The presence of a continuous flow across the coarctation is consistent with severe obstruction regardless of the peak pressure gradient. Transthoracic suprasternal notch (SSN) view with continuous Doppler in the upper descending aorta. The Doppler profile shows a high-velocity antegrade velocity of 316 cm/s consistent with a 40-mmHg systolic gradient. There is a lower velocity antegrade flow during diastole. These findings are consistent with coarctation of the aorta (see Figure 6.4).

19. c. The hallmark of coarctation is the presence of persistent antegrade flow in diastole. The image is a pulsed Doppler spectral recording from the abdominal aorta consistent with coarctation of the aorta. The findings consistent with coarctation are a blunted or low-velocity systolic flow and persistent antegrade flow in diastole (absent retrograde flow). The presence of early diastolic reversal excludes significant coarctation. Other findings consistent with coarctation include a low systolic-to-diastolic velocity ratio, decreased pulsatility, and a prolonged pulse delay. Transthoracic subcostal view with pulsed Doppler in the abdominal aorta. A blunted or low-velocity systolic flow and persistent antegrade flow in diastole (absent retrograde flow) are specific features consistent with coarctation of the aorta (see Figure 6.5).

20. c. Balloon angioplasty with or without stents is generally recommended. The patient has severe recoarctation of the aorta after surgical repair. The choice of intervention for coarctation remains controversial and should be made in a center experienced with congenital heart disease among a team of surgical and interventional specialists. However, for recurrent coarctation after surgical repair, catheter intervention with or without stents is generally preferred if the anatomy is suitable. Favorable anatomy is a discrete, nontortuous short segment of narrowing without aneurysms, pseudoaneurysm, or hypoplasia of the aorta. Additional consideration should be given to women considering pregnancy where there is concern regarding the tissue fragility and risk of aortic complications with residual coarctation tissue. In that setting, surgery may be considered. Cardiac MR angiography. Sagittal oblique maximum intensity projection showing a discrete, short region of coarctation in the upper descending aorta without associated dilatation of the adjacent segments (see Figure 6.6).

21. c. Asymptomatic patient with a peak-to-peak gradient across the coarctation site of 15 mmHg with extensive collaterals. According to the American College of Cardiology (ACC)/American Heart Association (AHA) 2008 guidelines for adults with congenital heart disease intervention for coarctation of the aorta is recommended if (a) peak-to-peak gradient across the coarctation is ≥20 mmHg or (b) peak-to-peak gradient across the coarctation is <20 mmHg but there is anatomic evidence of severe obstruction and radiologic evidence of collateral flow. For the patient undergoing aortic valve replacement for bicuspid severe aortic regurgitation, the coarctation of the aorta should be reassessed after surgery to determine whether it is clinically significant.

22. c. Osteogenesis imperfecta. The patient has osteogenesis imperfecta, a heritable disease of the connective tissue with mutations in procollagen that are associated with bone fragility (with multiple fractures), ocular changes (most notably blue sclerae), abnormal dentition, and hearing loss. Cardiovascular manifestations may occur and are similar to Marfan syndrome with aortic root dilatation, aortic regurgitation, and mitral valve prolapse.

23. b. Intravenous diltiazem. The initial management of aortic dissection is aimed at reduction in heart rate, BP, LV wall stress, and the force of LV contraction (d_p/d_t). The goals are a heart rate less than 60 bpm and BP less than 120 mmHg systolic. β-Blockers are the drug of choice if contraindications are not present. The patient described has severe COPD and therefore if a β-blocker is used it should be short-acting esmolol and not metoprolol. Otherwise, nondihydropyridine calcium-channel blocking agents such as diltiazem and verapamil are alternative options. Vasodilator therapy such as intravenous nitroprusside is contraindicated when initiated prior to atrioventricular blockade because of associated increase in reflex tachycardia, aortic wall stress, and LV force of contraction.

24. d. It is circumferential or crescentic. The CT demonstrates an intramural hematoma involving the descending aorta. The mechanism for intramural hematomas is thought due to rupture of the vasa vasorum in the media or small intimal tears. Typical features as seen by CT include the following: (a) absence of an intimal flap; (b) circumferential, focal, or crescentic appearance; (c) displacement of intimal calcium; and (d) high-attenuation thickening consistent with hematoma. Additional features that are seen by TEE include echolucent regions with flow consistent with intramural blood vessels.

Of note, the 2010 guidelines for thoracic aortic diseases state that intramural hematoma should be treated similar to aortic dissection in the corresponding segment of the aorta. Computed tomographic angiography axial image showing a descending thoracic aortic intramural hematoma. The intramural hematoma is evident given the circumferential appearance of high attenuation density of the aortic wall (see Figure 6.7).

25. d. TEE. A cardioembolic source of stroke is most likely given the territory of a middle cerebral artery event. The patient has a cholesterol level >300 suggestive of a heritable dyslipidemia and premature atherosclerosis and therefore aortic atheroma would be the most likely finding. A patent foramen ovale may be an alternative source of emboli in this young patient and would be the most likely etiology if the patient did not have a lipid disorder. Intracranial small-vessel disease detected by MRA would be less likely despite a dyslipidemic disorder. There is no information to suggest atrial fibrillation and therefore an event recorder would not likely be revealing.

26. a. Statin and aspirin. The TEE shows a large protruding sessile atheroma in the distal descending aorta/distal aortic arch. Treatment for aortic atheroma remains controversial. Antiplatelet therapies such as aspirin and statins are the mainstay of treatment. Systemic anticoagulation with warfarin or warfarin alternatives is unproven due to limited data. However, several observational reports particularly for aortic arch atheroma demonstrate resolution or reduction of large mobile thrombus/atheroma and embolic events in patients on warfarin. Transesophageal echocardiogram with a short-axis view of the upper descending aorta. A large sessile protruding atheromatous plaque is seen (see Figure 6.8).

27. a. 3-mm plaque with severe calcification and no mobile components. Predictors of embolic events in patients with aortic atheroma include (a) plaque thickness >4 mm, (b) mobile components, (c) ulceration, and (d) lack of calcification. Therefore, a smaller atheroma without mobile debris and with calcification is the least likely to be associated with an embolic event.

28. b. Alternative sites for cross-clamping or cannulation may reduce stroke risk. Alternative sites for cross-clamping and cannulation such as femoral and axillary arteries may reduce the risk of stroke in a patient with significant ascending aortic atheroma. Aortic arch endarterectomy has been found to increase the risk of perioperative stroke and is seldom recommended. Replacement of the ascending aorta is not generally recommended as a prophylactic measure to reduce the risk of stroke in patients with severe atheroma of the ascending aorta because of the additive surgical morbidity and mortality. Palpation of the aorta by the surgeon is usually not accurate in finding noncalcified atheroma that may be detected by TEE.

29. d. Williams syndrome. The physical examination findings are classic for supravalvular aortic stenosis, with a left-sided systolic ejection murmur (increase with expiration) heard best in the first right intercostal space, an increased intensity S_2/A_2 heart sound, increase in right-sided BP and pulses relative to the left side, and thrill in the suprasternal notch. Differential BP and pulses in the upper extremities is due to the Coanda effect with preferential deflection of blood flow toward the right brachiocephalic artery. Patent ductus arteriosus and severe coarctation of the aorta typically have continuous murmurs and would not typically have arm pulse differences. Supravalvular pulmonary stenosis would also not have pulse differences and the ejection murmur would decrease with expiration. Supravalvular aortic stenosis typically occurs in association with the Williams syndrome and associated mental retardation, and hypercalcemia. Supravalvular aortic stenosis is a form of aortopathy where obstruction occurs above the aortic sinuses usually at the sinotubular junction and is due to mutation in the elastin gene. The obstructive aortopathy is due either to a fibrous diaphragm, hour-glass deformity, or diffuse hypoplasia of the aorta.

30. **c.** Right-sided aortic arch. The CXR (Fig. 6.9) shows a right-sided aortic arch with the aortic knob on the right side and absence of a left-sided aortic knob. A bovine aortic arch is an anatomic variant where the origin of the innominate artery and the left carotid artery arises from a common origin or the left carotid artery arises from the innominate artery. This variant occurs in approximately 13% of individuals and has no clinical significance. A cervical arch refers to the takeoff of the aortic branch vessels above the sternum into the soft tissues of the neck before turning downward to the descending aorta. It may present as a pulsatile mass in the neck or supraclavicular region and be associated with compressive symptoms and other vascular anomalies.

31. **a.** Tetralogy of Fallot. A right-sided aortic arch is most commonly associated with tetralogy of Fallot, particularly for the mirror image form. There are several types of right-sided aortic arch, but the mirror image and the non-mirror image variety are the most common. With the non-mirror image type, the order of branches from left to right are as follows: left carotid, right carotid, right subclavian, and left subclavian artery. The left (aberrant) subclavian artery arises from the descending aorta. The mirror image type is much more frequently associated with congenital anomalies than the non-mirror image type. Chest X-ray PA projection shows tracheal deviation to the left and round opacity on the right with absence of a distinct aortic knob on the left. This is most consistent with a right-sided arch (see Figure 6.9).

32. **a.** Aberrant left subclavian artery and diverticulum of Kommerell. Aortic arch anomalies may result in dysphagia, stridor, or wheezing associated with vascular rings that compress the esophagus or trachea. With the non-mirror image right aortic arch, the left subclavian artery arises from the right side and crosses posterior to the esophagus and trachea. This causes a vascular ring that may cause compressive symptoms. Aberrant vessels such as the left subclavian artery may arise from an aneurysmal segment called a diverticulum of Kommerell. An aberrant right subclavian artery may be an isolated anomaly in a normal left-sided aortic arch and is the most common aortic arch abnormality. Although generally asymptomatic, it may also be associated with a vascular ring.

33. **d.** 24-Hour Holter monitoring. CTA or MRA of the aorta is required to assess postoperative complications of prior coarctation repair. Complications include recoarctation and aneurysms in the ascending aorta, aortic arch, or descending aorta in the region of the repair. In adults, a TTE does not adequately visualize the descending thoracic aorta, although gradients can be obtained to assess hemodynamic significance. Exercise-induced HTN may occur late after coarctation repair even among patients who are normotensive at rest and should be assessed for by exercise stress testing. TTE is important to assess the aortic valve and the possibility of a bicuspid valve, as well as associated structural abnormalities. Arrhythmias are an infrequent consequence of a corrected coarctation in an asymptomatic patient and therefore Holter monitoring is not necessary.

34. **a.** Generally every 5 years. The ACC/AHA 2008 guidelines for adults with congenital heart disease recommend at least a one-time CT or MR angiogram for repaired or unrepaired coarctation for complete evaluation of the thoracic aorta.

In addition, follow-up should be performed at intervals of 5 years or less depending on the prior findings.

35. **d.** Observation only. Based on examination and echocardiography, the patient has mixed but predominantly severe congenital bicuspid aortic regurgitation. Holodiastolic flow reversal in the descending aorta is the key confirmatory finding supporting severe aortic regurgitation. The three murmurs described include the systolic murmur of bicuspid aortic stenosis and the diastolic murmurs of aortic regurgitation with the associated Austin Flint murmur. There are no clinical or echocardiographic indications for surgery based on aortic valve or aortic disease. β-blockers for aortic root dimensions >4.0 cm should generally be used only if severe aortic regurgitation is not present because of concern of increasing regurgitant volume and fraction with slower heart rates.

36. **c.** Aortic valve replacement and aortic graft. Surgery is indicated in this patient both for symptomatic aortic regurgitation and because of significant progression in aortic size. ACC/AHA valvular heart disease guidelines for bicuspid aortic valves recommend replacement of the aortic root or ascending aorta if the diameter is greater than 4.5 cm at the time of aortic valve replacement. Aortic valve repair can be performed successfully in select patients with bicuspid aortic regurgitation but is usually not performed when stenosis is present or if there are unfavorable anatomic findings such as calcification. Therefore, aortic valve replacement with either a mechanical or bioprosthetic valve is indicated along with an aortic graft. The aortic graft may incorporate the aortic root or may be in the supracoronary position.

37. **b.** Screening men >65 years old is associated with a reduction in aneurysm-related deaths compared with unscreened men of similar ages. Guidelines to screen for AAA vary among different governing bodies. The United States Preventive Services Task Force (USPSTF) recommends one-time screening for any male former or present smoker between ages 65 and 75 years. They do not recommend screening in women based on the lower expected prevalence of AAA. Other vascular societies have less restrictive screening recommendations for men and women. However, screening in patients with first-degree relatives with AAA is recommended. Randomized controlled trials of ultrasound screening for AAA in predominantly men aged 65 to 75 years show a reduction in aneurysm-related mortality compared with unscreened age-matched controls. Ultrasound screening of at-risk patients in accredited laboratories is associated with sensitivities and specificities of over 90%, respectively. Repeat screening after a negative study is not recommended.

38. **c.** Inflammatory or infectious aneurysms should be repaired at any size. Two large trials of predominantly males showed that early elective AAA repair for aneurysms (4.0 to 5.5 cm) resulted in a similar mortality compared with medical therapy. Therefore, repair is generally indicated for asymptomatic AAA if (a) >5.5 cm; (b) increase in size ≥0.5 cm in 1 year; (c) inflammatory, traumatic, or infectious etiology; or (d) there is a family history of rupture. However, since AAAs may rupture at smaller sizes in women and smaller men, repair should be considered at 5.0 cm or even smaller in low-risk candidates for repair.

39. **b.** Open repair and EVAR are associated with similar long-term mortality. Endovascular repair of AAA is an alternative to open repair. Comparative trials including EVAR and DREAM have demonstrated a lower short-term morbidity and mortality (at 30 days) for EVAR compared with open repair. However, in long-term follow-up mortality was similar for the two procedures. EVAR is associated with more complications including endoleaks and need for repeat interventions and may require conversion to an open procedure.

40. b. Endoleaks may occur as a result of retrograde flow of small arterial branches back into the aneurysm sac. Endoleaks refer to the occurrence of repressurization of the excluded aneurysmal sac after an EVAR procedure. There are four main types: I—proximal or distal stent attachment site bleeding around the graft; II—leaking back into the sac from branch arterial vessels; III—mechanical failure of stent graft components; IV—leakage of blood through the graft material. Type II leaks are most common. Types I and III may require immediate reintervention, whereas type II can be monitored by repeat surveillance but may require repeat intervention if the aneurysm sac continues to expand.

41. d. CTA of the chest and aorta. The patient's history and examination has several features suggestive of Ehlers-Danlos syndrome. Since she has a low pre- and posttest probability of coronary ischemia, a cardiac catheterization is not advisable. The vascular type of Ehlers-Danlos syndrome (type IV) is associated with spontaneous or iatrogenic arterial or organ rupture (e.g., rupture of gravid uterus or intestines). Aortic complications including dissection and rupture can occur and therefore arterial puncture is generally contraindicated. A CTA of the chest and aorta would exclude pathologies found in Ehlers-Danlos syndrome, including aortic and pulmonary aneurysm and dissection.

42. b. DNA sequencing. Diagnosis of Ehlers-Danlos type IV is generally made based on clinical and family history and DNA sequencing for the COL3A1 gene mutations. However, a negative test does not definitively rule out disease since not all causative mutations are known. A punch biopsy of the skin to obtain fibroblasts for culture and detection of defective type III collagen can also be performed.

43. b. Loeys-Dietz syndrome. Loeys-Dietz is an autosomal dominant genetic aortic aneurysm syndrome. It predominantly involves children and young adults with risk of rapid progression to aneurysms, arterial tortuosity, and dissection. It is associated with a bifid uvula (shown in Fig. 6.10), cleft palate, and hypertelorism. Other clinical findings similar to Marfan syndrome may be present. Cogan syndrome is a rare large-vessel vasculitis that involves the aorta and is associated with vestibular and ocular abnormalities including uveitis and keratitis. Ormond disease is an inflammatory form of aortitis associated with retroperitoneal fibrosis. Behçet disease is an instead of a arteritis associated with oral and genital ulcers and skin lesions. Image of the oropharynx of a young boy with Loeys-Dietz syndrome showing a bifid uvula (see Figure 6.10).

44. b. TGFBR1 or TGFBR2. The genetic defect associated with Loeys-Dietz syndrome is a mutation in transforming growth factor β-receptor, TGFBR1 or TGFBR2. Table 6.5 shows the most common gene mutations associated with aortic diseases.

TABLE 6-5	**Most Common Mutations Associated with Aortic Diseases**
Condition	**Mutation**
Marfan syndrome	FBN1
Loeys-Dietz syndrome	TGFBR1/TGFBR2
Ehlers-Danlos syndrome	COL3A1
Familial aortic aneurysms/dissections	ACTA2

45. c. Recommend aortic repair. Because of high risk of aortic dissection in patients with Loeys-Dietz, surgery is recommended at smaller aortic sizes. The 2010 guidelines for thoracic aortic diseases recommend aortic repair based on CTA or MRA for a dimension ≥4.4 cm.

46. c. Descending aortic partial transection with pseudoaneurysm. The patient experienced blunt cardiac trauma with injury to the aorta. This type of deceleration MVA as occurs with a head-to-head car collision may result in catastrophic aortic transection, rupture, or pseudoaneurysm. The typical site of injury occurs at the aortic isthmus (level of the ligamentum arteriosum or junction of the aortic arch and descending thoracic aorta) as a result of fixation of the aorta to the spine by intercostal arteries. The favorable hemodynamics in this patient are not suggestive of either aortic transection or cardiac tamponade. The preserved upper extremity BP and reduced perfusion in the lower extremities are suggestive of partial transection of the descending aorta with a pseudoaneurysm. The pseudoaneurysm is suggested by the widening of the mediastinum on CXR.

47. c. Medical therapy is recommended. Medical therapy should be recommended for this patient. The timing of surgery for descending thoracic aneurysms is addressed by the 2010 guidelines for thoracic aortic diseases. Most descending thoracic aneurysms or chronic dissections (not including thoracoabdominal aneurysms) that are of degenerative, traumatic, or connective tissue etiologies should be repaired when the size is >5.5 cm if comorbidity-related risks are acceptable.

48. c. TEVAR is associated with a 30-day risk of endoleaks of 10%. There are no randomized trials comparing TEVAR with open aortic repair. However, non-randomized comparisons show a lower rate of hospital complications including paraplegia and death relative to open repair. Despite TEVAR patients generally being older with more comorbid conditions, long-term mortality seems similar. The estimated rate of type I endoleaks with TEVAR is approximately 10% due to difficulties achieving an adequate proximal anastomosis.

49. d. Aortic root localized dissection. Localized staining of contrast dye is seen in the region of the right sinus of Valsalva. This finding is consistent with an iatrogenic localized dissection. In this patient, it is likely due to either catheter trauma or retrograde propagation of the RCA dissection into the corresponding sinus of Valsalva. Coronary dissection is commonly associated with fibromuscular dysplasia. Contrast aortogram with staining of contrast seen in the right sinus of Valsalva that occurred post MI and following percutaneous coronary stenting in a young woman with fibromuscular dysplasia and RCA dissection. Contrast aortogram with staining of contrast seen in the right sinus of Valsalva that occurred post MI and following percutaneous coronary stenting in a young woman with fibromuscular dysplasia and RCA dissection (see Figure 6.11).

50. a. Observation and medical therapy. Most localized iatrogenic intramural hematomas or dissections occurring in the cardiac catheterization laboratory can be observed and managed medically even when involving the ascending aorta. In general, the site of tear seals and propagation or expansion does not occur. However, repeat aortic imaging should be performed to confirm stability.

SUGGESTED READINGS

Groenink M, den Hartog AW, Frankin R, et al. Losartan reduces aortic dilatation rate in adults with Marfan syndrome: a randomized controlled trial. *Eur Heart J.* 2013;34(45):3491–3500.

Hagan PG, Nienaber CA, Isselbacher EM, et al. The International Registry of Acute Aortic Dissection (IRAD): new insights into an old disease. *JAMA.* 2000;283:897–903.

Hiratzka LF, Bakris GL, Beckman JA, et al. 2010 ACCF/AHA/AATS/ACR/ASA/SCA/SCAI/SIR/STS/SVM guidelines for the diagnosis and management of patients with thoracic aortic disease: executive summary. *Circulation.* 2010;121:1544–1579.

Isselbacher EM, Cigarroa JE, Eagle KA. Cardiac tamponade complicating proximal aortic dissection: is pericardiocentesis harmful? *Circulation.* 1994;90:2375–2378.

Loeys BL, Dietz HC, Braverman AC, et al. The revised Ghent nosology for the Marfan syndrome. *J Med Genet.* 2010;47:476–485.

Loeys BL, Schwarze U, Holm T, et al. Aneurysm syndromes caused by mutations in the TGF-beta receptor. *N Engl J Med.* 2006;355: 788–798.

Maraj R, Rerkpattanapipat P, Jacobs LE, et al. Meta-analysis of 143 reported cases of aortic intramural hematomas. *Am J Cardiol.* 2000;86: 664–668.

Penn MS, Smedira N, Lytle B, et al. Does coronary angiography before emergency aortic surgery affect in-hospital mortality? *J Am Coll Cardiol.* 2000;35:889–894.

Pretre R, Chilcott M. Blunt trauma to the heart and great vessels. *N Engl J Med.* 1997;336:626–632.

Schermerhorn ML, O'Malley AJ, Jhaveri A, et al. Endovascular vs. open repair of abdominal aortic aneurysms in the medicare population. *N Engl J Med.* 2008;358:464–474.

Shores J, Berger KR, Murphy EA, et al. Progression of aortic dilatation and the benefit of long-term beta-adrenergic blockage in Marfan's syndrome. *N Engl J Med.* 1994;330:1335–1341.

Song JK, Kim HS, Kang DH, et al. Different clinical features of aortic intramural hematoma versus dissection involving the ascending aorta. *J Am Coll Cardiol.* 2001;37:1604–1610.

Svennson LG, Labib SB, Eisenhauer AC, et al. Intimal tear without hematoma: an important variant of aortic dissection that can elude current imaging techniques. *Circulation.* 1999;99:1331–1336.

Trimarchi S, Sangiorgi G, Sang X, et al. In search of blood tests for thoracic aortic diseases *Ann Thorac Surg.* 2010;90:1735–1742.

Tunick PA, Kronzon I. Atheromas of the thoracic aorta: clinical and therapeutic update. *J Am Coll Cardiol.* 2000;35:545–554.

Vilacosta I, San Roman JA, Aragoncillo P, et al. Penetrating atherosclerotic aortic ulcer: documentation by transesophageal echocardiography. *J Am Coll Cardiol.* 1998;32:82–89.

Warnes CA, Williams RG, Bashore TM, et al. ACC/AHA 2008 guidelines for the management of adults with congenital heart disease. *Circulation.* 2008;118:2395–2451.

chapter 7

Peripheral Vascular Disease

Douglas E. Joseph • Hemantha K. Koduri

QUESTIONS

1. A 53-year-old man with a history of obesity, obstructive sleep apnea, hypertension, and hypercholesterolemia presents to the clinic complaining of a non-healing ulcer on his left ankle present for the past month. His blood pressure is 160/78 mmHg. His physical examination is remarkable for mild bilateral lower leg edema as well as lipodermatosclerosis and hyperpigmentation around the ankles. A mildly tender, superficial ulceration is observed with an irregular pink base above his medial malleolus. His feet and toes are warm, pink, and have 2-second capillary refill and intact sensation. Laboratory tests on this patient include a random blood sugar of 160 mg/dL, creatinine of 1.1 mg/dL, calcium of 10.4 mg/dL, phosphorus of 4.4 mg/dL, and serum intact parathyroid hormone level of 50 pg/mL. What is the most likely etiology of the ulceration?

    a. Diabetes mellitus
    b. Chronic venous insufficiency
    c. Peripheral arterial disease (PAD)
    d. Calciphylaxis
    e. Brown recluse spider bite

2. A 49-year-old woman with a 60-pack per year history of smoking presents to the emergency department (ED) with complaints of constant, worsening right foot pain and tingling in the toes for several hours. She denies a history of trauma. On examination, she is in moderate distress from pain and has a regular cardiac rhythm at a rate of 104 bpm. Her right lower extremity has a palpable femoral pulse and cool, pale foot with nonpalpable pedal pulses. There is a faint dorsalis pedis arterial signal with continuous-wave handheld Doppler evaluation. Strength is intact in the foot and toes, but she reports pain during examination. What is the most appropriate next step?

    a. Admit to the hospital; begin a heparin infusion and antiplatelet therapy. Obtain an urgent echocardiogram to identify the source of embolism.
    b. Obtain urgent ankle–brachial indices (ABIs) and pulse volume recordings to determine the severity of disease and begin aggressive risk-factor–modifying medical therapy.
    c. Admit to the hospital for an urgent diagnostic abdominal aortogram with runoff and potential endovascular revascularization.

    d. Admit to the hospital for pain control and obtain a lumbar magnetic resonance imaging to evaluate for lumbar canal stenosis and pseudoclaudication.

    e. Obtain ABIs at rest and with exercise to assess for lower extremity PAD and a venous plethysmography of the lower extremities with exercise to evaluate for venous claudication.

3. A 65-year-old man presents with progressive, short-distance, intermittent claudication in his right leg and a declining ABI. He undergoes an abdominal aortic angiogram with runoff demonstrating a discrete 90% stenotic lesion of the superficial femoral artery. Percutaneous transluminal angioplasty followed by placement of a self-expanding nitinol mesh stent is performed with good postprocedural angiographic results. Which of the following is the most appropriate post-procedure surveillance program for this patient?

    a. Regular visits with assessment for interval change in symptoms, vascular examination, and ABI measurement beginning in the immediate post-procedure period and at intervals for at least 2 years

    b. Regular visits with assessment for interval change in symptoms, vascular examination, and arterial duplex at 1 month, 3 months, and at month 12

    c. Regular visits with assessment for interval change in symptoms, vascular examination, and ABI measurement at 3 months, 6 months, 9 months, and at month 12

    d. Regular visits with assessment for interval change in symptoms, vascular examination, and arterial duplex at 3 months, 6 months, 12 months, and 2 years

    e. Annual visits with assessment for interval change in symptoms, vascular examination, ABI measurement, and arterial duplex

Case 1 (Questions 4 and 5)

A 59-year old morbidly obese woman is admitted for cholecystectomy and postoperatively is placed on deep venous thrombosis (DVT) prophylaxis with mini-dose subcutaneous heparin. On hospital day 2, a peripherally inserted central venous catheter is placed in the right arm. The patient is discharged to a rehabilitation facility on hospital day 5 after removal of the venous catheter. Two days later she presents to the emergency room with right upper extremity pain and swelling. She reports she has not felt well enough to participate with physical therapy since being discharged from the hospital. Venous duplex of the right arm demonstrates acute thrombosis of the right cephalic vein. Complete blood count (CBC) and chemistries are within normal range with a platelet count of 180 K/μL.

4. What is the most appropriate management of this patient?

    a. Admit to the hospital and start on intravenous (IV) anticoagulation with heparin or a direct thrombin inhibitor (DTI).

    b. Prescribe enoxaparin 1 mg/kg every 12 hours and coumadin. Admit for 4 to 5 days of overlap and discontinue enoxaparin once the international normalized ratio (INR) is within therapeutic range for 2 consecutive days. Continue anticoagulant therapy for 3 months.

    c. Prescribe enoxaparin 1 mg/kg every 12 hours and coumadin. Discharge with instructions for 4 to 5 days of overlap and discontinue enoxaparin once the INR is within therapeutic range for 2 consecutive days. Continue anticoagulant therapy for 6 months.

    d. Prescribe enoxaparin 1 mg/kg every 12 hours and coumadin. Discharge with instructions for 4 to 5 days of overlap and discontinue enoxaparin once the INR is within therapeutic range for 2 consecutive days. Continue anticoagulant therapy for 12 months.

    e. Warm compresses and nonsteroidal anti-inflammatory drugs for pain.

5. What should the target activated partial thromboplastin time (aPTT) be to achieve optimal efficacy and safety if anticoagulation with a DTI were to be initiated in this patient?

   a. An aPTT of 3.0 to 4.0 times the baseline value
   b. An aPTT of 2.5 to 3.0 times the baseline value
   d. An aPTT of 2.0 to 3.0 times the baseline value
   e. An aPTT of 1.5 to 2.0 times the baseline value

Case 2 (Questions 6 to 8)

A 15-year-old man presents to the clinic accompanied by his mother for evaluation of "red hands." He earned money last winter clearing sidewalks of snow and plans to do so again in the upcoming weeks. He reports developing red discoloration of his hands after returning home from the cold. The discoloration persisted for a few minutes until his hands were rewarmed. He denies weakness, paresthesia, pain, or skin lesions. He is otherwise healthy. At the time of consultation, inspection of his hands is unrevealing. Radial and ulnar pulses are 2+/2 bilaterally. The Allen test and reverse Allen test reveal return of color to the hands in 7 seconds bilaterally. His mother reports that she and her mother both have Raynaud phenomenon. The patient's mother expresses concern that her son may have systemic lupus and she requests further testing.

6. What is the most likely diagnosis?

   a. Raynaud disease
   b. Raynaud phenomenon
   c. Normal physiologic cold response
   d. Acrocyanosis
   e. Thermal injury

7. Of the following, which is the most appropriate next step to objectively evaluate this patient?

   a. Obtain an upper extremity angiogram with selective imaging of the digital vessels and before and after administration of nitroglycerin.
   b. Obtain digital pulse volume recordings and transcutaneous partial pressure of oxygen measurements of the digits.
   c. Order a C-reactive protein level, erythrocyte sedimentation rate, and perform nailfold capillaroscopy.
   d. Order a C-reactive protein level, erythrocyte sedimentation rate, and plasma homocysteine level.
   e. Order antinuclear antibodies, erythrocyte sedimentation rate, and perform nailfold capillaroscopy.

8. When would be the most appropriate time to schedule a follow-up appointment?

   a. 5 years
   b. 3 years
   c. 2 years
   d. 1 year
   e. As needed

Case 3 (Questions 9 and 10)

A 49-year-old man presents to the clinic with complaints of progressive exertional dyspnea for several weeks. His speech is mildly breathless. Neck veins are distended bilaterally and there is moderate lower extremity edema. He denies chest pain. Electrocardiogram (ECG) shows sinus tachycardia without ST-segment abnormality. Physical examination reveals a parasternal heave and systolic ejection murmur. Past medical history is significant for splenectomy after a car accident several years ago.

9. Which of the following will most accurately confirm the underlying cause of this patient's symptoms?

   a. Chest computed tomography (CT) with IV contrast
   b. Transthoracic echocardiogram
   c. Transesophageal echocardiogram
   d. Pulmonary arteriogram
   e. Ventilation–perfusion scan

10. Which of the following statements is most accurate concerning this patient's underlying diagnosis?

   a. Inflammatory mechanisms have not been implicated in the pathogenesis.
   b. Patients should be anticoagulated with a vitamin K antagonist and target INR of 2.5 to 3.5.
   c. IV epoprostenol is an effective therapy in patients with advanced disease.
   d. Inhaled iloprost has been demonstrated to improve exercise capacity.
   e. Bosentan has been shown to improve exercise capacity in patients with mild-to-moderate liver disease.

11. You are consulted for recommendations regarding a deep vein thrombosis in a patient who is status post aortic valve replacement with a bioprosthetic valve 4 days prior. Earlier on the day of consult he complained of pain and was diagnosed with a partially occlusive left femoral vein thrombosis. His postoperative course has been otherwise uncomplicated. On examination, the patient is tender around the surgical site. There is moderate pitting edema in the legs bilaterally. He has palpable pulses in all extremities. What do you recommend?

   a. Bolus subcutaneous low-molecular-weight heparin (LMWH) 80 mg/kg, then dose at 1 mg/kg subcutaneously every 12 hours
   b. Placement of a retrievable inferior vena cava filter
   c. Catheter-directed thrombolysis
   d. Begin a DTI
   e. Begin a weight-based unfractionated heparin infusion

12. A patient with a history of heparin-induced thrombocytopenia (HIT) 8 years ago presents to your office for preoperative evaluation for bioprosthetic aortic valve replacement and coronary artery bypass grafting. He requires anticoagulation while on cardiopulmonary bypass pump during surgery. A recent ELISA (enzyme-linked immunosorbent assay) antiplatelet factor-4 antibody test is negative (<0.400 optical density). He has had no subsequent heparin exposures over the last 8 years. What is the most appropriate anticoagulation regimen you should recommend for this patient?

   a. Administration of IV fondaparinux intraoperatively with subsequent daily monitoring of platelet counts
   b. Administration of IV LMWH intraoperatively with subsequent daily monitoring of platelet counts
   c. Administration of IV argatroban intraoperatively with subsequent daily monitoring of platelet counts
   d. Administration of IV hirudin intraoperatively with subsequent daily monitoring of platelet counts
   e. Administration of IV unfractionated heparin intraoperatively with subsequent daily monitoring of platelet counts

13. A patient comes to your office 1 month after a hospital stay for gastric bypass surgery. She was diagnosed with a mesenteric vein thrombosis postoperatively. She denies a prior history of venous thromboembolism (VTE). She and her husband have questions about the duration of anticoagulant therapy. They bring copies of laboratory results showing she was checked for a hypercoagulable condition. One laboratory test indicates she is heterozygous for a mutation of the methylenetetrahydrofolate reductase (MTHFR) enzyme. All other laboratory tests are within normal range. She asks you how these results impact duration and intensity of anticoagulation. The most accurate reply is

a. all first-episode DVTs are treated similarly; thus, the discovery of this genetic mutation is of doubtful clinical significance.

b. given the clinical circumstances the laboratory finding is of doubtful clinical significance and you advise she should be anticoagulated with a vitamin K antagonist for 3 months with a target INR of 2.0 to 3.0.

c. she should be anticoagulated with a vitamin K antagonist for 3 months with an increased target INR of 2.5 to 3.5 because of increased thrombogenicity induced by the genetic mutation.

d. she should be anticoagulated with a vitamin K antagonist with a target INR of 2.0 to 3.0 for an extended duration of therapy to 6 months because of increased thrombogenicity induced by the genetic mutation.

e. she should be anticoagulated with a vitamin K antagonist with an INR target of 2.0 to 3.0 indefinitely because of the high rate of recurrent VTE associated with the heterozygous form of this genetic mutation.

14. A 34-year-old woman with a history of deep vein thrombosis who is chronically anticoagulated with warfarin discovers she is pregnant. Her due date is 34 weeks from now. Currently, she is on warfarin and has an INR of 2.2. She presents to the clinic for recommendations regarding her anticoagulation management. Which of the following is true regarding venous thromboembolic disease, anticoagulation therapy, and pregnancy?

a. When deep vein thrombosis of the lower extremities complicates a pregnancy, the right leg is affected significantly more often than the left, presumably because of exaggeration of the compressive effects of the left iliac artery compressing on the right iliac vein during pregnancy.

b. The incidence of teratogenic complications of pregnancy caused by warfarin, including nasal hypoplasia and stippled epiphyses, is greatest if warfarin exposure occurs during weeks 14 through 24.

c. Warfarin is contraindicated in the nursing mother because of a high incidence of inducing an anticoagulant effect in the infant fed with breast milk from a mother on warfarin therapy.

d. Fatal pulmonary embolism is a leading cause of maternal mortality in the Western world.

e. LMWHs have been proven safe and efficacious in pregnant woman with prosthetic heart valves, and supplanted unfractionated heparin as the standard of care in this setting.

Case 4 (Questions 15 and 16)

A 65-year-old man presents to the clinic with complaints of episodic burning pain involving the soles of his feet and toes. He reports symptoms are most severe when the weather becomes hot and generally occurs when he is outside in the heat. His feet and toes turn red and feel hot to touch during episodes. When he returns to an air-conditioned area, symptoms begin to dissipate or some episodes may take hours for complete resolution. Elevating his legs relieves symptoms as does walking barefoot on cold tile floors. His past medical history includes hypertension, well controlled with atenolol, and he takes once daily low-dose aspirin for primary prevention.

Physical Examination

> Blood pressure is 120/70 mmHg and pulse is 84 bpm.
>
> The cardiac and lung examinations are normal.
>
> The abdomen is soft and nontender with a normal-sized palpable aortic pulsation.
>
> No bruit can be heard over the neck, abdomen, or either groin.
>
> Radial, dorsalis pedis, and posterior tibial pulses are 2+/2 bilaterally.
>
> A mild erythema and increased warmth are noted in toes and soles of the feet.

15. Which of the following is the most likely diagnosis?

   a. Heat urticaria

   b. Erythromelalgia

   c. Chilblains (perniosis)

   d. Raynaud phenomenon

16. What laboratory values should be followed serially in patients with this condition?

   a. Electrolytes, blood urea nitrogen, and creatinine

   b. Erythrocyte sedimentation rate

   c. Ionic calcium

   d. Complete blood count with differential (CBC with diff)

17. A 17-year-old boy was involved in a motor vehicle accident, which resulted in multiple fractures as well as internal injuries that necessitated multiple abdominal surgeries over a 2-week period. He is expected to recover fully. An intraluminal filling defect was incidentally identified consistent with DVT of the right external iliac vein on a contrast-enhanced abdominal CT scan. Anticoagulation was contraindicated because of a retroperitoneal hemorrhage. It was determined that placement of an inferior vena cava filter was necessary. Of the following types of filters, which filter is most appropriate in this case?

   a. Bird's Nest vena cava filter

   b. Gunther Tulip retrievable vena cava filter

   c. TrapEase inferior vena cava filter

   d. Greenfield vena cava filter

   e. Simon Nitinol inferior vena cava filter

Case 5 (Question 18)

You are called to the bedside of a 68-year-old man in mild distress who underwent cardiac catheterization earlier in the day. He is complaining of increasing right groin pain. He complains of weakness and tingling in his foot and toes. He is presently on a heparin infusion because of atrial fibrillation. On inspection you note a large area of skin in his right groin and proximal thigh to be dark blue and there is a large, palpable, hard pulsatile mass. With ultrasound using color Doppler you note an irregular shaped area of flow measuring 4.0 cm × 3.3 cm near the common femoral artery, approximately 4.0-cm deep and connected to the artery by a 0.5-cm neck. There is surrounding hematoma observed. Spectral waveform analysis of the neck demonstrates a to-and-fro pattern.

18. What is the best treatment option for management of this patient's condition?

   a. Placement of a femoral compression device overnight and analgesics for pain

   b. Injection of thrombin by ultrasound guidance

   c. Ultrasound-guided compression for 30 minutes

   d. Surgical evacuation of the hematoma and suture repair of the artery

   e. Placement of a compression dressing with snugly applied bandages around the leg and serial duplex scans to monitor for resolution

19. A 74-year-old man is in the ICU (intensive care unit) recovering from coronary artery bypass surgery and has developed a hemorrhagic pericardial effusion. He is currently stable, but has noted swelling and pain in his left leg. An ultrasound is ordered and reveals acute thrombus in the left peroneal vein. Which of the following is the best management option?

   a. No action is required because calf vein thrombus is not clinically important

   b. Pneumatic compression stockings and enoxaparin 40 mg every 24 hours

   c. Follow up with serial duplex ultrasound scans

   d. Initiate a continuous unfractionated heparin infusion

   e. Proceed with placement of an inferior vena cava filter

Case 6 (Questions 20 and 21)

A 25-year-old man presents to the clinic with complaints of pain in his feet with walking. He reports this has been going on for several months and has progressively worsened in the past few weeks. He is beginning to develop symptoms in his right calf and earlier this week noticed a black area on his great toe. He has no medical problems, takes no medications, and is in good health overall. He is a smoker and works as a computer salesman. He reports a family history of VTE; his mother had a pulmonary embolism at the age of 50 and was diagnosed with the antiphospholipid antibody syndrome.

20. What is the most likely cause of his symptoms?

   a. Elevated anticardiolipin antibodies

   b. Thromboangiitis obliterans (TAO, Buerger disease)

   c. Takayasu arteritis

   d. Premature atherosclerosis

   e. Livedoid vasculitis (atrophie blanche)

21. What is the most important aspect of therapy for this patient?

   a. Anticoagulation with a vitamin K antagonist

   b. Cessation of exposure to all forms of tobacco

   c. Initiate immunosuppressive therapy with glucocorticoids

   d. Antiplatelet therapy with aspirin

   e. Admit to the hospital to begin tissue plasminogen activator therapy

Case 7 (Questions 22 and 23)

A 24-year-old woman presents with complaints of a swollen, painful left leg. She has a history of two episodes of deep vein thrombosis in the past. She recalls that they were both on the left side, but is unsure of which veins were involved. She was on warfarin in the past but discontinued it when she began attempting to conceive. Venous duplex demonstrates an acute deep vein thrombosis of the left femoral vein. You initiate treatment with LMWH.

22. What is the most likely diagnosis?

   a. Heterozygous prothrombin gene mutation

   b. Heterozygous factor V Leiden mutation

   c. May-Thurner syndrome

   d. Klippel-Trenaunay syndrome

   e. Klippel-Trenaunay-Weber syndrome

23. Which of the following is the best management option?

   a. Indefinite anticoagulant therapy with warfarin

   b. Indefinite monotherapy with enoxaparin

   c. Venography for thrombus removal and stent placement

d. Placement of an inferior vena cava filter and discontinue anticoagulants

e. Anticoagulate with either warfarin or enoxaparin for 6 months

24. A 68-year-old gentleman underwent coronary artery bypass surgery using the saphenous vein harvested from his left leg. He has done well postoperatively except for failure of the left leg incision to heal completely. Four months after surgery, his leg is still not fully healed and a peri-incisional ulcer is now present. He has significant edema in his leg, which was present prior to surgery. There are no symptoms or physical findings suggestive of infection. His ABI is 0.94 on the right and 0.89 on the left. You order an ultrasound, which is negative for acute thrombus but does reveal significant venous valvular incompetence in the deep veins. Which of the following is most likely to improve this patient's wound healing?

a. Whirlpool therapy

b. Antibiotics and topical steroids

c. Compression stockings

d. Plastic surgery consult

e. Revascularization

25. You are providing postoperative care for a patient who is in the cardiovascular surgery postoperative ICU, status post coronary artery bypass surgery. A venous duplex ultrasound was performed to evaluate for new-onset bilateral leg swelling. Results are reported as negative for DVT, but with monophasic flow noted within the bilateral common femoral veins. Which of the following is the next best step?

a. CT venogram of the lower extremities

b. CT venogram of the abdomen and pelvis

c. Enoxaparin therapy 1 mg/kg subcutaneous injections every 12 hours

d. Enoxaparin therapy 40 mg subcutaneous injections every 24 hours

Case 8 (Questions 26 and 27)

A 39-year-old man presents to the ED with shortness of breath and tachycardia. He eventually develops hypotension with a systolic blood pressure of 80 mmHg. A stat CT scan of the chest reveals a saddle pulmonary embolism involving the main pulmonary artery trunk.

26. Which of the following is the next most appropriate step?

a. Begin an IV unfractionated heparin infusion at 18 U/kg/h

b. Begin alteplase 100 mg IV over 2 hours

c. Begin enoxaparin subcutaneous injections 1 mg/kg every 12 hours

d. Insert an inferior vena cava filter

27. Which of the following findings or laboratory values could be used to predict his prognosis?

a. C-reactive protein

b. Atrial arrhythmia

c. Left ventricular dysfunction

d. Prolonged QT interval

e. Elevated serum myoglobin

28. A 52-year-old man with metastatic prostate cancer has developed left lower extremity swelling. You order an ultrasound and a left acute external iliac deep vein thrombosis is visualized. You hospitalize the patient and his initial labs

reveal hemoglobin 14.5 g/dL and creatinine 1.0 mg/dL. Which of the following treatment options is most appropriate?

a. Begin a weight-based unfractionated heparin infusion and bridge to warfarin.
b. Begin enoxaparin 1 mg/kg subcutaneous injections every 12 hours.
c. Place an inferior vena cava filter.
d. Begin unfractionated heparin 5,000 units subcutaneous injections every 8 hours.

29. A 55-year-old man is admitted to the hospital with upper gastrointestinal bleeding. He is transfused with 2 units of packed red blood cells and undergoes esophagogastroduodenoscopy. A bleeding gastric ulcer is discovered and treated with epinephrine injection. Several days into his admission he begins complaining of right calf discomfort. Venous duplex ultrasound is performed demonstrating acute deep vein thrombosis of the popliteal and posterior tibial veins. What is the next appropriate step in the management of this patient?

a. No action is required because calf vein thrombus is not clinically important.
b. Pneumatic compression stockings and enoxaparin 40 mg every 24 hours.
c. Follow up with serial duplex ultrasound scans.
d. Initiate a continuous unfractionated heparin infusion.
e. Proceed with placement of an inferior vena cava filter.

30. A 58-year-old man presents to the clinic with a complaint of bilateral lower extremity cramping muscular pain with exertion relieved after a few minutes of rest. His medical history includes coronary artery disease status post left anterior descending artery stent 2 years ago, diabetes mellitus type 2, and essential hypertension. An ABI is performed in your office demonstrating a right ABI of 1.10 and left ABI of 1.04. What is the most appropriate next step in the evaluation of this patient?

a. Reassurance and suggest low-impact exercise, i.e., swimming
b. Referral to a peripheral vascular interventionalist for lower extremity angiogram
c. Order bilateral ABI measurements in the vascular laboratory at rest and following an exercise protocol
d. Order magnetic resonance imaging of the lumbosacral spine to confirm the likely diagnosis of pseudoclaudication
e. Have him return in 6 months and repeat the resting ABI measurements

31. A 68-year-old woman recently diagnosed with PAD presents to the clinic for follow-up. A fasting lipid profile obtained prior to the appointment demonstrates a low-density lipoprotein (LDL) level of 145 mg/dL. You decide to initiate therapy with a hydroxymethyl glutaryl coenzyme-A reductase inhibitor (statin). Which of the following LDL target levels is most appropriate?

a. Less than 150 mg/dL
b. Less than 130 mg/dL
c. Less than 100 mg/dL
d. Less than 50 mg/dL
e. There is no defined LDL target

32. A 52-year-old woman with a history of PAD, diabetes mellitus type 2, and active smoking presents to the clinic with a blood pressure of 150/95 mmHg. What blood pressure target should you recommend for this patient?

a. Less than 150/90 mmHg
b. Less than 140/90 mmHg

   c. Less than 130/80 mmHg

   d. Less than 120/75 mmHg

   e. Less than 100/70 mmHg

33. For the above patient you decide to start her on a new antihypertensive medication. Which of the following class of medications are contraindicated?

   a. β-Adrenergic blockers

   b. Thiazide diuretics

   c. Angiotensin-converting enzyme inhibitors

   d. Angiotensin II receptor blockers

   e. None of the above

Case 9 (Questions 34 and 35)

A 68-year-old man with a 30 pack-year history of smoking is seen in the clinic for follow-up after a non-ST-elevation myocardial infarction (NSTEMI). Because of his smoking history and age you order an ultrasound of his abdomen to rule out abdominal aortic aneurysm (AAA). He is discovered to have an infrarenal AAA measuring 5.0 cm × 4.9 cm.

34. After this initial baseline study, how often should you repeat the ultrasound of the abdomen?

   a. Every 3 months

   b. Every 3 to 6 months

   c. Every 6 to 12 months

   d. Every 12 months

   e. Every 24 months

35. At what size measurement should you refer a patient for repair of an asymptomatic infrarenal AAA?

   a. 4.0 to 5.0 cm

   b. 4.5 to 5.0 cm

   c. 5.0 to 5.4 cm

   d. 5.5 cm or greater

   e. 6 cm or greater

36. Which of the following population groups is it appropriate to do a screening ultrasound of the abdomen for an AAA?

   a. Men >60 years of age with a first-degree relative with an AAA

   b. Women >60 years of age with a first-degree relative with an AAA

   c. Men 65 to 75 years of age with a smoking history

   d. Women 65 to 75 years of age with a smoking history

   e. All of the above groups are appropriate to screen for an AAA

Case 10 (Questions 37 and 38)

A 70-year-old man presents for follow-up in the clinic 1 month after undergoing right internal carotid artery stenting.

37. When should you get a post-procedure baseline carotid duplex ultrasound?

   a. Four weeks after the intervention

   b. Six weeks after the intervention

   c. Two months after the intervention

   d. Six months after the intervention

   e. Twelve months after the intervention

38. A baseline carotid duplex ultrasound demonstrates patency of the stent and no evidence of residual stenosis or restenosis of the right internal carotid artery after the procedure. One year after the carotid intervention, how often is it recommended to perform repeat carotid ultrasound surveillance in an asymptomatic patient?

    a. Every 6 months

    b. Every 12 months

    c. Every 18 months

    d. Every 24 months

    e. Every 36 months

Case 11 (Questions 39 to 42)

A 65-year-old man presents for a routine physical examination. During the interview he complains about swelling behind his right knee. You order an ultrasound of the area (findings illustrated in Fig. 7.1).

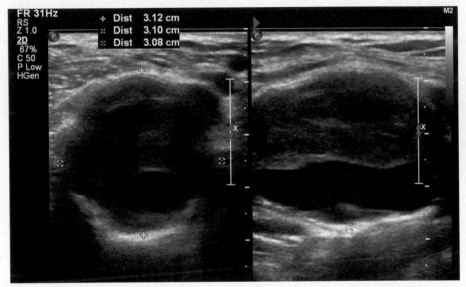

Figure 7.1

39. What is the most likely diagnosis?

    a. Abscess

    b. Baker cyst

    c. Popliteal artery aneurysm

    d. Enlarged lymph node

    e. Lipoma

40. What percentage of patients with a popliteal artery aneurysm have concomitant AAA?

    a. 10%

    b. 20%

    c. 40%

    d. 50%

    e. 60%

41. After finding the results illustrated in Figure 7.1 you refer the patient for ultrasound of the abdomen and contralateral popliteal artery. No additional abnormalities are discovered. What is the next appropriate step in his management?

    a. The finding is benign and no intervention is indicated.

    b. Repeat the ultrasound in 3 months.

  c. Repeat the ultrasound in 6 months.

  d. Repeat the ultrasound in 1 year.

  e. Refer for the repair of the aneurysm.

42. What is the most common complication of untreated, symptomatic popliteal artery aneurysms measuring more than 2.5 cm in greatest dimension?

  a. Rupture

  b. Thromboembolism

  c. Infection

  d. No complications

  e. Popliteal vein thrombosis

43. During rounds in the telemetry unit you evaluate a 55-year-old woman 1 day after she underwent a left heart catheterization. She complains of right groin pain and swelling at the vascular access site. You order a duplex ultrasound of the right groin. Findings of the ultrasound are illustrated in Figure 7.2A and B. What is your diagnosis?

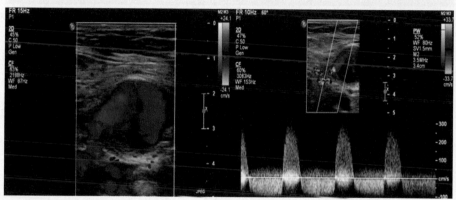

Figure 7.2

  a. Hematoma

  b. Arteriovenous fistula

  c. Abscess

  d. Pseudoaneurysm

  e. Enlarged lymph node

44. A 64-year-old woman presents to the clinic for evaluation prior to coronary artery bypass surgery. She underwent carotid duplex ultrasound demonstrating normal bilateral internal carotid arteries. Images from her scan are illustrated in Figure 7.3. What unexpected condition is demonstrated by her ultrasound images?

  a. Subclavian artery aneurysm

  b. Subclavian artery thrombosis

  c. Subclavian artery stenosis

  d. Subclavian vein thrombosis

  e. Hematoma surrounding the subclavian artery

45. A 55-year-old woman with a history of deep vein thrombosis 2 months ago for which she was on warfarin was admitted to the hospital for chest pain. She underwent chest CT angiography which was negative for pulmonary embolism. She underwent a left heart catheterization after her INR normalized. During her procedure she received IV heparin. Her coronary arteries were free of disease.

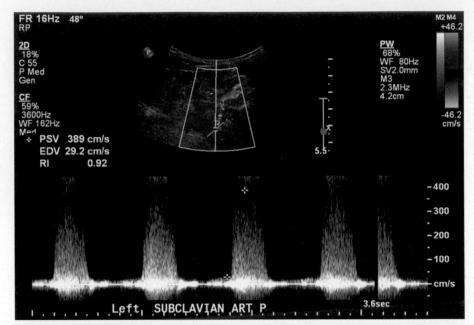

Figure 7.3

Following the procedure she was prescribed 10 mg of warfarin daily for 3 days. During this time her CBC was monitored and her hemoglobin and platelet counts showed minor fluctuations. A day later she developed a lesion on her abdomen illustrated in Figure 7.4. What is the likely cause of the skin lesion?

a. Heparin-induced skin necrosis

b. Vasculitis

c. Warfarin skin necrosis

d. Eczema

e. Allergic reaction

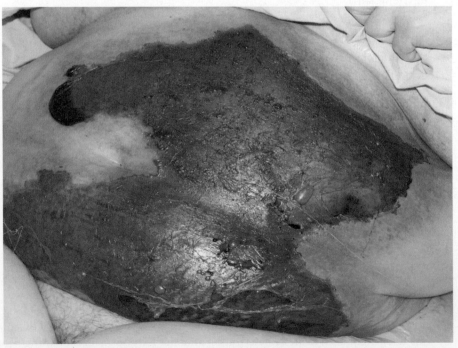

Figure 7.4

46. A 70-year-old man is admitted to the telemetry unit for workup of dizziness of 2 days' duration. He denies chest pain or shortness of breath. His heart rate is 60 bpm and blood pressure is 130/50 mmHg. On physical examination, a systolic murmur is heard over the left sternal border. Carotid duplex ultrasound is performed demonstrating the spectral waveforms of the bilateral internal carotid and vertebral arteries illustrated in Figure 7.5. Which of the following conditions is suggested by the carotid duplex waveforms?

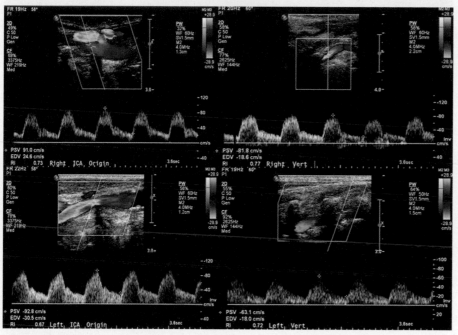

Figure 7.5

a. Pulmonary valve stenosis

b. Systolic heart failure

c. Pericardial tamponade

d. Aortic valve stenosis

e. Mitral regurgitation

47. A 55-year-old woman presents to the ED with precordial chest discomfort and shortness of breath. Her body mass index is 34. Her medical history includes essential hypertension, diabetes mellitus type 2, and a 30 pack-year smoking history. Laboratory results include a troponin of 2.4 mg/mL and a B-type natriuretic peptide of 840 pg/mL. An ECG reveals no ST-segment elevation and nonspecific ST-T wave changes. The ED physician requests cardiology consultation for an NSTEMI. When you arrive to see the patient you order an IV contrast-enhanced chest CT scan of the lungs. Findings are demonstrated in Figure 7.6. What is the diagnosis?

a. Type A aortic dissection

b. Myocarditis

c. Pneumonia

d. Saddle pulmonary embolism

e. Interstitial lung fibrosis

48. Which of the following cardiovascular risk factor assessment tools has not been demonstrated to be useful in the risk assessment for a first atherosclerotic cardiovascular event?

a. High-sensitivity C-reactive protein

b. Coronary artery calcium score

c. Carotid intima-media thickness

d. ABI

e. Family history of premature coronary vascular disease

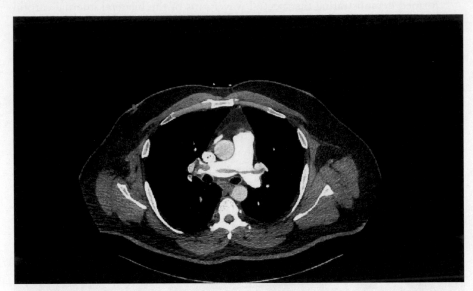

Figure 7.6

ANSWERS

1. **b.** Chronic venous insufficiency. This patient has no history of neuropathy and has intact sensation, making a neurotrophic ulcer often associated with diabetes unlikely. While his glucose is elevated, inadequate information is provided to make the diagnosis of diabetes mellitus. Bilateral leg edema, hyperpigmentation of the ankles, and the location of the ulcer over the medial malleolus ("gaiter distribution") are findings consistent with a venous stasis wound. Ulcers secondary to arterial disease are usually painful, involve the toes, and are well circumscribed. The information provided suggests adequate arterial supply. Wounds associated with calciphylaxis may be anywhere. They are usually very painful, involve large areas of skin, and are associated with black eschar formation. These wounds are most often seen in patients with renal impairment and hyperparathyroidism, neither of which is true in this case. Nothing in the clinical vignette is suggestive of a brown recluse spider bite.[11]

2. **c.** Admit to the hospital for an urgent diagnostic abdominal aortogram with runoff and potential endovascular revascularization. The patient described is suffering from acute critical limb ischemia. The hallmarks of acute limb ischemia are the five "P's", which are suggestive of impending tissue necrosis. They are pain, paralysis, paresthesia, pulseless, and pallor and some add poikilothermia (coldness) for a sixth "P." Our patient exhibits all but paralysis. Based on the Society for Vascular Surgery/International Society for Cardiovascular Surgery classification scheme for clinical categories of acute limb ischemia, her limb is marginally to intermediately threatened. Acute limb ischemia requires prompt diagnosis and intervention to avoid limb loss and life-threatening systemic illness resulting from tissue gangrene.[12]

3. **a.** Regular visits with assessment for interval change in symptoms, vascular examination, and ABI measurement beginning in the immediate post-procedure period and at intervals for at least 2 years. Unlike follow-up of autologous vein bypass grafts, well-established evidence-based guidelines for surveillance of post-endovascular revascularization patients do not exist. However, it is considered standard of care to evaluate these patients with interval history, examination, and measurement of the ABI regularly for at least 2 years after their percutaneous revascularization procedure.[13]

4. **e.** Warm compresses and nonsteroidal anti-inflammatory drugs for pain. Empiric anticoagulation, including outpatient anticoagulation, for superficial vein thrombosis is not routinely recommended. The clinical scenario may represent HIT and she should have a follow-up platelet count in 2 days. Her prior platelet counts from her recent hospitalization should be evaluated for a drop in platelets of ≥50% from baseline.[15]

5. **e.** An aPTT prolongation of 1.5 to 2.0 times the baseline value. Although the recommended range for therapeutic anticoagulation for VTE with a DTI is 1.5 to 2.5 times the baseline, which is not given as an option, published data indicate that anticoagulation with a DTI target aPTT of 1.5 to 2.0 times the baseline is just as efficacious and is associated with less bleeding risk.[16]

6. **c.** Normal physiologic cold response. This patient is exhibiting a normal response to prolonged exposure to cold. The diagnosis of Raynaud phenomenon is clinical and includes the presence of pallor or acrocyanosis and pain with cold exposure. Redness of the hands with warming after prolonged cold exposure, without concomitant pain, may be a normal response in a healthy young individual. He should be counseled to wear gloves and report any change in his symptoms, as his family history does predispose him to development of Raynaud phenomenon.[17]

7. e. Order antinuclear antibodies, erythrocyte sedimentation rate, and perform nailfold capillaroscopy. If all these tests are normal, it is very unlikely that this patient has secondary Raynaud phenomenon and no further testing is necessary.[18]

8. e. As needed. Although the patient does not have Raynaud phenomenon, he should be encouraged to follow up as needed because of his family history. Patients who have primary Raynaud phenomenon should have clinical follow-up for a minimum of 2 years after diagnosis.[17]

9. d. Pulmonary arteriogram. An arteriogram is the test most likely to confirm pulmonary artery hypertension in this patient presenting with cor pulmonale, although a right heart catheterization is usually done first. This patient most likely has chronic thromboembolic pulmonary hypertension (CTEPH), a condition seen in otherwise healthy postsplenectomy patients. Other predisposing conditions include history of pulmonary embolism, myeloproliferative disorders, and chronic inflammatory conditions.[19]

10. c. IV epoprostenol is an effective therapy in patients with advanced disease. Patients with CTEPH may be bridged to pulmonary endarterectomy with IV epoprostenol. The other answers are incorrect. Anticoagulation with a vitamin K antagonist is indicated; however, the INR target of 2.0 to 3.0 is recommended. The Aerosolized Iloprost Randomization (AIR) study did not demonstrate improved exercise capacity with inhaled iloprost. Bosentan does improve exercise capacity and decreases pulmonary vascular resistance, but is not advocated for use in patients with moderate-to-severe hepatic dysfunction.[19]

11. e. Begin a weight-based unfractionated heparin infusion. Although LMWH may be appropriate as the initial anticoagulant of choice for the treatment of an acute DVT in the ambulatory as well as hospitalized patient, it does not require a bolus. In the setting of the postoperative state where rapid reversal of anticoagulation may be required, unfractionated heparin is favored. An inferior vena cava filter would be an appropriate recommendation if anticoagulation could not be administered at therapeutic levels. Thrombolytic therapy is contraindicated in the setting of recent open heart surgery. Use of a DTI is not indicated for routine anticoagulation.[22]

12. e. Administration of IV unfractionated heparin intraoperatively with subsequent daily monitoring of platelet counts. The nature of immune response to heparin is anamnestic; this means a second exposure in the absence of positive antibodies is not associated with the development of a clinical hyperacute immune response. Perioperatively, heparin products should be avoided in patients with a history of HIT even with undetectable antiplatelet antibodies prior to cardiac surgery or vascular surgery. Nevertheless, heparin is favored over DTIs in cardiac and vascular surgery because of its reversibility and relative ease of use. Acute HIT is unlikely to occur even in patients who have a remote history of HIT as long as there has been no heparin exposure within the previous 100 days. This recommendation is based on expert opinion (level 1C) and not on randomized controlled trials.[15]

13. b. Given the clinical circumstances the laboratory finding is of doubtful clinical significance and you advise she should be anticoagulated with a vitamin K antagonist for 3 months with a target INR of 2.0 to 3.0. While the site of thrombosis is somewhat out of the ordinary, it was in the setting of abdominal surgery and was her first episode; therefore, a routine course of 3 months of anticoagulation with a vitamin K antagonist and an INR target of 2.0 to 3.0 is appropriate. All first-episode venous thrombotic events are not treated the same. Patients with malignancy-related thrombosis, idiopathic events, and those with certain thrombophilic conditions such as the antiphospholipid antibody syndrome require a longer duration of therapy relative to patients with transient risk factors for VTE. The MTHFR genetic mutation in the absence of hyperhomocysteinemia is not associated with increased risk of recurrence after discontinuation of anticoagulant therapy and has not been shown to increase thrombogenicity requiring a higher than usual INR target.[23]

14. **d.** Fatal pulmonary embolism is a leading cause of maternal mortality in the Western world. Thromboembolism is clearly the leading direct cause of maternal mortality according to the Seventh Report of the Confidential Enquiries into Maternal Deaths in the United Kingdom. The May-Thurner syndrome involves compression of the left iliac vein by the right iliac artery. The greatest teratogenicity of warfarin is seen during weeks 6 through 12. Use of LMWH in pregnant women who have prosthetic heart valves is highly controversial and certainly not the standard of care.[24]

15. **b.** Erythromelalgia. The name of this condition is based on three Greek words: *erythro* meaning red, *melos* meaning extremity, and *algos* meaning pain. It is uncommon, affecting about 1 in 40,000. It may be primary or secondary. Primary erythromelalgia is usually bilateral, not associated with gangrene, and patients have normal pulses. Secondary erythromelalgia is often unilateral, can be associated with gangrene, and patients have variable pulses. Secondary erythromelalgia can be associated with medications including bromocriptine, nifedipine, nicardipine, and verapamil. It may also herald the onset of a myeloproliferative disease such as polycythemia vera or essential thrombocythemia.[24]

16. **d.** Complete blood count with differential (CBC with diff). Patients with this condition should have a CBC with diff checked periodically for at least 2 to 3 years. It is important for treating physicians to recognize that erythromelalgia can precede the laboratory manifestations of a myeloproliferative disorder by up to 2 to 3 years.[28]

17. **b.** Gunther Tulip retrievable vena cava filter. This patient is young and his deep vein thrombosis is situational. He is expected to recover fully with no sequelae; thus he does not require placement of a permanent inferior vena cava filter. Proximal iliac thrombus in the setting of a hospitalized trauma patient following multiple abdominal surgeries is a very high-risk scenario for development of serious, life-threatening VTE. Anticoagulation is the treatment of choice when it can be safely administered; however, when contraindicated an inferior vena cava filter should be placed without delay. Patients with a temporary contraindication for anticoagulants should be reassessed at short intervals and, if circumstances permit, anticoagulants should be instituted for treatment of their VTE and to prevent recurrence. Of the filter types listed, only the Gunther Tulip is approved in the United States for retrieval. The OptEase is also approved for retrieval. The Bird's Nest filter is the only filter available for use in patients with a so-called megacava (vena cava greater than 28 mm). The Bird's Nest filter can be placed into an inferior vena cava of up to 42 mm in diameter. The TrapEase, Greenfield, and Simon Nitinol filters were not designed to have the option of retrieval.[25]

18. **d.** Surgical evacuation of the hematoma and suture repair of the artery. The patient complains of developing numbness in the setting of developing a large hematoma and pseudoaneurysm. To relieve the compressive effect of the hematoma, prevent irreversible injury, and relieve pain, the most appropriate method of repair in this patient is to evacuate the hematoma. Most small to moderately sized pseudoaneurysms can be treated with either ultrasound-guided compression, thrombin injection, or when very small may be observed for spontaneous resolution. Placement of a femoral compression device (Fem-Stop) is not appropriate in this setting, and bandages should not be wrapped proximally around the thigh as this will cause worsening swelling and pain.[26]

19. c. Follow up with serial duplex ultrasound scans. The peroneal vein is a calf vein with less propensity for clinically significant sequelae. Anticoagulant therapy for calf vein DVT is controversial. However, in this setting there is a clear contraindication to anticoagulate. Even prophylactic doses of anticoagulants are not advisable in patients with hemorrhagic pericardial effusions status post open heart surgery. Serial ultrasound scans have been studied as an alternative to anticoagulant therapy. If no propagation after several weeks, no anticoagulant therapy is necessary. If propagation occurs, then anticoagulation versus placement of an inferior vena cava should be considered.[27]

20. b. Thromboangiitis obliterans (TAO, Buerger disease). TAO classically manifests in young, male patients with a recent history of heavy tobacco use. The clinical presentation is consistent with ischemia, beginning distally and involving the small- and medium-sized arteries. Usually the lower extremities are involved, with ischemia or claudication of the feet or legs. Foot or arch claudication is typical. Occasionally, the hands are involved. If the disease progresses with continued exposure to tobacco, patients are at significant risk for progressive ischemia, ulceration, gangrene, and eventually amputation. Antiphospholipid antibody syndrome is certainly possible, but it is not a hereditary condition and most often manifests with venous thrombosis. Takayasu arteritis does not usually present in this way. Nothing is suggestive of atrophie blanche, and premature atherosclerosis presenting in a 25-year-old man with claudication and ischemia would be highly unusual.[28]

21. b. Cessation of exposure to all forms of tobacco. The strong link between tobacco abuse and TAO is well recognized. There have been suggestions that some patients may demonstrate an abnormal sensitivity to a component of tobacco, which leads to small vessel occlusive disease. It has been shown that patients with TAO have higher tobacco consumption as well as higher carboxyhemoglobin levels than do patients with atherosclerosis.[28]

22. c. May-Thurner syndrome. Also known as iliac vein compression syndrome, Cockett syndrome, or iliocaval compression syndrome, May-Thurner syndrome is caused by compression of the left common iliac vein by the right common iliac artery and the underlying vertebral body. A history of chronic left lower extremity edema with or without the presence of DVT is suggestive of May-Thurner syndrome, especially in a female population. This phenomenon causes a partial obstruction caused by physical entrapment of the vein under the artery as well as by repetitive pulsatile force resulting in intimal hyperplasia of the vein. It has been estimated that this condition occurs in 2% to 5% of patients who are evaluated for lower extremity venous problems.[29]

23. c. Venography for thrombus removal and stent placement. May-Thurner syndrome is an anatomical anomaly that results in repeated venous trauma and often subsequent thrombus formation. Removal of thrombus followed by angioplasty, if needed, and placement of a stent is a potentially definitive treatment that could avoid the need for indefinite anticoagulant therapy in the young woman presented in this case.[29]

24. c. Compression stockings. The importance of edema control is often underestimated for wound healing. This patient has deep system venous reflux. He has no signs of infection complicating the healing of his incision, so antibiotics are unlikely to be helpful. Topical steroids offer no benefit in this case. His ABIs suggest adequate arterial inflow for wound healing. Whirlpool therapy is helpful in select cases, most often when multiple small wounds are present, which need cleansing and gentle debridement. Although the size of the wound is not clearly stated, these wounds are most often small and referral for skin grafting is not indicated.[30]

25. **b.** CT venogram of the abdomen and pelvis. Monophasic (loss of respiratory phasicity) flow is suggestive of proximal venous obstruction, especially in a patient with swollen limbs and under high-risk circumstances for VTE. Monophasicity is not specific to thrombosis. Other potential causes include obesity, pregnancy, and a pelvic mass. Respiratory or cardiac dysfunction may also produce an abnormal venous flow pattern.[31]

26. **b.** Begin alteplase 100 mg IV over 2 hours. The patient presented has a clinically massive pulmonary embolism with hemodynamic compromise; thus thrombolytic therapy is indicated.[32]

27. **b.** Atrial arrhythmia. There have been many laboratory, ECG, and echocardiogram findings shown to be predictive of mortality and prognosis. Right ventricular dysfunction, particularly when accompanied by hypotension, is predictive of pulmonary embolism–related hospital mortality. Elevated serum troponin and elevated brain natriuretic peptide have also been shown to predict an increased risk of death. Additional findings associated with a poorer prognosis include atrial arrhythmia, right bundle branch block, inferior Q waves and precordial T-wave inversions, and ST-segment changes. The other distracters have not been shown to predict prognosis.

28. **b.** Begin enoxaparin 1 mg/kg subcutaneous injections every 12 hours. Cancer patients are at a sixfold increased risk of developing VTE. Patients with active cancer make up about 20% of all new VTE diagnosed in the community. The risk, however, varies somewhat with cancer type, and those that incur a higher risk include malignant brain tumors and adenocarcinoma of the ovary, pancreas, colon, stomach, lung, prostate, and kidney. Several studies have demonstrated a benefit to treatment with LMWH when compared with coumadin in this patient population. One study, which compared dalteparin with coumadin, reported 27 of 336 patients in the LMWH group had recurrent VTE when compared with 53 of 336 in the coumadin group in a 6-month follow-up period. There was no increased risk of bleeding in the LMWH group.[33,34]

29. **e.** Proceed with placement of an inferior vena cava filter. The patient has a proximal DVT with a contraindication for anticoagulation. This scenario represents an absolute indication for the placement of an inferior vena cava filter. Pneumatic compression stockings are indicated for the prevention of VTE but not for treatment. Serial duplex ultrasound scans may be an acceptable strategy for management of isolated acute calf vein thrombosis but not for proximal DVT. IV unfractionated heparin or enoxaparin 1 mg/kg subcutaneous injections would be appropriate treatment options if the patient did not have a recent gastrointestinal bleed requiring transfusion.[35]

30. **c.** Order bilateral ABI measurements in the vascular laboratory at rest and following an exercise protocol. The patient in the clinical vignette presented with classic intermittent claudication symptoms suggestive of PAD. A normal resting ABI does not rule out PAD in a patient presenting with ambulatory symptoms.[36] Performing the test following exercise often unmasks significant disease revealing markedly lower ABI values. Exercise may be an appropriate suggestion but it will not help to establish the diagnosis of this patient's presenting problem. It would be premature to refer this patient for intervention. Pseudoclaudication may present similarly, but this patient has risk factors for PAD; therefore, a post exercise ABI would be the most appropriate next step in their workup. Repeating the resting ABI in 6 months is not likely to provide new information.

31. **c.** Less than 100 mg/dL. The most recent practice guidelines for the management of PAD, updated in March 2013, recommend a target LDL of less than 100 mg/dL for patients with an established diagnosis of PAD.[36]

32. c. Less than 130/80 mmHg. The most recent practice guidelines for the management of PAD, updated in March 2013, recommend a target blood pressure of less than 140/90 mmHg for patients with PAD. The guidelines recommend a lower target, less than 130/80 mmHg, for patients with PAD and concomitant diabetes mellitus or renal insufficiency.[36]

33. e. None of the above. Thiazide diuretics, angiotensin-converting enzyme inhibitors, angiotensin II receptor blockers, and β-adrenergic blockers are all acceptable medications to achieve blood pressure targets in patients with PAD.[36]

34. c. Every 6 to 12 months. According to the appropriate use criteria published by the intersocietal committee on peripheral vascular testing and the American College of Cardiology Foundation/American Heart Association practice guidelines for PAD, patients with an asymptomatic AAA measuring 4.0 to 5.4 cm should have surveillance imaging every 6 to 12 months in the first year.[36,37]

35. d. 5.5 cm or greater. The patient should be referred for repair once the infrarenal AAA reaches a diameter of 5.5 cm or greater due to an increased risk of spontaneous rupture.[36] Surveillance imaging is advised at regular intervals for aneurysms less than 5.5 cm.

36. e. All of the above groups are appropriate to screen for an AAA. According to the appropriate use criteria published by intersocietal committee on peripheral vascular testing all of the groups listed are appropriate for AAA screening.[37]

37. a. Four weeks after the intervention. All patients should get a baseline carotid duplex ultrasound within 4 weeks after a carotid artery stenting or endarterectomy procedure.[37]

38. b. Every 12 months. It is recommended to repeat carotid duplex ultrasound every 12 months after the first year following carotid artery stenting to assess for evidence of in-stent restenosis.[37]

39. c. Popliteal artery aneurysm. Shown is a transverse and longitudinal image of a large popliteal artery aneurysm containing mural thrombus. The appearance is not suggestive of an abscess, Baker cyst, lymph node, or lipoma.

40. d. 50%. A large number of patients with a popliteal artery aneurysm will also have an AAA. Furthermore, 50% of patients with a popliteal artery aneurysm will have an aneurysm of the contralateral popliteal artery.[38]

41. e. Refer for repair of the aneurysm. Popliteal artery aneurysms measuring greater than 2.5 cm are at risk for thrombosis, embolism, or rupture and therefore should be repaired.[36] Popliteal artery aneurysms measuring less than 2.5 cm are imaged at regular intervals.

42. b. Thromboembolism. Popliteal artery aneurysms most commonly cause thromboembolism that can lead to popliteal artery occlusion or painful distal embolic lesions. Rupture of popliteal artery aneurysms occurs infrequently.[38,39]

43. d. Pseudoaneurysm. The spectral Doppler waveform shown is a typical to-and-fro signal seen within the neck of the pseudoaneurysm. The incidence of pseudoaneurysm complicating percutaneous arterial procedures ranges between 0.2% and 0.5%. Patients typically present post catheter-based procedure with a painful pulsatile mass. When small these may resolve spontaneously, while others require intervention such as ultrasound-guided thrombin injection or surgical repair.[5]

44. c. Subclavian artery stenosis. Color Doppler imaging shows significant color aliasing, spectral broadening, and turbulent high-velocity flow within the subclavian artery. It is important to recognize severe subclavian artery stenosis prior to coronary artery bypass surgery in which the internal mammary artery may be utilized. Severe subclavian artery stenosis can lead to retrograde flow in the internal mammary artery predisposing to early graft failure. In an aneurysm usually the velocities are decreased.

45. c. Warfarin skin necrosis. Pictured is a large erythematous lesion with surrounding violaceous borders. Given the history of several days of high doses of warfarin without parental anticoagulation makes warfarin skin necrosis the most correct response. Heparin skin necrosis has been described but usually occurs at the site of subcutaneous injections.

HIT can rarely be associated with necrotic skin lesions but in this case her platelets remained stable. A vasculitis can cause skin necrosis but is unlikely in the given scenario.

46. d. Aortic valve stenosis. The waveforms in the bilateral internal carotid and vertebral arteries have a Tardus-Parvus morphology. They have a blunted and slow upstroke, suggesting more proximal or central narrowing. In this patient, these findings along with a systolic murmur are suggestive of aortic valve stenosis.

47. d. Saddle pulmonary embolism. This patient has a pulmonary embolism involving both main pulmonary arteries. Massive and submassive pulmonary embolism can cause an increase in troponin and B-type natriuretic peptide as seen in acute myocardial infarction. The image shown illustrates a filling defect within the main pulmonary artery at the bifurcation. There are no findings suggestive of aortic dissection, pneumonia, or interstitial fibrosis.

48. c. Carotid intima-media thickness. According to the latest American College of Cardiology/American Heart Association cardiovascular risk assessment guidelines, there is insufficient evidence available to recommend use of carotid intima-media thickness, ApoB, albuminuria, glomerular filtration rate, or cardiorespiratory fitness in cardiovascular risk assessment. There is adequate evidence to recommend use of high-sensitivity C-reactive protein, ABI, coronary artery calcium score, and a family history of premature cardiovascular disease for refinement of cardiovascular risk assessment.[40]

REFERENCES

1. Dziewas R, Konrad C, Drager B, et al. Cervical artery dissection. *J Neurol.* 2003;250(10):1179–1184.

2. Mafee MF, Raofi B, Kumar A, et al. Glomus faciale, glomus jugulare, glomus tympanicum, glomus vagale, carotid body tumors, and simulating lesions. Role of MR imaging. *Radiol Clin North Am.* 2000;38(5):1059–1076.

3. Wilgis EF. Evaluation and treatment of chronic digital ischemia. *Ann Surg.* 1981;193(6):693–698.

4. Slovut DP, Olin JW. Fibromuscular dysplasia. *N Engl J Med.* 2004;350 (18):1862–1871.

5. Ferguson JD, Whatling PT, Martin V, et al. Ultrasound guided percutaneous thrombin injection of iatrogenic femoral artery pseudoaneurysms after coronary angiography and intervention. *Heart.* 2001;85(4):e5.

6. Kelm M, Perings SM, Jax T, et al. Incidence and clinical outcome of iatrogenic femoral arteriovenous fistulas, implications for risk stratification and treatment. *J Am Coll Cardiol.* 2002;40(2):291–297.

7. McEllistrem RF, O'Toole DP, Keane P. Post cannulation radial artery aneurysm—a rare complication. *Can J Anaesth.* 1990;37:907–909.

8. Podlaha J, Holub R, Konecny Z, et al. 20 year experience with operations for popliteal artery aneurysm. *BMJ/Bratisl Lek Listy.* 2005;106(12): 421–422.

9. TASC Guidelines. Management of PAD. *J Vasc Surg.* 2000;31:S1–S296.

10. Criqui MH, Fronek A, Klauber MR, et al. The sensitivity, specificity, and predictive value of traditional clinical evaluation of peripheral arterial disease: results from noninvasive testing in a defined population. *Circulation.* 1985;71:516–522.

11. Hirsch AT, Haskal ZJ, Hertzer NR, et al. ACC/AHA 2005 practice guidelines for the management of patients with peripheral arterial disease (lower extremity, renal, mesenteric, and abdominal aortic): a collaborative report from the American Association for Vascular Surgery/ Society for Vascular Surgery, Society for Cardiovascular Angiography and Interventions, Society for Vascular Medicine and Biology, Society of Interventional Radiology, and the ACC/AHA Task Force on Practice Guidelines (Writing Committee to Develop Guidelines for the Management of Patients with Peripheral Arterial Disease). *Circulation.* 2006;21(113):e471–e486.

12. Hirsch AT, Haskal ZJ, Hertzer NR, et al. ACC/AHA 2005 practice guidelines for the management of patients with peripheral arterial disease (lower extremity, renal, mesenteric, and abdominal aortic): a collaborative report from the American Association for Vascular Surgery/ Society for Vascular Surgery, Society for Cardiovascular Angiography and Interventions, Society for Vascular Medicine and Biology, Society of Interventional Radiology, and the ACC/AHA Task Force on Practice Guidelines (Writing Committee to Develop Guidelines for the Management of Patients with Peripheral Arterial Disease). *Circulation.* 2006;21(113):e525–e557.

13. Hirsch AT, Haskal ZJ, Hertzer NR, et al. ACC/AHA 2005 practice guidelines for the management of patients with peripheral arterial disease (lower extremity, renal, mesenteric, and abdominal aortic): a collaborative report from the American Association for Vascular Surgery/ Society for Vascular Surgery, Society for Cardiovascular Angiography and Interventions, Society for Vascular Medicine and Biology, Society of Interventional Radiology, and the ACC/AHA Task Force on Practice Guidelines (Writing Committee to Develop Guidelines for the Management of Patients with Peripheral Arterial Disease). *Circulation.* 2006;21:e527–e533.

14. Hirsch AT, Haskal ZJ, Hertzer NR, et al. ACC/AHA 2005 practice guidelines for the management of patients with peripheral arterial disease (lower extremity, renal, mesenteric, and abdominal aortic): a collaborative report from the American Association for Vascular Surgery/ Society for Vascular Surgery, Society for Cardiovascular Angiography and Interventions, Society for Vascular Medicine and Biology, Society of Interventional Radiology, and the ACC/AHA Task Force on Practice

Guidelines (Writing Committee to Develop Guidelines for the Management of Patients with Peripheral Arterial Disease). *Circulation.* 2006;21(113):e547–e557.

15. Warkentin TE, Greinacher A. Review heparin-induced thrombocytopenia: recognition, treatment, and prevention: the Seventh ACCP Conference on Antithrombotic and Thrombolytic Therapy. *Chest.* 2004;126;311S–317S.

16. Warkentin TE, Greinacher A. Heparin-induced thrombocytopenia: recognition, treatment, and prevention: the Seventh ACCP Conference on Antithrombotic and Thrombolytic Therapy. *Chest.* 2004;126;311–337.

17. Wigley FM. Raynaud's phenomenon. *N Engl J Med.* 2002;347:1001–1008.

18. Creager MA, Dzau VJ, Loscalzo J. *Vascular Medicine: A Companion to Braunwald's Heart Disease.* Philadelphia, PA: Elsevier Health Sciences; 2006:689–706.

19. Hoeper MM, Mayer E, Simonneau G, et al. Chronic thromboembolic pulmonary hypertension. *Circulation.* 2006;113:2011–2020.

20. Ely JW, Osheroff JA, Chambliss ML, et al. Approach to leg edema of uncertain etiology. *J Am Board Fam Med.* 2006;19:148–160.

21. Eberhardt RT, Raffetto JD. Chronic venous insufficiency. *Circulation.* 2005;111:2398–2409.

22. Buller HR, Agnelli G, Hull RD, et al. Antithrombotic therapy for venous thromboembolic disease: the Seventh ACCP Conference on Antithrombotic and Thrombolytic Therapy. *Chest.* 2004;126:401S–428S.

23. Bates SM, Greer IA, Hirsh J, et al. See use of antithrombotic agents during pregnancy: the Seventh ACCP Conference on Antithrombotic and Thrombolytic Therapy, Section 5.0. *Chest.* 2004;126:627S–644S.

24. Young JR, Olin JW, Bartholomew JR, eds. *Peripheral Vascular Diseases,* 2nd ed. St. Louis, MO: Mosby; 1996:614–617.

25. Hann CH, Streiff MB. The role of vena cava filters in the management of venous thromboembolism. *Blood Rev.* 2005;19:179–202.

26. Creager MA, Dzau VJ, Loscalzo J, eds. *Vascular Medicine: A Companion to Braunwald's Heart Disease.* Philadelphia, PA: Saunders; 2006:159–160.

27. The Sixth ACCP Conference on Antithrombotic and Thrombolytic Therapy: evidence-based guidelines. *Chest Suppl.* 2001;119:176S–193S.

28. Creager MA, Dzau VJ, Loscalzo J, eds. *Vascular Medicine: A Companion to Brunwald's Heart Disease.* Philadelphia, PA: Saunders; 2006:641–654.

29. Cil BE, Akpinar E, Karcaaltincaba M, et al. Case 76: May-Thurner syndrome. *Radiology.* 2004;233:361–365.

30. Takahaski PY, Kiemele LJ, Jones JP. Wound care for elderly patients: advances and clinical applications for practicing physicians. *Mayo Clin Proc.* 2004;79:260–267.

31. Dewald CL, Jensen CC, Park YH, et al. Vena cavography with CO_2 versus iodinated contrast material for IVC filter placement: a prospective evaluation. *Radiology.* 2000;216:752–756.

32. The Seventh ACCP Conference on Antithrombotic and Thrombolytic Therapy: evidence-based guidelines. *Chest Suppl.* 2004;126:413S.

33. Lee AYY, Levine MN, Baker RI, et al. Low-molecular-weight heparin versus coumadin for the prevention of recurrent venous thromboembolism in patients with cancer. *N Engl J Med.* 2003;349:146–153.

34. The Seventh ACCP Conference on Antithrombotic and Thrombolytic Therapy: evidence-based guidelines. *Chest Suppl.* 2004;126:371S.

35. Kearon C, Akl EA, Comerota AJ, et al. Antithrombotic therapy for VTE disease: antithrombotic therapy and prevention of thrombosis, 9th ed: American College of Chest Physicians evidence-based clinical practice guidelines. *Chest.* 2012;141:e419S–e494S.

36. Anderson JL, Halperin JL, Albert NM, et al. Management of patients with peripheral artery disease (compilation of 2005 and 2011 ACCF/ AHA guideline recommendations): a report of the American College of Cardiology Foundation/American Heart Association Task Force on Practice Guidelines. *Circulation.* 2013;127:1425–1443.

37. Mohler III ER, Gornik HL, Gerhard-Herman M, et al. ACCF/ACR/AIUM/ASE/ASN/ICAVL/SCAI/SCCT/SIR/SVM/SVS 2012 appropriate use criteria for peripheral vascular ultrasound and physiological testing part I: arterial ultrasound and physiological testing. *J Am Coll Cardiol.* 2012;60:242–276.

38. Huang Y, Gloviczki P, Noel AA, et al. Early complications and long-term outcome after open surgical treatment of popliteal artery aneurysms: is exclusion with saphenous vein bypass still the gold standard? *J Vasc Surg.* 2007;45:706–713.

39. Dawson I, Sie RB, van Bockel JH, et al. Atherosclerotic popliteal aneurysm. *Br J Surg.* 1997; 84:293–299.

40. Goff Jr DC, Lloyd-Jones DM, Bennett G, et al. 2013 ACC/AHA guideline on the assessment of cardiovascular risk. *J Am Coll Cardiol.* 2013. doi:10.1016/j.jacc.2013.11.005

chapter 8

Congestive Heart Failure

Miriam S. Jacob • Gary S. Francis • Leslie Cho

QUESTIONS ● ● ● ○

1. Your patient is a 50-year-old woman with nonischemic cardiomyopathy who just received an orthotopic heart transplant. Which of the following is NOT important to help prevent transplant vasculopathy?

   a. Empirically starting statin therapy
   b. Strict control of hypertension (HTN) and diabetes
   c. Use of rapamycin as part of the immunosuppressive regimen
   d. Abstinence from smoking

2. You are taking care of a 65-year-old man with history of coronary artery disease and prior bypass surgery. He is currently taking carvedilol and lisinopril at maximum doses. He was recently hospitalized for heart failure 3 months ago. Which of the following criteria would make it reasonable to add eplerenone to his regimen?

   a. Ejection fraction (EF) of 15% with creatinine clearance of 20 mL/min/1.73 m^2
   b. EF of 20% and dyspnea while doing chores at home (New York Heart Association [NYHA] class II symptoms)
   c. EF of 35% with QRS >130 milliseconds
   d. EF of 45% and dyspnea with walking less than a block

3. For a patient with heart failure, coronary artery bypass grafting (CABG) is not reasonable for a patient with severe three-vessel coronary artery disease and

   a. chest pain on exertion.
   b. no viability found on dobutamine echo with EF of 15%.
   c. recent ST-elevation myocardial infarction (MI).
   d. heart failure with preserved EF.
   e. systolic heart failure with EF of 30% and viable myocardium.

4. A 60-year-old African American man comes to your clinic with few months' history of fatigue, dyspnea on exertion, and lower extremity edema. He has no history of prior coronary artery disease or heart failure. What features on an echo would not be consistent with amyloid heart disease?

   a. Presence of a pericardial effusion
   b. Biatrial enlargement

   c. Normal tissue Doppler measurement of the left ventricular (LV) lateral and septal walls

   d. LV hypertrophy

   e. Grade 3 diastolic dysfunction

5. Which of the following characterizes heart failure?

   a. Downregulation of β_1- and β_2-receptors

   b. Downregulation primarily of β_1-receptors with little change in β_2-receptors

   c. Downregulation of G proteins and β_1- and β_2-receptors

   d. Increase in myocardial norepinephrine stores

   e. Intact baroreceptor function

6. In the Veterans Administration Heart Failure Trial II (V-HeFT II), which combination of medications improved LV function and exercise tolerance?

   a. Angiotensin-converting enzyme (ACE) inhibitors

   b. Hydralazine plus nitrates

   c. ACE inhibitor plus hydralazine plus nitrates

   d. ACE inhibitor plus nitrates

7. A 56-year-old man presents to your clinic for follow-up after being discharged from the hospital 6 weeks ago. He underwent a successful primary angioplasty for acute anterior MI; however, his EF is now 40%. He is currently taking simvastatin (Zocor), acetylsalicylic aspirin, clopidogrel bisulfate (Plavix), metoprolol tartrate (Lopressor), and losartan (Cozaar). He states that he cannot afford all of these medications. He would like to know which medications are essential for a longer life. Which medications should you tell him are essential?

   a. All of them

   b. All of them except clopidogrel bisulfate

   c. All of them except losartan

   d. All except clopidogrel bisulfate and losartan

8. A 78-year-old woman with congestive heart failure (CHF) (EF, 25%), chronic atrial fibrillation (AFib), gastroesophageal reflux disease, HTN, hyperlipidemia, diabetes, and osteoporosis takes 12 different pills. At the recent senior citizen day at the local church, a nurse told her that she does not need to take digoxin because she is on amiodarone. She wants to eliminate digoxin from her medication regimen, and she wants to know why you put her on it in the first place. What is your answer?

   a. Digoxin improves survival.

   b. Digoxin reduces hospitalization.

   c. Digoxin improves contractility.

   d. Digoxin decreases the volume of distribution of amiodarone.

   e. Digoxin reduces sympathetic nervous system activity.

9. Recently, a 43-year-old lawyer received heart transplantation. His hospital course was unremarkable, and he was discharged. He found out from the heart failure nurses that allograft vasculopathy is the leading cause of long-term morbidity and mortality in transplant patients. He wants to know what proven treatments prevent allograft vasculopathy. Which of the following treatments should you recommend?

   a. Annual cardiac catheterization, intravascular ultrasound, and percutaneous coronary intervention (PCI), as needed

   b. Annual stress test

    c. Biannual stress test

    d. Statins

    e. No known treatment

10. A 72-year-old woman is transferred from another hospital. She was initially admitted with palpitation, diagnosed with AFib, and treated with amiodarone. A transthoracic echocardiogram (TTE) showed an EF of 10% with a regional wall motion abnormality. She underwent cardiac catheterization and was found to have a heavily calcified 80% lesion in the mid–left anterior descending artery (LAD), a 40% lesion in a nondominant circumflex, and an 80% lesion in the posterior descending artery. Her children want to know what you plan to do for her. What should you recommend?

    a. She has terrible EF and should be on medication only because CABG would be of too high risk.

    b. She should undergo PCI because she is too high risk for CABG.

    c. She should undergo CABG because this is the definitive treatment.

    d. She should have a positron emission tomography (PET) scan to assess the area of viability before proceeding with CABG or PCI.

11. A 53-year-old woman with a history of CHF presents to the emergency room (ER). She is cool and clammy. She reports being short of breath. Her blood pressure (BP) is 71/40 mmHg, her heart rate (HR) is 110 bpm, and her respiratory rate is 30. She has elevated neck veins and a prominent S_3. Her echocardiogram (ECG) shows sinus tachycardia. She is admitted to the CCU (coronary care unit) with heart failure. A pulmonary artery (PA) catheterization is performed, and her hemodynamics are as follows: right atrial (RA) pressure, 12 mmHg; PA pressure, 62/30 mmHg; cardiac output, 1.9 L/min/m^2; pulmonary capillary wedge pressure (PCWP), 36 mmHg; and systemic vascular resistance (SVR), 2,000 dyne/s/cm^5. Which of the following is your next step?

    a. Start furosemide (Lasix).

    b. Start dopamine.

    c. Insert intra-aortic balloon pump (IABP).

    d. Begin dobutamine.

    e. Start nesiritide.

12. This patient continues to deteriorate after your initial treatment. Her BP is 64/32 mmHg, and her HR is 132 bpm. She is now intubated on maximal pressor support and has an IABP in place. Which of the following should be your next therapeutic option?

    a. There is no option. She is on maximal therapy.

    b. Consider emergent cardiac transplant.

    c. Consider LV assist device.

    d. Consider cardiopulmonary bypass.

13. A 35-year-old man with a history of HTN presents to the ER in respiratory distress. He is intubated in the ER for respiratory distress. His BP is 73/48 mmHg, his HR is 130 bpm, and his respiratory rate is 20. He is taken to the medical ICU (intensive care unit), and a PA catheterization is performed. His hemodynamics are as follows: RA pressure, 22 mmHg; PA pressure, 20/10 mmHg; cardiac output, 3.5 L/min/m^2; PCWP, 12 mmHg; and SVR, 1,690 dyne/s/cm^5. What is your diagnosis?

    a. Pulmonary embolism

    b. Cardiogenic shock

    c. Acute right ventricular (RV) failure

   d. Decompensated heart failure

   e. Hypovolemic shock

14. You receive a call from a cardiologist in a small community hospital regarding a patient in heart failure. She states that the patient was admitted last night with heart failure and was started on intravenous (IV) nitroglycerin; IV furosemide infusion; captopril, 12.5 mg t.i.d.; and digoxin. There has been no improvement; therefore, the cardiologist placed a Swan-Ganz catheter this morning. The patient's hemodynamics are as follows: BP, 120/89 mmHg; HR, 89 bpm; cardiac output, 2.0 L/min/m^2; PCWP, 29 mmHg; and SVR, 1,766 dyne/s/cm^5. The cardiologist also added dobutamine. Which of the following additional therapies should you recommend to the cardiologist for this patient?

   a. Begin patient transfer arrangement.

   b. Suggest nitroprusside.

   c. Suggest nesiritide.

   d. Suggest dopamine.

   e. Suggest IABP.

15. A 57-year-old woman, who experienced inferior wall MI in 1992, has an EF of 30% and was diagnosed with nonsustained ventricular tachycardia (VT) (four beats of VT) at another hospital on a routine ECG that she needed before cataract surgery. She has been in excellent health and has never been hospitalized for CHF. She has never had palpitation or syncopal episodes. Her doctors advised her that she would need an implantable defibrillator. She does not agree and wants a second opinion. She wants to know whether there is any evidence to support the implantable defibrillators. What is your advice?

   a. Place an implantable defibrillator.

   b. Do not place an implantable defibrillator: A single episode is probably insignificant.

   c. Perform an electrophysiologic (EP) study.

   d. Begin β-blockers with amiodarone.

16. A 49-year-old man is admitted with new-onset heart failure. He is diagnosed with dilated cardiomyopathy with an EF of 20%. On hospital day 1, he is diuresed and started on a regimen of furosemide, digoxin, acetylsalicylic aspirin, captopril, and simvastatin. A medical student wants to know why you did not start him on a β-blocker. What is your explanation?

   a. β-Blockers have not been shown to decrease mortality in dilated cardiomyopathy patients. Only ischemic cardiomyopathy patients have derived benefit.

   b. There have been several conflicting results from randomized trials; therefore, β-blockers are not recommended as the first line of therapy.

   c. β-Blockers have been shown to improve survival but should only be used in patients with an EF greater than 25%.

   d. β-Blockers should be started in stable CHF patients.

17. The same medical student wants to know whether the patient should also be started on calcium channel blockers. What is your answer?

   a. There has never been a study to demonstrate the benefit of calcium channel blockers.

   b. Diltiazem has proved to be of small but significant benefit in nonischemic cardiomyopathy patients and should be started.

   c. Calcium channel blockers should be started after discharge once the patient has been stabilized.

d. Felodipine has proved to be of small benefit only in ischemic cardiomyopathy patients. This patient does not fit this criterion.

e. Amlodipine proved to be of small benefit in a NYHA class III or IV patient with an EF <30%. This benefit was seen more in dilated cardiomyopathy patients.

18. A 24-year-old female medical student presents to urgent care with 5 days of fever and shortness of breath. She is diagnosed with a viral infection and sent home. Five months later during her physical examination class, she is found to have an S_3 by her fellow students. She presents to your office for a second opinion. On examination, she appears healthy and in no distress. Her BP is 96/50 mmHg, with an HR of 71 bpm and a respiratory rate of 12. Her neck veins are not distended, and her examination is unremarkable except for an enlarged heart. You do not appreciate an S_3. You order a TTE, which shows an EF of 20% with a dilated heart. There is no valvular abnormality. Which of the following is your recommendation?

    a. Begin ACE inhibitor, β-blockers, and steroid.

    b. Begin ACE inhibitor and β-blockers.

    c. Begin ACE inhibitor, β-blockers, diuretics, and digoxin.

    d. Begin ACE inhibitor, β-blockers, diuretics, and spironolactone.

    e. She is well compensated; nothing needs to be done.

19. A 79-year-old man with diabetes, HTN, chronic renal insufficiency, and ischemic cardiomyopathy was recently admitted with CHF exacerbation. At home, he takes captopril, 75 mg t.i.d.; digoxin, 0.125 mg per day; furosemide, 60 mg b.i.d.; aspirin; and atorvastatin calcium (Lipitor). When admitted, he was in heart failure with elevated neck veins and S_3. During his admission, he was diuresed with IV furosemide and metolazone. His baseline creatinine was 1.7 and now is 2.5, with blood urea nitrogen of 100. What is your next step?

    a. Stop captopril.

    b. Stop diuretics.

    c. Rule out renal artery stenosis.

    d. Stop aspirin and ACE inhibitor.

20. The severity of symptomatic exercise limitation in heart failure

    a. is caused by elevated PCWP.

    b. is caused by reduced blood flow to skeletal muscles.

    c. bears little relation to the severity of LV dysfunction.

    d. can be reversed by inotropic therapy.

    e. is related to markers of central hemodynamic disturbance.

21. A 59-year-old woman with CHF and an EF of 30% comes to your office for follow-up. She is on carvedilol (Coreg), enalapril, aspirin, atorvastatin calcium, digoxin, and furosemide. She has been doing well without any rehospitalization. However, she wants to improve her exercise tolerance. What should you recommend?

    a. Cardiac transplantation

    b. IV dobutamine

    c. Higher doses of ACE inhibitor

    d. Adding spironolactone

    e. Enrolling her in an exercise training program

22. Prognosis in heart failure correlates best with which of the following?

    a. Peak $\dot{V}O_2$ during exercise

    b. $\dot{V}_E/\dot{V}O_2$ slope during exercise

    c. EF at rest

   d. Blood gases during exercise

   e. Myocardial contractility measurements

23. An 86-year-old woman is transferred from a nursing home in respiratory distress. She was found to be short of breath. On examination, she has labored breathing, and her BP is 62/34 mmHg with an HR of 60 bpm. She is intubated in the ER and admitted to the CCU. She is started on norepinephrine and dopamine at high doses without significant effect. Her ECG shows sinus bradycardia but is otherwise unremarkable. Her chest X-ray (CXR) shows pulmonary edema. The nursing home calls and says that she has mistakenly received 100 mg IV metoprolol tartrate. Which of the following should be your next step?

   a. Glucagon and milrinone

   b. Glucagon and dobutamine

   c. IABP

   d. Fluid resuscitation

   e. Transvenous pacemaker

24. A 62-year-old man with an EF of 20% and chronic renal insufficiency presents to your office for follow-up. He has non-insulin-dependent diabetes mellitus and has developed worsening renal failure caused by diabetes. His medication regimen includes a β-blocker that is significantly affected by reduced renal function. Which of the following β-blockers is he taking?

   a. Propranolol

   b. Atenolol

   c. Carvedilol

   d. Metoprolol

   e. Sotalol

25. A 38-year-old patient with CHF is transferred from another hospital. You are doing rounds in the CCU while the clinicians are performing a TTE. They ask you to assess his LV function. You notice that the E:A wave ratio is greater than 1.5, with an E-wave deceleration time of 120 milliseconds. Which of the following do you guess is his PCWP?

   a. PCWP is 12 mmHg.

   b. PCWP is 18 mmHg.

   c. PCWP is 26 mmHg.

   d. You cannot tell from the E:A wave ratio and deceleration time.

26. For the patient in the previous question, the E:A wave ratio and the E-wave deceleration time indicate which of the following?

   a. Low filling pressure and reduced LV compliance

   b. High filling pressure and increased LV compliance

   c. Low filling pressure and increased LV compliance

   d. High filling pressure and reduced LV compliance

27. A 67-year-old patient with HTN, hyperlipidemia, and an EF of 45% comes to your office for a second opinion. He had an exercise test and was told that his HR recovery was abnormal. His physician told him not to worry *unless* his heart function deteriorates. He is not convinced and wants your opinion and treatment. What should you recommend?

   a. Abnormal HR recovery does not predict mortality in patients with an EF greater than 35%; therefore, no treatment is needed.

   b. Abnormal HR recovery predicts mortality only in patients after MI; therefore, no treatment is needed.

c. Abnormal HR recovery predicts mortality in all patients; however, there is no treatment.

d. Abnormal HR recovery predicts mortality in all patients, and exercise training is the treatment of choice.

28. A 41-year-old man presents to the CCU with CHF symptoms. On examination, he has elevated neck veins, severe peripheral edema, and S_3 gallop. He is started on medication and has improvement in all of his symptoms. He has a PET scan, which shows a large area of hibernating myocardium. His cardiac catheterization reveals mild disease in the right coronary artery, a focal 80% lesion in the circumflex, and a focal 70% lesion in the LAD. All of his lesions are type A American College of Cardiologists/American Heart Association score. His EF is 15%. According to randomized clinical trials, which of the following is the best treatment for this patient?

    a. Percutaneous transluminal coronary angioplasty (PTCA)/stent with abciximab and clopidogrel bisulfate

    b. PTCA/stent with cardiothoracic surgery backup

    c. CABG

    d. PTCA/stent with abciximab and IABP

29. A 28-year-old woman comes to your office for a second opinion. She had peripartum cardiomyopathy and wants to get pregnant again. You obtain a TTE, which shows a normal LV. What should you recommend?

    a. She should not have another pregnancy because she is likely to have recurrent cardiomyopathy.

    b. She may conceive again because her LV is normal. Her chance of having recurrent cardiomyopathy is less than 5%.

    c. She may conceive again because her LV is normal. However, her chance of having recurrent cardiomyopathy is 30% to 50%.

    d. She should undergo exercise testing for better assessment.

30. A 78-year-old retired federal judge comes to your office for follow-up. He has long-standing HTN and has undergone PTCA/stent for a mid-LAD lesion. He has normal LV function and is active and healthy. Currently he is on ramipril (Altace), atorvastatin, and aspirin. He heard on television that the combination of aspirin and ramipril increases mortality. He wants your opinion. What is your answer?

    a. These are only observational studies, and they have not been proven. Continue the current regimen.

    b. There are randomized studies to support this; however, the sample size was too small to make any conclusive recommendations. Continue the current regimen.

    c. This has been shown in large trials; we should change aspirin to clopidogrel bisulfate or ramipril to metoprolol tartrate.

    d. Although this has been seen in retrospective trials, it has not been validated in a randomized trial; therefore, continue the current regimen.

31. A 56-year-old man with dilated cardiomyopathy with an EF of 15% comes to your office for an opinion regarding medication. He is in NYHA class II and wants to know about biventricular pacing. He heard on television news that this may save lives. His ECG shows a sinus rate of 71, a PR interval of 210 milliseconds, a QRS duration of 188 milliseconds, and a QT/QT_C of 364:427 milliseconds. What should you recommend?

    a. Refer the patient for biventricular pacing based on PR interval.

    b. Refer the patient for biventricular pacing based on QRS duration.

   c. Refer the patient for biventricular pacing based on QT/QT_C interval.

   d. Refer the patient for exercise test to further assess.

32. A 31-year-old woman with hypertrophic cardiomyopathy presents to your office for follow-up. She has been doing well. She denies any palpitation or syncope. She has researched her disease on the Web and found out that most people die of arrhythmia. She would like to have an EP study. Which of the following is the predictive value of the EP study for ventricular arrhythmia?

   a. 20%

   b. 40%

   c. 50%

   d. 80%

   e. 100%

33. A 61-year-old woman with an EF of 50% is admitted with an AFib with rapid ventricular response. She is started on metoprolol tartrate with excellent rate control and heparin. Her daughter, who is a nurse, wants to know why you did not start her on dofetilide because this is the best new drug. What is your response?

   a. Dofetilide showed increased mortality when compared with amiodarone and would be a bad choice for her mother.

   b. Dofetilide had safety and efficacy comparable to those of β-blockers.

   c. Dofetilide was used in patients with an EF less than 35%.

   d. Dofetilide has safety and efficacy comparable to those of calcium channel blockers.

   e. Dofetilide is reserved for patients with chronic renal insufficiency.

34. A 79-year-old woman with HTN and non-insulin-dependent diabetes mellitus comes to your office for a second opinion. She is doing well and is currently on enalapril, aspirin, simvastatin, glipizide, and metformin. She read in her monthly American Association of Retired Persons newsletter that losartan is better than enalapril. She wants you to change her prescription. Based on trial data, which of the following is your recommendation?

   a. Losartan did not show mortality benefit but did show reduced hospitalization; because she has no history of CHF, there is no reason to change her medication.

   b. Losartan showed neither mortality benefit nor reduced hospitalization.

   c. Losartan did not show mortality benefit but decreased the risk of MI; therefore, she should have her prescription changed.

   d. Losartan did show mortality benefit, but only in patients younger than 60 years.

35. A 61-year-old woman with CHF and an EF of 25% is admitted with CHF exacerbation to your partner's service. On the day of discharge, your partner is sick, and you must explain her discharge medications. You explain to her the benefits of lisinopril, simvastatin, aspirin, digoxin, and furosemide. Finally, you want to explain the benefit of spironolactone (Aldactone) to her. What is your explanation?

   a. Spironolactone in addition to standard therapy (ACE inhibitor, diuretic) does not decrease mortality or morbidity.

   b. Spironolactone in addition to standard therapy only decreases rehospitalization—it does not improve NYHA functional class.

   c. Spironolactone in addition to standard therapy decreases mortality and rehospitalization.

   d. Spironolactone only benefits those not on standard therapy.

36. A 63-year-old man with non-insulin-dependent diabetes mellitus, HTN, hyperlipidemia, and chronic renal insufficiency is admitted with acute anterior wall MI 10 hours after symptom onset. He is taken emergently to the cardiac catheterization laboratory. He is noted to have proximal LAD occlusion, and he undergoes a successful PTCA/stent to the LAD with abciximab and heparin. His EF is noted to be 30% on a TTE performed 3 days later. On hospital day 4, he reports chest pain and is found to be in AFib with an HR of 121. His BP is 90/44 mmHg, and he is short of breath and anxious. Which of the following should you administer next?

    a. Procainamide

    b. Lidocaine

    c. Amiodarone

    d. Metoprolol tartrate

    e. Cardioversion

37. An LV pressure–volume loop is shown in Figure 8.1. Label 1, 2, 3, and 4.

    a. Mitral valve opening

    b. End diastole

    c. Aortic valve opening

    d. End systole

38. A 57-year-old man with a history of CHF presents with acute pulmonary edema. His BP is 110/60 mmHg with an HR of 92 bpm. His examination is consistent with heart failure. His hemodynamics are as follows: PA pressure, 62/27 mmHg; PCWP, 12 mmHg; cardiac output, 1.8 L/min/m^2; and SVR, 1,968 dyne/s/cm^5. Which way should the LV pressure–volume loop be shifted?

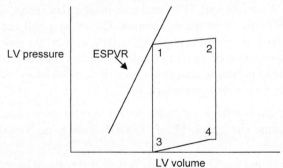

Figure 8.1 • ESPVR, end-systolic pressure–volume relation (From Little WC, Braunwald E. Assessment of cardiac function. In: Braunwald E, ed. *Heart Disease: A Textbook of Cardiovascular Medicine*, 5th ed. Philadelphia, PA: WB Saunders; 1997, with permission.)

    a. To the right

    b. To the left

    c. Up

    d. Down

Questions 39 to 43

Figures 8.2, 8.3, 8.4, 8.5, and 8.6 are schematic illustrations of the carotid pulse. Match the diagnosis with the pulse.

    a. Normal

    b. Aortic stenosis

    c. Aortic regurgitation

    d. Hypertrophic cardiomyopathy

    e. Severe CHF decompensation

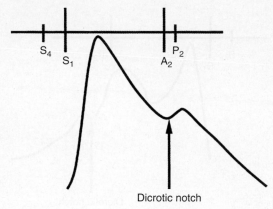

Figure 8.2 • (From Chatterjee K. Physical examination. In: Topol EJ, ed. *Textbook of Cardiovascular Medicine*, 2nd ed. Philadelphia, PA: Lippincott Williams & Wilkins; 2002: Fig. 15.2, with permission.)

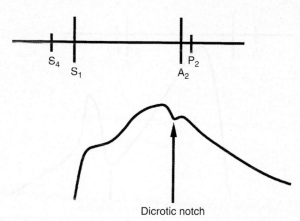

Figure 8.3 • (From Chatterjee K. Physical examination. In: Topol EJ, ed. *Textbook of Cardiovascular Medicine*, 2nd ed. Philadelphia, PA: Lippincott Williams & Wilkins; 2002: Fig. 15.2, with permission.)

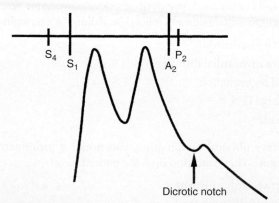

Figure 8.4 • (From Chatterjee K. Physical examination. In: Topol EJ, ed. *Textbook of Cardiovascular Medicine*, 2nd ed. Philadelphia, PA: Lippincott Williams & Wilkins; 2002: Fig. 15.2, with permission.)

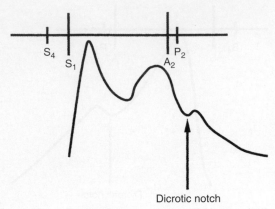

Dicrotic notch

Figure 8.5 • (From Chatterjee K. Physical examination. In: Topol EJ, ed. *Textbook of Cardiovascular Medicine*, 2nd ed. Philadelphia, PA: Lippincott Williams & Wilkins; 2002: Fig. 15.2, with permission.)

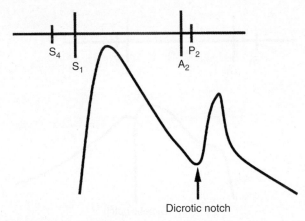

Dicrotic notch

Figure 8.6 • (From Chatterjee K. Physical examination. In: Topol EJ, ed. *Textbook of Cardiovascular Medicine*, 2nd ed. Philadelphia, PA: Lippincott Williams & Wilkins; 2002: Fig. 15.2, with permission.)

44. During physical examination, you notice an elevated systemic *venous* pressure with sharp *y*-descent Kussmaul sign and quiet pericardium. What might the patient have?

  a. Constrictive pericarditis
  b. Restrictive myocardial disorder
  c. Tricuspid regurgitation
  d. Pulmonary HTN
  e. Tamponade

45. During another physical examination, you notice a prominent v wave with a sharp *y* descent. What condition does the patient have?

  a. Constrictive cardiomyopathy
  b. Restrictive cardiomyopathy
  c. Tricuspid regurgitation
  d. Pulmonary HTN
  e. Tamponade

46. Again you notice an elevated systemic *venous* pressure without obvious *x* or *y* descent and quiet precordium and pulsus paradoxus. What does the patient have?

    a. Constrictive cardiomyopathy

    b. Restrictive cardiomyopathy

    c. Tricuspid regurgitation

    d. Pulmonary HTN

    e. Tamponade

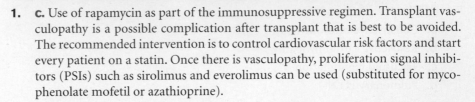

ANSWERS

1. **c.** Use of rapamycin as part of the immunosuppressive regimen. Transplant vasculopathy is a possible complication after transplant that is best to be avoided. The recommended intervention is to control cardiovascular risk factors and start every patient on a statin. Once there is vasculopathy, proliferation signal inhibitors (PSIs) such as sirolimus and everolimus can be used (substituted for mycophenolate mofetil or azathioprine).

2. **b.** EF of 20% and dyspnea while doing chores at home (New York Heart Association [NYHA] class II symptoms). Based on the results of Emphasis-HF trial, patients with NYHA class II symptoms and EF <30% are eligible for adding eplerenone to their regimen if they were hospitalized in the last 6 months or had an elevated brain natriuretic peptide. This extended the patients who could be placed on an aldosterone blocker. Previous studies studied the benefit of spironolactone in patients with NYHA class IV symptoms in the last 6 months and EF ≤35% and eplerenone in patients 2 weeks post-MI with EF ≤40% and signs of heart failure. Aldosterone antagonists should not be used in patients with creatinine clearance <30 mL/min/1.73 m². EF or QRS alone are not enough to determine patients who would benefit. Functional class assessment is important.

3. **b.** No viability found on dobutamine echo with EF of 15%. The use of surgical revascularization of coronary disease and systolic heart failure is reasonable in patients with acute coronary syndrome and symptomatic angina. Although in the STITCH (Surgical Treatment for Ischemic Heart Failure) trial, a study of medical therapy versus CABG in patients with EF ≤35%, there was no difference in all-cause mortality, there was a suggestion of a trend toward patients with CABG having fewer hospitalizations for heart failure or death from cardiovascular causes. The choice of CABG in a patient with no viability and very low EF is unlikely to be successful in improving morbidity or mortality from heart failure.

4. **c.** Normal tissue Doppler measurement of the left ventricular (LV) lateral and septal walls. Patients with amyloid heart disease usually show restrictive pattern of diastology with low tissue Doppler of the LV myocardium.

5. **b.** Downregulation primarily of β_1-receptors with little change in β_2-receptors. In the cardiac myocyte, there are 3 adrenergic receptors (α_1, β_1, and β_2). In a normal heart the predominant β receptor is β_1. In a failing heart there is selective down-regulation of β_1 receptors not β_2 receptors.

6. **b.** Hydralazine plus nitrates. In the V-HeFT II trial, although ACE inhibitors improved survival, it was hydralazine in combination with nitrates that had greater improvement in LV function and exercise tolerance.

7. **c.** All of them except losartan. There is no trial evidence that angiotensin II receptor blocker improved mortality in post-MI patients. The Studies of Left Ventricular Dysfunction (SOLVD) prevention used ACE inhibitors in patients with an EF less than 35%.

8. **b.** Digoxin reduces hospitalization. In the large Digitalis Investigation Group study, digitalis only improved hospitalization. It had no effect on survival.

9. **e.** No known treatment. Allograft vasculopathy is the leading cause of long-term morbidity and mortality for cardiac transplant patients. Routine cardiac catheterization has been advocated for these patients but has not shown survival benefit with revascularization. Statin therapy appears to improve long-term survival in these patients and should be used for all heart transplant patients. However, its effect on allograft vasculopathy is unknown.

10. **d.** She should have a positron emission tomography (PET) scan to assess the area of viability before proceeding with CABG or PCI. This patient is at high risk for any type of intervention because of her low EF. However, if there are areas of viability on the PET scan, her EF might improve with complete revascularization. Studies have consistently shown that patients with low EF do better with CABG than with PCI.

11. **b.** Start dopamine. This patient is in cardiogenic shock. She needs BP support before all else. In these patients, dopamine is the first line of choice, followed by norepinephrine. If there is no change with dopamine and norepinephrine, then dobutamine may be added while the patient is being prepared for IABP placement.

12. **c.** Consider LV assist device. This is a relatively young patient with no contraindication to cardiac transplant. However, in the current state, she is not eligible for transplantation. LV assist device as a bridge to transplant has been performed with success.

13. **c.** Acute right ventricular (RV) failure. His hemodynamic pressures are characteristic of acute RV failure. He needs aggressive fluid resuscitation.

14. **b.** Suggest nitroprusside. This patient is in heart failure and needs to have her BP and SVR lowered. BP is adequate and does not need vasopressor or IABP support. Although nesiritide has been approved for use in acute heart failure, it only mildly lowers the BP.

15. **a.** Place an implantable defibrillator. She fits the criteria of the initial Multicenter Automatic Defibrillator Trial (MADIT). Therefore, based on randomized clinical trial data, she would benefit from an implantable defibrillator. Also, secondary prevention trials such as the Antiarrhythmics Versus Implantable Defibrillators Trial, the Canadian Implantable Defibrillator Study, and the Cardiac Arrest Study Hamburg trial also support an implantable defibrillator in this patient.

16. **d.** β-Blockers should be started in stable CHF patients. They should not be started when the patient is congested. Although nonselective agents with vasodilating effects may be preferred, this is not clear at this time.

17. **e.** Amlodipine proved to be of small benefit in a NYHA class III or IV patient with an EF <30%. This benefit was seen more in dilated cardiomyopathy patients. In the Prospective Randomized Amlodipine Survival Evaluation Trial, in which NYHA class III or IV patients with an EF less than 30% were enrolled, there was a statistically insignificant reduction in the combined mortality and morbidity in the amlodipine group. However, the benefit appeared to be greater in patients with nonischemic cardiomyopathy.

18. **b.** Begin ACE inhibitor and β-blockers. She has well-compensated cardiomyopathy. Only medication that prolongs her life needs to be started. She does not need medication for symptom relief; therefore, ACE inhibitor and β-blockers should be started.

19. **b.** Stop diuretics. This patient has prerenal azotemia caused by aggressive diuresis. His renal function should recover.

20. **c.** Bears little relation to the severity of LV dysfunction. Short-term administration of positive inotropic agents and vasodilators does not improve maximal exercise capacity in patients with CHF. Moreover, ACE inhibitors have failed to show consistent improvement in exercise tolerance. Numerous studies have not shown a correlation between LV function and exercise tolerance.

21. **e.** Enrolling her in an exercise training program. As stated, there is no medication that has consistently shown improvement in exercise tolerance; exercise training is the only method that has shown consistent improvement in these patients.

22. **b.** $\dot{V}_E/\dot{V}O_2$ slope during exercise. This is the best correlate of prognosis. There is a higher ventilation for any given CO_2 production ($\dot{V}_E/\dot{V}O_2$ slope), which reflects the severity of heart failure and prognosis.

23. **a.** Glucagon and milrinone. Milrinone is a second-generation phosphodiesterase inhibitor. It has no β-effect; therefore, it is an ideal vasopressor in the setting of β-blocker overdose. Although a pacer is a good idea and should be placed, giving medication is faster and should be instituted first.

24. **b.** Atenolol. Atenolol is most affected by reduced renal function. Depending on how severe his creatinine clearance is, he should have his medication dose or frequency adjusted.

25. **c.** PCWP is 26 mmHg. Restrictive mitral inflow pattern in the presence of a short E-wave deceleration time has been shown to correlate with high pulmonary capillary pressure, impaired functional class, and bad prognosis in postinfarction patients.

26. **d.** High filling pressure and reduced LV compliance. These conditions are indicated by a restrictive mitral inflow pattern with short E-wave deceleration time.

27. **c.** Abnormal HR recovery predicts mortality in all patients; however, there is no treatment. A delayed decrease in HR after exercise or an abnormal HR recovery predicts all-cause mortality in healthy adults and in patients referred for exercise testing—independent of ischemia. However, at this time, there is no treatment to improve abnormal HR recovery.

28. **c.** CABG. This patient has left main trunk equivalent with low EF. He is a candidate for CABG with left internal mammary artery to the LAD. CABG will prolong his long-term survival compared with PTCA/stent.

29. **d.** She should undergo exercise testing for better assessment. Recurrent peripartum cardiomyopathy occurs in 20% of patients with normal resting LV function but abnormal stress ventricular response. Recurrent peripartum cardiomyopathy with decompensation occurred in 41% of patients with abnormal resting LV function.

30. **d.** Although this has been seen in retrospective trials, it has not been validated in a randomized trial; therefore, continue the current regimen. In a substudy done by the Gruppo Italiano per lo Studio della Sopravvivenza nell'Infarto Miocardico, aspirin did not decrease the mortality benefit of lisinopril after MI or increase the risk of adverse clinical events. There have been some retrospective studies to assess this question that have had conflicting results; therefore, it is best to stay with the current regimen.

31. **b.** Refer the patient for biventricular pacing based on QRS duration. Patients with QRS duration greater than 150 to 160 milliseconds derived the greatest benefit from biventricular pacing.

32. **a.** 20%. There is no role for routine EP study in the asymptomatic hypertrophic cardiomyopathy patient.

33. **c.** Dofetilide was used in patients with an EF less than 35%. The study compared dofetilide with amiodarone. Dofetilide did not increase mortality. It has not been studied against β-blockers or calcium channel blockers in patients with normal EF.

34. **b.** Losartan showed neither mortality benefit nor reduced hospitalization. In the large Evaluation of Losartan in the Elderly II study, losartan did not show mortality benefit or reduced hospitalization. Losartan was better tolerated than captopril. Because the patient has no side effects with enalapril, her prescription should not be changed.

35. **c.** Spironolactone in addition to standard therapy decreases mortality and rehospitalization. In the Randomized Aldactone Evaluation Study, patients with

NYHA class III or IV with an EF less than 35% had improvement in mortality, reduction in hospitalization, and improvement in functional class when spirono-lactone was taken in addition to standard therapy (ACE inhibitor and diuretic).

36. **e.** Cardioversion. This patient has post-MI AFib. He has LV dysfunction and renal insufficiency. Procainamide should be used in patients with normal LV and renal clearance. Amiodarone would take too long to work, and he is already in distress. Lidocaine is not used in AFib. Metoprolol tartrate would exacerbate his heart failure; therefore, cardioversion is the only choice.

37. An LV pressure–volume loop.
    a. = 1. Mitral valve opening
    b. = 2. End diastole
    c. = 3. Aortic valve opening
    d. = 4. End systole

38. **c.** Up. The response of the LV to increased afterload is to shift the loop up. Increased preload would shift the loop to the right.

39. **a.** Normal. The initial peak of the carotid puse waveform reflects the ejection of the blood from the LV into the aorta before it goes into the periphery. After the pressure peaks, it begins a decline as ejection slows and blood continues to flow to the periphery. There is a reversal of blood flow from the compliant central arteries back toward the ventricle. With this reversal of flow, the aortic valves close. A notch on the descending limb of the aortic pressure curve is associated with this transient reversal of blood flow. The smaller secondary positive wave is attributed to the elastic recoil of the aorta and aortic valve.

40. **b.** Aortic stenosis. Pulsus parvus et tardus which is characteristic of aortic steno-sis. Small and delayed carotid pulse.

41. **c.** Aortic regurgitation. Pulsus bisferiens or bifid arterial pulse.

42. **d.** Hypertrophic cardiomyopathy. This can also be characterized by a bisferiens carotid pulse with rapid fall in first wave with rapid rise of the second.

43. **e.** Severe CHF decompensation. Demonstrates the dicrotic pulse which can occur in diastole in patients with low stroke volume being ejected. This can occur in severe heart failure, cardiac tamponade, and hypovolemic shock.

44. **a.** Constrictive pericarditis. The high initial venous wave (a wave) is characteristic of atrial contraction. The rapid y descent is suggestive of rapid ventricular filling.

45. **c.** Tricuspid regurgitation. The v wave is a reflection of ventricular contraction and the pressure that is transmitted back to the atrium from a tricuspid valve that pushes back into the atrium. In the tricuspid regurgitation, there is increased pressure during ventricular systole.

46. **e.** Tamponade. There is constant pressure from the pericardium that does not allow for atrial relaxation so the y descent is blunted.

SUGGESTED READINGS

Greenberg B, Kahn AM. Chapter 26: Clinical assessment of heart failure. In: Braunwald E, ed. Heart Disease: A Textbook of Cardiovascular Medicine, 9th ed. Elsevier Saunders.

Chatterjee, K. Chapter 16: Physcial examniation. In: Topol EJ, Califf RM, eds. Textbook of Cardiovascular Medicine, 3rd ed. Philadelphia, PA: Lippincott Williams & Wilkins; 2007.

Costanzo MR, Dipchand A, Starlin R, et al. The International Society of Heart and Lung Transplantation guidelines for the care of heart transplant recipients. *J Heart Lung Transplant*. 2010;29(8):914–956.

Francis G. Pathophysiology of the heart failure clinical syndrome. In: Topol EJ, ed. *Textbook of Cardiovascular Medicine*, 2nd ed. Philadelphia, PA: Lippincott Williams & Wilkins; 2002.

Iyengar S, Haas GJ, Young JB. Chapter 86: Acute heart failure management. In: Topol EJ, Califf RM, eds. Textbook of Cardiovascular Medicine, 3rd ed. Philadelphia, PA: Lippincott Williams & Wilkins; 2007.

Mann D. Chapter 28: Management of heart failure with reduced ejection fraction. In: Braunwald E, ed. Heart Disease: A Textbook of Cardiovascular Medicine, 9th ed. Elsevier Saunders.

Tang WHW, Young JB. Chapter 87: Chronic heart failure management. In: Topol EJ, Califf RM, eds. Textbook of Cardiovascular Medicine, 3rd ed. Philadelphia, PA: Lippincott Williams & Wilkins; 2007.

chapter 9

Adult Congenital Heart Disease

Luke J. Burchill

Adult Congenital Heart Disease Source Material

Published guidelines for the management of adult congenital heart disease (ACHD) patients provide an excellent overview of ACHD and are a rich source of questions for the cardiology boards.[1-5] The questions in this section relate directly to existing guidelines for the care of ACHD patients, with particular emphasis given to the American Heart Association (AHA) guidelines.

QUESTIONS

1. A 55-year-old woman with a history of unrepaired ventricular septal defect (VSD) and Eisenmenger physiology presents to your clinic. Her most recent hemoglobin measured 17.5 g/dL (11.5 to 15.0), hematocrit 55% (36 to 46), mean corpuscular volume (MCV) 76 (83 to 99), and platelet count 140×10^3 cells/μL (150 to 400). She reports New York Heart Association class III limitations with increasing fatigue and infrequent headaches over the last 6 months. Blood pressure (BP) 110/70 mmHg, heart rate (HR) 70 BPM, and regular, O_2 saturation 77% on room air. Cardiac examination reveals peripheral clubbing and cyanosis, a parasternal heave, loud P_2, and a murmur of tricuspid regurgitation (TR). Electrocardiogram (ECG) shows sinus rhythm. She has had repeat phlebotomy for treatment of presumed hyperviscosity syndrome but does not feel any better. What of the following options is the most appropriate next step in management?

    a. Phlebotomy should continue until symptoms improve.

    b. Refer for heart–lung transplantation.

    c. Measure serum erythropoietin.

    d. Commence a pulmonary vasodilator.

    e. Obtain iron studies.

2. A 25-year-old man presents to your clinic with 48-hour history of documented fever and chills. He has a history of a "hole in the heart" and examination reveals a 4/6 systolic murmur heard loudest at the lower left sternal edge. A restrictive

muscular VSD is confirmed on echocardiogram. Which of the following is the most appropriate next step?

a. Oral antibiotics
b. Intravenous (IV) antibiotics
c. Blood cultures
d. Transesophageal echocardiogram
e. Cardiac surgery consult

3. Blood cultures are positive for *Streptococcus viridans* and the patient is treated for infective endocarditis (IE). A small mobile echodensity is noted adjacent to the VSD. At clinic review 3 months later he is much improved, repeat blood cultures are negative, and transesophageal echocardiography (TEE) is negative for vegetations. The patient asks whether his VSD should now be closed. What is the best answer?

a. Closure is indicated in those with a VSD complicated by IE.
b. VSD closure is NOT indicated in those with a VSD complicated by IE.
c. VSD closure is only indicated in the presence of a significant shunt (Q_p/Q_s, pulmonary to systemic blood flow ratio ≥ 2.0).
d. VSD closure is only indicated in the presence of a significant shunt accompanied by symptoms.

4. For which of the following conditions is IE prophylaxis not required prior to extensive dental procedures (more than one option may be correct)?

a. Ebstein anomaly without prior intervention
b. 4 weeks following percutaneous closure of a secundum atrial septal defect (ASD)
c. Mechanical aortic valve replacement (AVR) for bicuspid aortic valve disease
d. Eisenmenger syndrome
e. Tetralogy of Fallot (TOF) with residual VSD at the site of prior surgical repair

5. With which of the following adult congenital heart conditions can the following ECG tracing be seen (Fig. 9.1)?

a. Primum ASD
b. Congenitally corrected transposition
c. Ebstein anomaly
d. VSD
e. Coarctation of the aorta

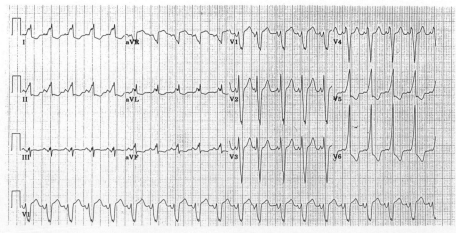

Figure 9.1

6. Which of the following is an absolute contraindication to pregnancy?
    a. Surgically corrected transposition of great arteries
    b. Congenitally corrected transposition of great arteries
    c. Ebstein anomaly
    d. Eisenmenger syndrome
    e. Status post Fontan operation

Questions 7 to 11

Match the following conditions with their corresponding surgical procedures. There may be more than one answer for each question.

7. Pulmonary atresia

8. D-transposition of great vessels

9. Tricuspid atresia

10. Congenitally corrected transposition of the great arteries

11. Aortic stenosis
    a. Ross
    b. Blalock-Taussig
    c. Senning or Mustard
    d. Arterial switch
    e. Fontan
    f. Rashkind
    g. None of the above

Questions 12 to 16

Match the following disease conditions with their gender preponderance.

12. VSD

13. ASD

14. Bicuspid aortic valve

15. Coarctation of the aorta

16. Pulmonary atresia with an intact ventricular septum
    a. Predominantly male
    b. Predominantly female
    c. Equal preponderance

Questions 17 to 21

Match the following cardiac catheterization still-frame slides (Figs. 9.2, 9.3, 9.4, 9.5, and 9.6) to their respective diagnoses.

17. Figure 9.2

18. Figure 9.3

19. Figure 9.4

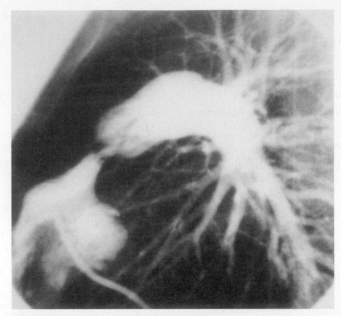

Figure 9.2

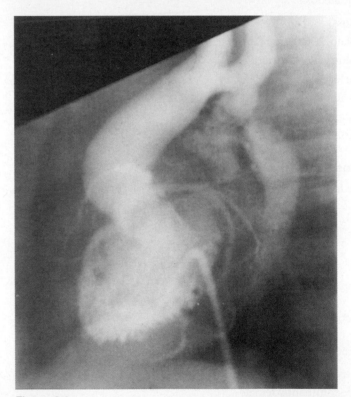

Figure 9.3

20. Figure 9.5

21. Figure 9.6

    a. Coarctation of the aorta

    b. Patent ductus arteriosus (PDA)

    c. Hypertrophic cardiomyopathy

    d. Pulmonic stenosis

    e. VSD

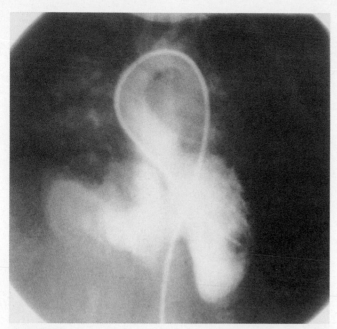

Figure 9.4

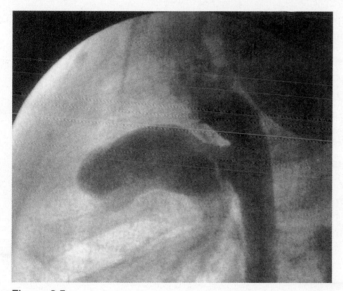

Figure 9.5

Questions 22 to 26

Match the physical examination findings with the corresponding adult congenital heart disorder.

22. Right ventricular (RV) lift with a loud systolic ejection murmur along the left sternal border, with a single S_2

23. Systolic ejection click, loud S1, holosystolic murmur, split S2 and hepatomegaly

24. Weak or delayed femoral arterial pulses, harsh systolic ejection murmur in the back, and a systolic ejection click in the aortic area

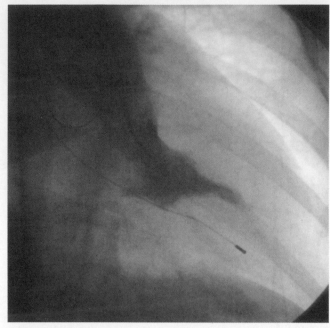

Figure 9.6

25. Cyanosis, digital clubbing, loud P_2, and a variable Graham Steell murmur

26. Wide pulse pressure, prominent left ventricular (LV) impulse, and a continuous machinery murmur enveloping S_2

   a. Eisenmenger syndrome

   b. Coarctation of the aorta

   c. PDA

   d. Ebstein anomaly

   e. TOF

Questions 27 to 31

Match the following congenital defects with their associated disease conditions. (more than one may apply)

27. Ostium primum ASD

28. Noonan syndrome

29. Coronary sinus ASD

30. Williams syndrome

31. Sinus venosus ASD

   a. Supravalvular aortic stenosis

   b. Supravalvular pulmonic stenosis

   c. Cleft mitral valve

   d. Anomalous pulmonary venous drainage

   e. Persistent left superior vena cava (SVC)

Questions 32 to 36

Match the characteristic chest radiography findings with the corresponding congenital disorder.

32. Prominent central pulmonary arteries (PAs) (possible calcifications) and peripheral pruning

33. Right aortic arch, RV enlargement, and a "boot-shaped" heart

34. Marked cardiomegaly, severe right atrial (RA) enlargement, and normal lung fields

35. Posterior rib notching and a "reverse E" or "3" sign

36. Pulmonary plethora, prominent ascending aorta, proximal PA dilatation, and opacity at the confluence of the aortic knob and descending aorta

   a. Eisenmenger syndrome
   b. Coarctation of the aorta
   c. PDA
   d. Ebstein anomaly
   e. TOF

Questions 37 to 41

Match the following congenital cardiac disorder with the characteristic transthoracic echocardiogram (TTE) finding (Figs. 9.7, 9.8, 9.9, 9.10, and 9.11).

37. Bicuspid aortic valve

38. Cor triatriatum

39. Ostium primum ASD

40. Quadricuspid aortic valve

41. Subaortic valve stenosis

   a. Figure 9.7
   b. Figure 9.8
   c. Figure 9.9
   d. Figure 9.10
   e. Figure 9.11

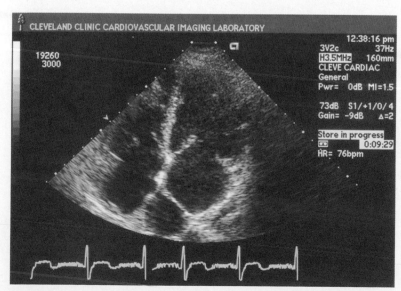

Figure 9.7

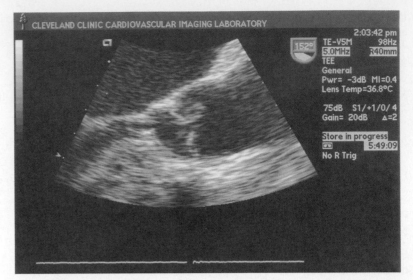

Figure 9.8

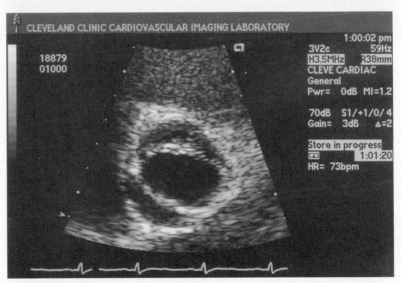

Figure 9.9

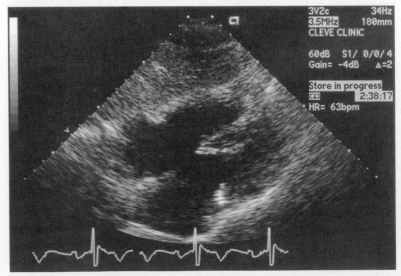

Figure 9.10

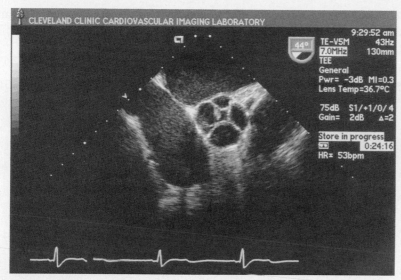

Figure 9.11

Intracardiac Shunts

42. Which of the following are associated with patent foramen ovale (PFO)?

a. Migraine

b. Platypnea-orthodeoxia

c. Decompression sickness

d. Paradoxical embolism & stroke

e. All of the above

43. A 25-year-old man is referred to you for an abnormal heart sound. The patient is asymptomatic and very active. BP is 130/50 mmHg. He has a continuous murmur at the left upper sternal border. A TTE reveals a small PDA with mildly dilated left atrium (LA) and mildly dilated LV but normal RV size and normal pulmonary pressures. How would the patient be best managed?

a. Ligation or percutaneous closure of the PDA

b. Repeat TTE in 1 year

c. Stress echocardiography to determine LV enlargement or dysfunction postexercise

d. Pulmonary vasodilator

e. TEE

44. Which of the following is **most** commonly associated with a sinus venosus ASD?

a. Coarctation of the aorta

b. Bicuspid aortic valve

c. Anomalous right pulmonary venous connection

d. Inlet VSD

e. Persistent left SVC

45. The best echocardiographic scan plane for demonstrating a secundum ASD is

a. apical four-chamber view.

b. parasternal long-axis view.

c. parasternal short-axis view.

d. subcostal four-chamber view.

e. suprasternal long-axis view.

46. Review the image taken at the time of percutaneous closure of an intracardiac shunt in a 25-year-old patient (Fig. 9.12). Which of the following defects was closed in this patient?

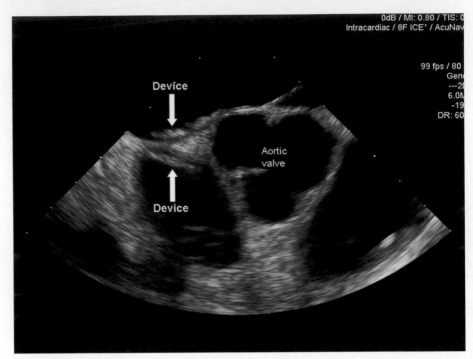

Figure 9.12

    a. Primum ASD

    b. Secundum ASD

    c. Sinus venosus ASD

    d. Unroofed coronary sinus

    e. Atrioventricular septal defect (AVSD)

47. Secundum ASDs may be associated with

    a. pulmonary hypertension.

    b. mitral valve prolapse.

    c. partial anomalous pulmonary venous connection.

    d. pulmonic stenosis.

    e. all of the above.

48. Which type of VSD is demonstrated in Figure 9.13?

    a. Type 1/supracristal

    b. Type 2/perimembranous

    c. Type 3/inlet

    d. Type 4/muscular

49. Percutaneous VSD closure is approved by the U.S. Food and Drug Administration for which type of VSD?

    a. Type 1/supracristal

    b. Type 2/perimembranous

    c. Type 3/inlet

    d. Type 4/muscular

    e. None: Surgery is the only approved treatment for VSD closure

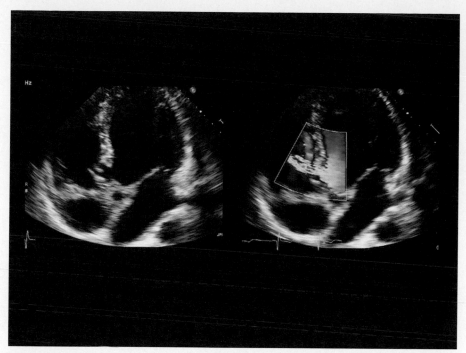

Figure 9.13

Left-Sided Lesions

50. What is the most common coexisting congenital anomaly in patients with coarctation of the aorta?

   a. Cleft mitral valve

   b. Bicuspid aortic valve

   c. Ebstein anomaly

   d. VSD

   e. PDA

51. A 20-year-old man is referred for further evaluation of hypertension. He has remained hypertensive despite a 12-week trial of β-blocker treatment. Examination reveals a right upper extremity BP of 150/100 mmHg and a right lower extremity BP of 130/90 mmHg. HR is 88 bpm. There is brachial–femoral pulse delay. The rest of the physical and neurologic examinations are within normal limits. A TTE confirmed a diagnosis of coarctation of the aorta, with a maximum gradient of 30 mmHg. He is referred for cardiac catheterization. Intervention for coarctation is recommended when the coarctation gradient is greater than which of the following?

   a. 10 mmHg

   b. 20 mmHg

   c. 40 mmHg

   d. 60 mmHg

   e. None of the above; indications for intervention in coarctation are determined by symptoms and not the coarctation gradient

52. Which of the following is the most common coronary artery anomaly?

   a. Bland-Garland-White syndrome (left main coronary arising from the PA)

   b. Coronary arteriovenous fistula

   c. Left circumflex artery arising from the right coronary artery

    d. Left coronary artery arising from the right sinus of Valsalva

    e. Coronary cameral fistula

53. Which of the following statements about coronary arteriovenous fistula is *true*?

    a. The left coronary artery is most commonly involved.

    b. The fistula most commonly empties into the LV.

    c. Despite the success of surgical closure, the prognosis is still poor.

    d. Spontaneous closure rarely occurs.

    e. A large right-to-left shunt may cause congestive heart failure (CHF).

54. Which of the following differentiates valvular aortic stenosis from subvalvular aortic stenosis?

    a. Male preponderance

    b. Surgical risk of repair

    c. Dilatation of the ascending aorta

    d. Aortic regurgitation

    e. Valvular calcification

55. Echocardiography in a 20-year-old asymptomatic man reveals a subaortic membrane with a peak gradient of 20 mmHg. The aortic valve remains mobile, but there is associated mild to moderate aortic valve insufficiency. LV size is normal ejection fraction is 60%. What should you advise this patient?

    a. There is no indication for intervention at this time.

    b. Surgical resection of the membrane and debridement of the aortic valve to reduce aortic regurgitation is indicated.

    c. Transluminal balloon dilatation is the best treatment option in this case.

    d. AVR and membrane resection is indicated.

56. The peak age range for surgical intervention for patients with a bicuspid aortic valve is

    a. 10 to 20 years.

    b. 20 to 40 years.

    c. 40 to 60 years.

    d. 60 to 80 years.

Right-Sided Lesions

57. A 45-year-old man with known Ebstein anomaly seeks your advice with regard to optimal management. He is asymptomatic and has an active lifestyle without any limitations. His physical examination is remarkable for the absence of cyanosis. He has a loud holosystolic murmur at the left lower sternal border that is accentuated with respiration. He has no organomegaly or peripheral edema. His TTE reveals moderately severe 3+ TR with an RV systolic pressure of 35 mmHg and normal LV and RV systolic function. There is no evidence of interatrial communication. Which of the following should you recommend?

    a. Furosemide and digoxin

    b. Tricuspid valve repair

    c. Tricuspid valve replacement

    d. Dual-chamber pacemaker

    e. Regular follow-up with repeat TTE in 6 months

58. The most common problem in adults with surgically repaired TOF is

    a. ventricular tachycardia.

    b. pulmonary hypertension.

    c. pulmonary regurgitation.

    d. cyanosis.

    e. residual VSD.

59. A 34-year-old gentleman reports a history of TOF, Blalock-Taussig shunt at 10 months, and complete repair at age 3. Although he has been reasonably active for several years, he has noted progressive exercise intolerance in recent months. Examination reveals a III/VI systolic ejection murmur loudest at the second left intercostal space and a II/IV diastolic murmur along the left sternal edge. Jugular venous pulse is not elevated. Lungs are clear and there is no hepatomegaly or peripheral edema. An echocardiogram demonstrates RV dilatation, moderate-to-severe pulmonic regurgitation but no significant TR. The ECG shows sinus rhythm and right bundle branch block with a QRS duration of 160 milliseconds. The most reasonable next step in the evaluation of this patient would be

    a. repeat echocardiogram with a saline bubble study.

    b. electrophysiologic study for ventricular arrhythmias.

    c. cardiac catheterization.

    d. cardiac magnetic resonance imaging study.

    e. diuretics and digitalis.

60. A 35-year-old man is referred for evaluation of dyspnea and a loud cardiac murmur. Examination reveals an RV lift, a palpable systolic thrill at the second left intercostal space, and a widely split second heart sound. There is a loud and harsh ejection systolic murmur heard loudest at the second left intercostal space. BP is 130/80 mmHg, HR 90 bpm, and regular, oxygen saturation 98% on room air. What is the most likely diagnosis?

    a. Unrepaired TOF

    b. ASD

    c. VSD

    d. PDA

    e. Pulmonary stenosis

61. Echocardiography confirms doming valvular pulmonary stenosis with a mean Doppler gradient of 40 mmHg. There is no significant pulmonary regurgitation or TR. ECG is normal. The patient undergoes cardiac catheterization (results below):

	Pressure	Saturation
SVC		82
IVC		78
RA	Mean 15	
RV	70/15	
PA	23/15 mean 19	82
PCWP	Mean 6	
Aorta	130/80 mean 90	98

What is the most appropriate management for this patient?

    a. Referral to a pulmonary hypertension specialist

    b. Repeat cardiac catheterization with vasodilator challenge

    c. Balloon valvotomy

    d. Surgical repair

    e. Diuretics

62. Which complications are seen in adults late after the atriopulmonary Fontan procedure among those born with tricuspid atresia?

   a. Protein-losing enteropathy

   b. Thromboembolic events

   c. Intra-atrial reentrant tachycardia (IART)

   d. All of the above

Syndromes

63. Which of the following syndromes is associated with pulmonary arteriovenous fistula?

   a. Williams syndrome

   b. Weber-Osler-Rendu syndrome

   c. Bland-Garland-White syndrome

   d. Kartagener syndrome

   e. Crouzon syndrome

64. What is the most common cardiac defect seen in patients with Noonan syndrome?

   a. AVSD

   b. Pulmonary stenosis

   c. Coarctation of the aorta

   d. Hypertrophic cardiomyopathy

   e. Mitral valve prolapse

65. The most common chromosomal abnormality associated with TOF is

   a. 22q11.2 microdeletion.

   b. 7q11.23 microdeletion.

   c. missense mutations in the PTPN11 gene on chromosome 12.

   d. Trisomy 21.

   e. Monosomy X (45, X).

66. Which of the following is true for Loeys-Dietz syndrome (LDS)?

   a. Inheritance is autosomal recessive.

   b. FBN1 mutations have been implicated.

   c. The risk of aortic dissection is lower than for patients with Marfan syndrome.

   d. Patients are characteristically tall with long extremities.

   e. Hypertelorism, bifid uvula, and arterial tortuosity are common features.

67. Which of the following syndromes is/are NOT associated with pulmonary stenosis?

   a. Noonan syndrome

   b. Williams syndrome

   c. Shone syndrome

   d. Congenital rubella syndrome

   e. LEOPARD syndrome

ANSWERS

1. **e.** Obtain iron studies. Eisenmenger syndrome is the most extreme manifestation of pulmonary arterial hypertension associated with any nonrestrictive congenital heart defect that exposes the pulmonary vascular bed to systemic pressures. The development of pulmonary obstructive arteriopathy and increased pulmonary vascular resistance leads to shunt reversal and cyanosis. Secondary erythrocytosis is a physiologic response to chronic hypoxemia. Eisenmenger syndrome is a multisystem disease that also results in abnormal clotting, impaired renal function, altered uric acid and bilirubin metabolism, and musculoskeletal disease including gout. A common misconception in the management of patients with cyanotic coronary heart disease (CHD) is that an increased hematocrit level alone is an indication for phlebotomy. In fact, therapeutic phlebotomy has a very limited role in patient management and should only be performed if the hemoglobin is more than 20 mg/dL and the hematocrit is greater than 65% *with* symptoms of hyperviscosity and no evidence of dehydration. Symptoms of hyperviscosity include headache, fainting/dizziness, altered mentation, altered vision, tinnitus, myalgias, and restless legs. Hyperviscosity symptoms should disappear after adequate phlebotomy.

    Eisenmenger patients with a history of repeat phlebotomies are at increased risk for iron deficiency anemia, which itself is associated with increased stroke risk.[6] The patient's history of phlebotomies, persistent fatigue, low MCV, and low hemoglobin (relative to oxygen saturation) are all suggestive of iron deficiency anemia. Iron studies are the most appropriate next investigation in this context. Pulmonary vasodilator therapy has been shown to improve 6-minute walk distance in patients with Eisenmenger physiology[7]; however, further investigations are generally indicated prior to commencement (e.g., pulmonary function tests with volumes and CO_2 diffusion, computed tomography for exclusion of pulmonary emboli, cardiac catheterization with vasodilator challenge). Heart–lung transplantation may be considered in Eisenmenger patients with severe limitations; however, long-term survival after heart–lung transplantation is often inferior to continuing conservative management in this population.

2. **c.** Blood cultures. The incidence of IE in young adults with CHD is almost 35-fold that of the general population.[8] Hence, a high index of suspicion for IE is required in these patients. ACHD patients who present with fever and potential IE should have blood cultures drawn before antibiotic therapy is initiated to avoid subsequent false-negative blood cultures and, in the instance of positive blood cultures, to guide antibiotic treatment. In this case, blood cultures should be taken as the first step in the patient's management and prior to commencement of antibiotic therapy. Since the sensitivity of TTE is too low to exclude IE, TEE should be performed after multiple sets of blood cultures are taken. Surgery for IE is indicated in patients with recurrent emboli, medically uncontrolled infection, prosthetic material infection, CHF, and development of heart block.

3. **a.** Closure is indicated in patients with a VSD complicated by IE (AHA guidelines, class I recommendation, level of evidence C[1]). VSD closure is also indicated in the following circumstances:

    *   Patients with attributable symptoms; LV volume overload; deteriorating ventricular function due to volume (LV) or pressure (RV) overload; and/or a Q_p/Q_s (pulmonary-to-systemic blood flow ratio) $\geq$1.5:1 in the absence of advanced pulmonary vascular disease
    *   Significant RV outflow tract (RVOT) obstruction (catheter gradient > 50 mmHg)
    *   VSD closure may also be considered in patients with a perimembranous or subarterial VSD and more than mild or progressive aortic regurgitation[3]

In deciding whether to close a defect, TTE ± TEE is essential to define the size and location of the defect and to identify coexisting septal defects as more than one muscular defect is common.

4. **a.** Ebstein anomaly without prior intervention. Current AHA guidelines for ACHD patients recommend antibiotic prophylaxis before dental procedures in the following patient subgroups[1]:

- Prosthetic cardiac valve or prosthetic material used for cardiac valve repair
- Prior IE
- Unrepaired and palliated cyanotic congenital heart disease, including surgically palliated constructed palliative shunts and conduits
- Completely repaired CHD with prosthetic materials, whether placed by surgery or by catheter intervention, during the first 6 months after the procedure
- Repaired CHD with residual defects at the site or adjacent to the site of a prosthetic patch or prosthetic device that inhibits endothelialization

5. **c.** Ebstein anomaly. The ECG demonstrates a short PR interval, presence of delta waves, and wide QRS interval that are all consistent with preexcitation and Wolff-Parkinson-White syndrome. Wolff-Parkinson-White syndrome is commonly associated with Ebstein anomaly. Catheter ablation can be beneficial for treatment of recurrent supraventricular tachycardia in some patients, although recurrence is common due to the presence of multiple accessory pathways.[9] (see also question 57).

6. **d.** Eisenmenger syndrome. Eisenmenger syndrome is one of few conditions that pose an absolute contraindication to pregnancy[1–3] due to very high maternal mortality and fetal loss.

7. **b, e.** Blalock-Taussig and Fontan (see also Table 9.1).

8. **c, d, f.** Senning or Mustard, arterial switch, and Rashkind.

9. **e, f.** Fontan and Rashkind.

10. **g.** None of the above.

11. **a.** Ross. Please refer to Table 9.1, which provides a complete overview of common surgical procedures for congenital heart disease.

12. **c.** Equal preponderance.

13. **b.** Predominantly female.

14. **a.** Predominantly male.

15. **a.** Predominantly male.

16. **c.** Equal preponderance.

17. **Figure 9.2, d.** Pulmonic stenosis. A left lateral right ventriculogram demonstrates pulmonic stenosis with dilatation of the proximal main PA.

18. **Figure 9.3, a.** Coarctation of the aorta. Left lateral view of the LV and aorta. The catheter was advanced from the femoral vein and crossed a large patent foramen ovale to reach the left side of the heart. A discrete area of narrowing (coarctation) is seen in the upper descending aorta.

19. **Figure 9.4, e.** VSD. A left ventriculogram obtained in the left anterior oblique view allows optimal visualization of the interventricular septum and demonstrates a large VSD with significant left-to-right shunt of contrast.

| TABLE 9-1 | Common Surgical Procedures for Congenital Heart Disease |

Procedure	Description	Intent	Result
Blalock-Taussig	Subclavian artery to PA anastomosis	PAL	Increases PBF
Central shunt	Conduit or anastomosis between the aorta and PA	PAL	Increases PBF
Fontan	Anastomosis or conduit between the right atrium and PA	PAL	Increases PBF in cases of univentricular heart or tricuspid atresia
Hemi-Fontan	SVC to PA anastomosis with baffle placed in the right atrium so that inferior vena cava blood flow goes across ASD to left heart	PAL	Increases PBF and sets the stage for Fontan completion
Glenn (bidirectional Glenn)	SVC to PA anastomosis	PAL	Increases PBF
Jatene arterial switch	Transection of the aorta and PA with reimplantation onto the proper ventricles, coronary arteries reimplanted	COR	Creates normal relationship between the ventricles and great arteries in d-TGA
Konno	Replacement of aortic valve with aortic valve annular enlargement	COR	Alleviates subaortic obstruction and replaces abnormal aortic valve
Mustard/Senning	Atrial switch with intra-atrial baffle made of pericardium (Mustard) or atrial wall flaps (Senning)	COR	Reestablishes proper flow sequence to PA and aorta in d-TGA
Norwood (first stage)	PA anastomosis to aorta, conduit from the aorta to main PA	PAL	Increases flow to aorta for subaortic obstruction with single ventricle
PA band	Constrictive band around main PA	PAL	Decreases PBF
Potts	Descending aorta-to-PA shunt	PAL	Increases PBF (rarely done anymore)
Rashkind	Atrial septostomy with catheter balloon	PAL	Increases mixing of blood for d-TGA or tricuspid atresia
Rastelli	Closure of VSD + valved conduit from RV to PA	COR	Increases PBF, may reestablish proper sequence of flow to aorta and PA
Ross	Pulmonary autograft to aorta, pulmonary homograft	COR	Correction for aortic stenosis; avoids mechanical and bioprosthetic valves
Waterston	Ascending aorta to right pulmonary anastomosis	PAL	Increases PBF (rarely done anymore)

ASD, atrial septal defect; COR, total correction; d-TGA, D-transposition of the great arteries; PA, pulmonary artery; PAL, palliation; PBF, pulmonary blood flow; RV, right ventricle; SVC, superior vena cava.

From *ACC Current Journal Review*. March/April 1996:46, with permission.

20. **Figure 9.5, b.**   Patent ductus arteriosus (PDA). An aortogram in straight lateral view. There is a large abnormal communication between the upper descending aorta and the main PA, confirming the diagnosis of PDA.

21. **Figure 9.6, c.**   Hypertrophic cardiomyopathy. A left ventriculogram in right anterior oblique projection demonstrates a small ventricle with marked ventricular hypertrophy and narrow left ventricular outfl ow tract (LVOT).

22. **e.**   TOF. On cardiac palpation and auscultation, patients with TOF demonstrate RV lift (RV hypertrophy) and a systolic ejection murmur over the

pulmonic region caused by RVOT obstruction. A soft, short systolic ejection murmur suggests severe obstruction. The intensity and severity of the ejection murmur are inversely related to the severity of RV obstruction. P_2 is absent, and only the aortic component of S_2 is audible.

23. **d.** Ebstein anomaly. Patients with Ebstein anomaly have a widely split S_1 (reflecting delayed closure of the anterior tricuspid leaflet) and split S_2 (delayed closure of the pulmonary valve due to associated right bundle branch block). The "sail sound" contributes to a loud S_1 and reflects increased tension in the large mobile anterior leaflet as it reaches the limits of its systolic excursion. The systolic murmur of TR is typically grade 2/6 to 3/6 and heard loudest overlying the tricuspid area. Ejection clicks, opening snaps, and diastolic murmurs may be heard. Hepatomegaly caused by passive congestion and elevated RA pressure may be present.

24. **b.** Coarctation of the aorta. Patients with coarctation of the aorta have systolic hypertension and higher BP in their arms than in their legs, resulting in delayed femoral arterial pulses. Because many patients also have bicuspid aortic valve, a systolic ejection click is frequently present, and the aortic component of S_2 is accentuated. A harsh systolic ejection murmur is audible along the left sternal border and radiates to the back, especially over the point of discrete coarctation.

25. **a.** Eisenmenger syndrome. Patients with Eisenmenger syndrome demonstrate cyanosis and digital clubbing, the severity of which depends on the magnitude of right-to-left shunting. An RV lift and loud P_2 caused by pulmonary hypertension are usually present. The murmur caused by ASD, VSD, or PDA is no longer present when Eisenmenger syndrome develops because left- and right-sided pressures have equalized. Many patients will have a tricuspid or pulmonary regurgitation murmur, or both.

26. **c.** PDA. Patients with PDA exhibit hyperdynamic LV impulse with wide pulse pressure. A continuous machinery murmur, heard best in the pulmonic region, is a characteristic finding.

27. **c.** Cleft mitral valve. (see also question 45).

28. **b.** Supravalvular pulmonic stenosis.

29. **e.** Persistent left SVC. (see also question 45).

30. **a.** Supravalvar aortic stenosis and b.   Supravalvar pulmonary stenosis

31. **d.** Anomalous pulmonary venous drainage. (see also question 44).

32. **a.** Eisenmenger syndrome.

33. **e.** TOF.

34. **d.** Ebstein anomaly.

35. **b.** Coarctation of the aorta.

36. **c.** PDA.

37. **c.** Figure 9.9. This is a parasternal short-axis view at the aortic valve level using TTE. Two leaflets showing a "fish-mouth" opening during systole are seen instead of three leaflets.

38. **a.** Figure 9.7. This is an apical four-chamber view using TTE. There is a membrane separating the LA into a posterior chamber, usually where the pulmonary veins empty, and an anterior chamber that contains the mitral valve.

39. d. Figure 9.10. Subcostal TTE view showing the ASD in the lower atrial septum, with downward displacement of the atrioventricular (AV) valve. (see also question 45).

40. e. Figure 9.11. This is a parasternal short-axis view at the aortic valve level, using TTE. There are four visible leaflets.

41. b. Figure 9.8. A magnified TEE long-axis view of the LVOT, aortic valve, and ascending aorta. There is a membrane visible in the LVOT, consistent with a sub-aortic membrane.

42. e. All of the above. The foramen ovale is the interface between the septum primum and septum secundum and in utero provides an important route for blood as it bypasses the collapsed fetal lungs (oxygenation being achieved via the placenta). In about 25% of humans the flap of tissue making up the foramen ovale does not fuse after birth and results in a PFO. Stroke patients with PFO and atrial septal aneurysm (ASA) have an average annual risk of recurrent stroke of 4.4%.[10] PFO is also associated with decompression sickness, platypnea-orthodeoxia, and migraine. Factors associated with a greater risk of paradoxical embolism are large PFO size and the presence of an ASA. Though several management strategies exist for patients with cryptogenic stroke and PFO, including anticoagulation, antiplatelet therapy, and closure via percutaneous or surgical means, no clear consensus regarding therapy exists.

43. a. Ligation or percutaneous closure of the PDA. PDA is the persistence after birth of an in utero communication between the aorta and the left PA, which, along with the foramen ovale, is designed to bypass blood away from the collapsed fetal lungs. It is the third most common congenital heart defect in adults and is generally found in isolation in the adult. Frequently, this lesion is discovered by the unusual quality of a continuous "machinery" murmur at the left upper sternal border. Because a patent ductus is an aortopulmonary communication, the pulse pressure frequently is widened and the pulses are brisk to bounding.

Closure of a PDA either percutaneously or surgically is indicated for LA and/or LV enlargement or in patients with prior endarteritis.[1] It is reasonable to close a small asymptomatic PDA by catheter device so as to decrease the future risk of endarteritis (0.45% per year after the second decade of life); however, this is somewhat controversial. Surgical repair is recommended in those who meet indications and with PDAs too large for device closure or distorted ductal anatomy. Pulmonary vasodilators are not indicated in this patient due to the absence of pulmonary hypertension. By lowering pulmonary vascular resistance, pulmonary vasodilators could conceivably increase left-to-right shunting in those with moderate-to-large PDAs. Endocarditis prophylaxis is recommended for ACHD patients with a residual shunt including PDA.

44. c. Anomalous right pulmonary venous connection. Sinus venosus ASDs constitute 2% to 3% of interatrial communications. Strictly speaking, this defect lies outside the true atrial septum and is an abnormality of the venous connections. These defects are located on the right side of the upper or posterior atrial septum, most commonly at the SVC/RA junction and less commonly at the level of the inferior vena cava (IVC). Because of their superior location, sinus venosus defects are easily missed on TTE. Partial anomalous venous return of the right upper pulmonary vein is a common association (seen in up to 85% of patients). A bicaval view on TEE or demonstration by CT/MRI is diagnostic.

45. d. Subcostal four-chamber view. ASDs and anomalous pulmonary venous return should be suspected in patients with unexplained RV dilatation and volume/pressure overload (Fig. 9.14).

A secundum ASD is the common type of ASD and is located centrally in the interatrial septum at the site of the fossa ovalis. The defect may be single, multiple, or fenestrated. This defect is best viewed by transthoracic echocardiography in the subcostal view (due to ultrasound waves being better reflected off

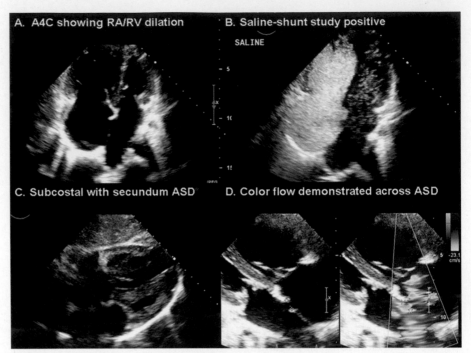

Figure 9.14 • The findings of RA and RV dilatation in the apical four-chamber (A4C) view (**A**) and significant right-to-left shunting of agitated saline (**B**) are highly suggestive of an ASD ± anomalous pulmonary venous return. A secundum ASD is confirmed as a defect in the mid-portion of the interatrial septum, best seen in subcostal scan plane (**C**) and with color flow Doppler (**D**). ASD, atrial septal defect; RA, right atrium; RV, right ventricle.

the interatrial septum in this view). Coexisting partial anomalous pulmonary venous drainage is seen in 5% of patients with a secundum ASD. The atrial septal defect occurs when the interatrial septum is deficient at the crux of the heart/ level of the atrioventricular valves.

A primum ASD occurs as part of the spectrum of AVSD. Partial AVSD commonly describes a primum ASD in combination with a so-called cleft mitral valve, more correctly described as a trileaflet left-sided AV valve. Primum ASDs are often well demonstrated from the apical four-chamber view (± subcostal) in association with mitral regurgitation from a trileaflet left-sided AV valve (Fig. 9.15).

A coronary sinus defect is located in the wall that separates the coronary sinus from the LA. It may be fenestrated or completely absent. There is an associated left-sided SVC contributing to dilatation of the coronary sinus seen best on parasternal long-axis views. A coronary sinus defect should be suspected in a patient who has evidence of RV volume or pressure overload but no suggestion of a defect in the central portion of the atrial septum. Injection of agitated saline into the left arm leads to contrast in the coronary sinus, then the RA and finally the RV. An unroofed coronary sinus contains fenestrations such that bubbles travel from the left sided SVC and into the left atrium.

46. b.   Secundum ASD. The majority of secundum ASDs can be closed with a percutaneous catheter technique. ASD closure is indicated for RA and RV enlargement with or without symptoms. Small ASDs (<5 mm) with no evidence of volume overload do not require closure unless associated with cryptogenic paradoxical embolism. Sinus venous, coronary sinus, and primum defects are not amenable to device closure (Fig. 9.16; see also Question 3).

47. e.   All of the above. Large ASDs can lead to RV volume overload, excessive blood flow to the pulmonary circulation, and pulmonary hypertension. Associated lesions are listed in Table 9.2 for each ASD type.

48. b.   Type 2/perimembranous. See Table 9.3.

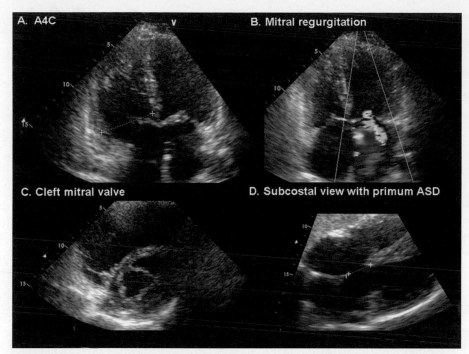

Figure 9.15 • Primum ASD and its associated features. Note that the septal leaflet of the tricuspid valve is on the same plane as the mitral valve (**A**). Normally the septal leaflet of the tricuspid leaflet is apically displaced compared with the mitral valve. Mitral regurgitation frequently coexists with primum (**B**). (**C**) Short-axis views of the mitral valve show a "cleft" pointing toward the septum (*). (**D**) The cleft is more accurately characterized as a commissure between the superior and inferior bridging leaflets of the common AV canal. Additional echocardiographic features of AVSD (not demonstrated here) include elongation of the LV outflow tract (gooseneck deformity) ± LVOT obstruction. A4C, apical 4 chamber; ASD, atrial septal defect.

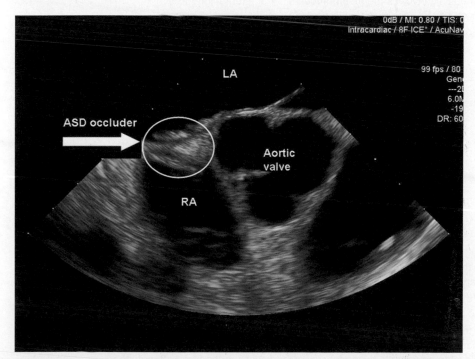

Figure 9.16 • An atrial septal defect (ASD) occlusion device is seen positioned across a secundum ASD. The image was acquired using intracardiac echocardiography and consists of a short-axis view of the heart demonstrating the aortic valve and the interatrial septum dividing the left atrium (LA) and right atrium (RA).

TABLE 9-2 Atrial Septal Defects and Associated Lesions

Type of Atrial Septal Defect	Associated Lesions
Secundum	Pulmonic stenosis
	Mitral valve prolapse
	Partial anomalous pulmonary venous connection (5%)
Primum	Trileaflet left-sided AV valve aka "cleft" mitral valve
	LVOT obstruction / RVOT obstruction
	Pulmonary vascular disease risk highest in Trisomy 21[11]
Sinus venosus	Partial anomalous pulmonary venous connection (right upper pulmonary vein in 80%)
Coronary sinus	Persistent left-sided SVC
	Partial anomalous pulmonary venous connection

AV, atrioventricular; LVOT, left ventricular outflow tract; RVOT, right ventricular outflow tract; SVC, superior vena cava.
Modified from Warnes et al.[1]

TABLE 9-3 Classification of Ventricular Septal Defects

VSD Type	Synonyms	Location	Echocardiographic Views and Associated Features
Type 1	Conal Supracristal Subarterial Doubly committed juxta-arterial	Below the aortic and pulmonary valves in the conal/outlet septum	Short-axis view VSD flow in the RVOT and just below the aortic valve annulus Aortic valve prolapse is most common in this group due to progressive prolapse of the aortic valve
Type 2	Perimembranous Paramembranous Membranous	Involves the membranous septum and is bordered by an AV valve (commonly the aortic valve)	Parasternal long-axis Aortic valve prolapse may be present Aneurysm formation involving the septal leaflet of the tricuspid valve can accompany complete or partial closure of the VSD
Type 3	Inlet AV canal type	In the inlet portion of the RV septum inferior to the AV valve apparatus	Apical four-chamber/subcostal Left- and right-sided AV valves on the same level Primum ASD + "cleft" mitral valve with mitral regurgitation Gooseneck deformity (elongation) of the LVOT ± LVOT obstruction
Type 4	Muscular	A VSD completely surrounded by muscle Single or multiple Apical, posterior, or anterior	Apical four-chamber/subcostal/PLAX VSDs may occur in association with left-sided obstructive lesions such as bicuspid aortic valve, subaortic stenosis, aortic coarctation

Small VSDs ≤25% of the aortic annulus diameter/main PA <20 mmHg/Q_p:Q_s < 1.2:1. Usually restrictive and do not cause pulmonary arterial, left atrial, or LV dilatation.

Moderate VSDs 25–75% of the aortic annulus diameter/main PA = 35 mmHg/Q_p:Q_s > 1.2:1. Moderately restrictive but can lead to mild-to-moderate pulmonary/LA/LV dilatation.

Large VSDs ≥75% of the aortic diameter are usually nonrestrictive and the LV pressure is directly transmitted to the RV and pulmonary vascular bed. Significantly elevated pulmonary pressures. The majority of patients with large VSDs will develop irreversible pulmonary vascular disease in the first 1–2 y of life.

ASD, atrial septal defect; AV, atrioventricular; LA, left atrium; LV, left ventricle; LVOT, left ventricular outflow tract; PA, pulmonary artery; RV, right ventricle; RVOT, right ventricular outflow tract; VSD, ventricular septal defect.

49. d.   Type 4/muscular. When indicated (see also Question 9), percutaneous device closure of a muscular VSD may be performed in VSDs remote (>4 mm) from the tricuspid and aortic valves. Percutaneous VSD closure is NOT approved by the U.S. Food and Drug Administration in the presence of the following:

- High pulmonary vascular resistance and/or irreversible pulmonary vascular disease
- Perimembranous or post-infarction VSDs
- Sepsis or an active bacterial infection
- Contraindications to antiplatelet therapy
- Weight < 5.2 kg

50. b.   Bicuspid aortic valve. Aortic coarctation is a common congenital defect that usually occurs in the region of the ligamentum arteriosus. It is most often discrete but may be associated with diffuse hypoplasia of the aortic arch and isthmus. Bicuspid aortic valve is the most common coexisting anomaly. However, the presence of VSD, PDA, and malformations of the mitral valve apparatus is well documented. Intracranial aneurysms have been reported in 3% to 10% of patients with coarctation of the aorta.[12] There is no association between aortic coarctation and Ebstein anomaly (the latter being associated with right-sided lesions).

51. b.   20 mmHg. Intervention for coarctation is recommended in those with a peak-to-peak coarctation gradient greater than or equal to 20 mmHg.[1,4] In the presence of significant collateral vessel blood flow, catheter-based and Doppler systolic gradients may underestimate the degree of obstruction and intervention may be considered with gradients <20 mmHg in this setting.

The most appropriate intervention for adults with native coarctation of the aorta remains controversial and either surgical or percutaneous intervention may be considered according to anatomy, comorbidities, center outcomes, and patient preference. In most ACHD centers, stenting has replaced balloon dilatation as the percutaneous intervention of choice, although this is not recommended in those with long segments of coarctation, vessel tortuosity, and transverse arch hypoplasia. Early mortality is usually less than 1% for primary operation in aortic coarctation.

52. d.   Left coronary artery arising from the right sinus of Valsalva.

53. d.   Spontaneous closure rarely occurs. Coronary fistulae rarely close spontaneously. The most common origin of coronary arteriovenous fistula is the right coronary artery, with a fistulous communication into the RV, RA, or coronary sinus (appearance on echocardiography demonstrated on the next page). Less commonly, it empties into the LV, LA, or PA. Complications may include CHF from left-to-right shunt, bacterial endocarditis, coronary ischemia, and rupture or thrombosis of the fistula. Surgical closure is associated with a good outcome (Fig. 9.17).

54. e.   Valvular calcification. Both valvular and subvalvular aortic stenoses have male preponderance and may be associated with dilatation of the ascending aorta. The indications and risk of operation are similar. Although aortic regurgitation is more common in subvalvular aortic stenosis, it may also occur in valvular aortic stenosis. Valvular calcification is usually not observed in subvalvular aortic valve stenosis.

55. c.   Transluminal balloon dilatation is the best treatment option in this case. Subaortic valve stenosis involves the presence of a membranous diaphragm in the LVOT that creates a turbulent flow across the LVOT. This frequently causes damage to the aortic valve and may cause aortic valve insufficiency. Surgical intervention is recommended for patients with subaortic stenosis and a peak

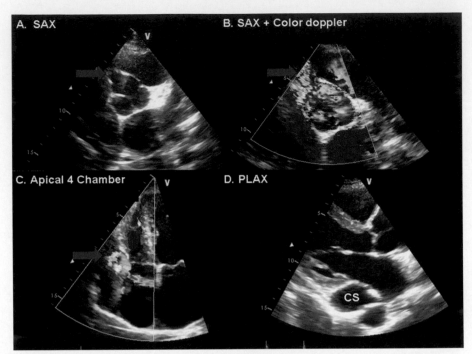

Figure 9.17 • The right coronary artery fistula (red arrow) is seen in transthoracic short-axis (SAX) views arising from the right coronary cusp of the aortic valve (**A**) confirmed with color flow Doppler (**B**). In this case, the right coronary fistula drained into the right atrium (**C**) via a dilated coronary sinus (**D**). PLAX, parasternal long axis.

instantaneous gradient of 50 mmHg or mean gradient of 30 mmHg on echo Doppler.[1] Elective surgical resection is also indicated with lesser gradients <30 mmHg in the presence of progressive aortic regurgitation, LV systolic dysfunction (<55%), or dilatation (end-systolic diameter >50 mm). Although recurrences occur, surgical resection is frequently curative. Patients with aortic regurgitation may undergo valve repair at the time of subaortic stenosis resection. AVR would best be avoided unless the valve is severely damaged as it would involve the patient having to have further surgery if a biologic valve or be on long-term anticoagulation if a mechanical valve.

56. **d.** 60 to 80 years. Bicuspid aortic valve is the most common congenital cardiac anomaly with an incidence of 1% to 2% and a male predominance (4:1 sex ratio). Bicuspid aortic valve is sometimes inherited as an autosomal dominant trait with variable penetrance. Three morphologic types are recognized on the basis of commissural fusion: fusion of the left and right coronary cusps (most common), fusion of the right and non-coronary cusps, and fusion of the left and non-coronary cusps (least common). Sclerosis of the bicuspid aortic valve begins in the second decade and calcification may appear as early as the fourth decade.[13] The peak age range for surgical intervention is between 60 and 80 years.[14] Bicuspid aortic valve disease is associated with intrinsic abnormalities of the aortic media that predisposes to aortic root dilatation/aneurysm/rupture, and/or dissection. Other left-sided lesions associated with bicuspid aortic valve include coarctation of the aorta, subaortic stenosis, parachute mitral valve, VSD, and PDA.

57. **e.** Regular follow-up with repeat TTE in 6 months. Ebstein anomaly is characterized by apical displacement of the septal tricuspid leaflet of >8 mm/m² and the presence of an elongated anterior tricuspid leaflet. The clinical presentation of Ebstein anomaly is influenced by numerous factors including the extent of tricuspid leaflet distortion and regurgitation, the degree of pulmonary stenosis, RA pressure, right heart size, and the presence of a right-to-left shunt. More than

50% of patients have a shunt at the atrial level with either a PFO or secundum ASD. Tricuspid valve repair or replacement is recommended by the AHA for the following indications[1]:

- Symptoms or deteriorating exercise capacity
- Cyanosis (saturations < 90%) due to right-to-left shunting
- Paradoxical embolism
- Progressive RV dilatation or reduction in RV systolic function

The patient has moderately severe TR with preserved RV systolic function. He has no symptoms and no evidence of CHF. There is no indication for intervention at this time.

58. c. Pulmonary regurgitation. TOF comprises (1) RVOT obstruction, (2) a VSD, (3) an aorta that overrides the VSD, and (4) RV hypertrophy. Primary repair in the first year of life consists of VSD closure and relief of RVOT obstruction, the latter achieved by increasing the RVOT diameter through patch augmentation or placement of a transannular patch. The integrity of the pulmonary valve is frequently disrupted at the time of repair and predisposes patients to pulmonary regurgitation, the most common residual abnormality seen in adults with repaired TOF.

Although less common than pulmonary regurgitation, ventricular tachycardia is an important cause of late mortality in adults with repaired TOF. TOF patients at highest risk for ventricular tachycardia and sudden death include those with significant residual pulmonary regurgitation/RVOT obstruction, reduced RV or LV function, QRS duration >180 milliseconds, high-grade ectopy on Holter monitoring, and inducible ventricular tachycardia.[15–17]

59. d. Cardiac magnetic resonance imaging study. Pulmonary valve replacement is recommended in adults with repaired TOF, severe pulmonary regurgitation, and any of the following[1]:

- Moderate-to-severe RV dysfunction
- Moderate-to-severe RV enlargement (generally defined as >160 to 170 mL/m^2)
- Development of symptomatic or sustained atrial and/or ventricular arrhythmias
- Moderate-to-severe TR

Surgery in adults with repaired TOF may also be considered for residual RVOT obstruction (peak gradient >50 mmHg), residual VSD with shunt greater than 1.5:1, and severe aortic regurgitation with associated symptoms or more than mild LV dysfunction.

Due to the complex geometry of the RV and limitations of echocardiography, cardiac magnetic resonance imaging is the gold standard investigation for assessment of RV dimensions and function in repaired TOF. Further evaluation of pulmonary regurgitation is also possible.

A positive bubble study would be helpful in confirming the presence of an ASD but would not help in deciding timing of pulmonary valve replacement. An ASD is unlikely to explain the degree of RV dilatation seen in this patient, particularly in the presence of a clear etiology (severe pulmonary regurgitation). Formal electrophysiologic testing is not indicated in TOF patients without a history of presyncope or palpitations. Invasive hemodynamics would not provide additional diagnostic or prognostic information. Since there is no evidence of volume overload, the initiation of diuretics and digoxin would not be recommended.

60. e. Pulmonary stenosis. The clinical findings (RV lift, a palpable systolic thrill at the second left intercostal space, a widely split second heart sound, and harsh ejection systolic murmur heard loudest at the second left intercostal space) are consistent with significant pulmonary stenosis. The RV lift is evidence of a pressure-loaded RV. The second heart sound is split due to delayed closure of the pulmonary valve. Pulmonary valve stenosis is heard loudest at the second left intercostal space and may be associated with a palpable thrill.

61. c. Balloon valvotomy. Echocardiography (TTE ± TEE) generally provides a definitive diagnosis in most patients with pulmonary stenosis. Doppler gradients from echo are adequate for deciding on the timing of intervention. Cardiac catheterization may be used to confirm the diagnosis of pulmonary stenosis and to exclude pulmonary hypertension in cases where this is a concern.

The cardiac catheterization results confirm RV hypertension (RV systolic pressure 70 mmHg) with a slightly elevated end-diastolic RV pressure (15 mmHg). RV hypertension should be differentiated from pulmonary hypertension: The finding of normal main PA pressures distal to the site of valvar stenosis (+ normal transpulmonary gradient) excludes pulmonary hypertension in this patient. Hence, vasodilator challenge and referral to a pulmonary hypertension are not indicated.

For patients with domed valvular pulmonary stenosis, balloon valvotomy is the treatment of choice. Balloon valvotomy is recommended in patients with a peak instantaneous Doppler gradient greater than 60 mmHg or a mean gradient greater than 40 mmHg (assuming less than moderate pulmonary regurgitation).[1] There is no role for medical therapy in valvular pulmonary stenosis patients who meet criteria for intervention.

62. d. All of the above. Protein-losing enteropathy is a condition diagnosed in <5% of Fontan patients,[18] in which protein is lost via the gut resulting in ascites, peripheral edema, and pleural and pericardial effusions. The precise cause of protein-losing enteropathy is unknown, although elevated systemic venous pressures appear to play a role. The diagnosis is made by measuring increased a1-antitrypsin in the stool.

Thromboembolic complications occur in up to 20% of patients with the slow passive flow in the Fontan circuit and the coagulation abnormalities consequent on liver congestion both playing a role.

Atrial tachyarrhythmias are very common in adults after the Fontan operation,[19] the most common type being an atypical form of atrial flutter called "intra-atrial reentrant tachycardia" or IART. IART arises from macroreentrant circuits around surgical scars and patches and tends to be slower than typical flutter. Early recognition and treatment of IART is important for preventing complications such as thromboembolism, hemodynamic instability, syncope, and death. Unfortunately, recurrence of IART is common even in the setting of chronic antiarrhythmic medications and catheter-based ablation.

63. b. Weber-Osler-Rendu syndrome. Pulmonary arteriovenous fistula involves direct communication between pulmonary arteries and veins. Most patients have associated Weber-Osler-Rendu syndrome, a condition associated with the presence of multiple telangiectasias. Williams syndrome is associated with mental retardation, elfin facies, and supravalvular aortic and pulmonic stenosis. Bland-Garland-White syndrome involves the anomalous origin of the left coronary artery from the PA. Kartagener syndrome is associated with situs inversus, sinusitis, and bronchiectasis. Crouzon syndrome is associated with PDA and aortic coarctation (see also Table 9.4).

64. b. Pulmonary stenosis. Pulmonary stenosis is the most common cardiac abnormality (40%) seen in patients with Noonan syndrome. Other associations include AVSDs (13.8%), coarctation of the aorta (12.5%), and hypertrophic cardiomyopathy (8.8%).[20] Although less common in Noonan syndrome patients, LVOT obstruction may be due to asymmetric hypertrophy and valvular or supra-valvar aortic stenosis.[21]

65. a. 22q11.2 microdeletion. See Table 9.4.

TABLE 9-4	Common Chromosomal Abnormalities Seen in Adult Congenital Heart Disease		
Chromosomal Abnormality	**Syndrome**	**Cardiac Defects**	**Extracardiac Manifestations**
22q11.2 microdeletion Autosomal dominant	22q11.2 microdeletion syndrome Previously called DiGeorge/CATCH-22	Conotruncal defects Tetralogy of Fallot Truncus arteriosus Interrupted aortic arch Double outlet right ventricle	C—Cardiac defects A—Abnormal facies* T—Thymic hypoplasia C—Cleft palate H—Hypocalcemia + Psychiatric conditions (schizophrenia)
7q11.23 microdeletion Autosomal dominant Defects involving the elastin gene	William syndrome	Pulmonary artery stenosis Supravalvar LVOTO	Elfin facies (small chin, patulous lips, upturned nose, broad forehead), infantile hypercalcemia Short stature "Cocktail" personality
Chromosome 12/PTPN11 gene Autosomal dominant	Noonan syndrome	Dysplastic pulmonary valve stenosis Pulmonary artery stenosis TOF ASD Hypertrophic cardiomyopathy	Short stature, ptosis, hypertelorism, webbed neck, flat chest, pectus deformity, lymphedema, inguinal hernia, undescended/cryptorchid testes Intellectual impairment in 1/3
Trisomy 21	Down syndrome	AVSD VSD Mitral valve prolapse Aortic regurgitation Pulmonary HT	Short stature, characteristic facial appearance Intellectual impairment Atlantoaxial instability Thyroid disorders White blood cell disorders
Monosomy X (45, X) 45 XO karyotype in 50% 45XO/XX mosaics and other X-chromosome abnormalities in the remainder	Turner syndrome	Coarctation of the aorta (postductal) Left-sided obstructive lesions PAPVR without ASD Aortic dissection/rupture Systemic HT	Short stature, webbing of the neck, wide set nipples, small chin, prominent ears, absent pubic hair Intellectual function is grossly intact

ASD, atrial septal defect; AVSD, atrioventricular septal defect; HT, hypertension; LVOTO, LV outflow tract obstruction; PAPVR, partial anomalous pulmonary venous return; TOF, tetralogy of Fallot; VSD, ventricular septal defect.

*hypertelorism, low set ears, micrognathia, small mouth, malformed nose, and down-slanting palpebral fissures

66. e. Hypertelorism, bifid uvula, and arterial tortuosity are common features. LDS is an autosomal dominant syndrome caused by transforming growth factor-fl receptor gene mutations and characterized by the triad of (a) arterial tortuosity and aneurysms, (b) hypertelorism, and (c) bifid uvula or cleft palate.[22] Almost all patients with LDS will develop aortic root dilatation that requires early surgical intervention due to the increased risk of dissection and rupture in these patients. Surgical intervention is recommended once the aortic root (or other aortic segments) is >4.0 cm or rapidly expanding (>0.5 cm over 1 year).[23] Other aortic segments and branch vessels may also be involved. While there is overlap in the skeletal manifestations of Marfan syndrome and LDS (both demonstrate joint hyperlaxity, arachnodactyly, pectus deformity, and scoliosis), long limbs and tall stature are not characteristic of LDS.

67. c. Shone syndrome. The key learning point is that Shone syndrome/complex describes left-sided obstructive lesions and is therefore not implicated in pulmonary stenosis (Table 9.5).

TABLE 9-5	Adult Congenital Heart Disease Syndromes Associated with Pulmonary Stenosis
Syndrome	**Cardiac Defects**
Noonan syndrome	Dysplastic pulmonary valve stenosis, pulmonary artery stenosis
	Tetralogy of Fallot, atrial septal defect, hypertrophic cardiomyopathy[21]
Williams syndrome	Pulmonary artery stenosis
	Supravalvar aortic stenosis[24,25]
Shone syndrome	Multilevel obstruction of left ventricular inflow and outflow
	Mitral stenosis (parachute mitral valve, supramitral ring)
	Subvalvular left ventricular outflow tract obstruction
	Valvular outflow tract obstruction
	Coarctation of the aorta[26]
	May be familial
Congenital rubella syndrome	Pulmonary artery stenosis, peripheral pulmonary artery stenosis
	Patent ductus arteriosus
	Non-cardiac: Cataracts, retinopathy, deafness, intellectual impairment[27]
LEOPARD syndrome	Pulmonary stenosis
	Non-cardiac: Café-au-lait spots and multiple lentigines[28]

REFERENCES

1. Warnes CA, Williams RG, Bashore TM, et al. ACC/AHA 2008 guidelines for the management of adults with congenital heart disease: a report of the American College of Cardiology/American Heart Association Task Force on Practice Guidelines (Writing Committee to Develop Guidelines on the Management of Adults with Congenital Heart Disease). *Circulation.* 2008;118:e714–e833.

2. Baumgartner H, Bonhoeffer P, De Groot NM, et al. ESC guidelines for the management of grown-up congenital heart disease (new version 2010). *Eur Heart J.* 2010;31:2915–2957.

3. Silversides CK, Dore A, Poirier N, et al. Canadian Cardiovascular Society 2009 Consensus Conference on the management of adults with congenital heart disease: shunt lesions. *Can J Cardiol.* 2010;26:e70–e79.

4. Silversides CK, Kiess M, Beauchesne L, et al. Canadian Cardiovascular Society 2009 Consensus Conference on the management of adults with congenital heart disease: outflow tract obstruction, coarctation of the aorta, tetralogy of Fallot, Ebstein anomaly and Marfan's syndrome. *Can J Cardiol.* 2010;26:e80–e97.

5. Silversides CK, Salehian O, Oechslin E, et al. Canadian Cardiovascular Society 2009 Consensus Conference on the management of adults with congenital heart disease: complex congenital cardiac lesions. *Can J Cardiol.* 2010;26:e98–e117.

6. Ammash N, Warnes CA. Cerebrovascular events in adult patients with cyanotic congenital heart disease. *J Am Coll Cardiol.* 1996;28:768–772.

7. Galie N, Beghetti M, Gatzoulis MA, et al. Bosentan therapy in patients with Eisenmenger syndrome: a multicenter, double-blind, randomized, placebo-controlled study. *Circulation.* 2006;114:48–54.

8. Hayes CJ, Gersony WM, Driscoll DJ, et al. Second natural history study of congenital heart defects. Results of treatment of patients with pulmonary valvar stenosis. *Circulation.* 1993;87:I28–I37.

9. Oh JK, Holmes DR Jr, Hayes DL, Porter CB, Danielson GK. Cardiac arrhythmias in patients with surgical repair of Ebstein's anomaly. *J Am Coll Cardiol.* 1985;6:1351–1357.

10. Lamy C, Giannesini C, Zuber M, et al. Clinical and imaging findings in cryptogenic stroke patients with and without patent foramen ovale: the PFO-ASA Study. Atrial septal aneurysm. *Stroke.* 2002;33:706–711.

11. Rowland TW, Nordstrom LG, Bean MS, Burkhardt H. Chronic upper airway obstruction and pulmonary hypertension in Down's syndrome. *Am J Dis Child.* 1981;135:1050–1052.

12. Connolly HM, Huston J 3rd, Brown RD Jr, Warnes CA, Ammash NM, Tajik AJ. Intracranial aneurysms in patients with coarctation of the aorta: a prospective magnetic resonance angiographic study of 100 patients. *Mayo Clin Proc.* 2003;78:1491–1499.

13. Beppu S, Suzuki S, Matsuda H, Ohmori F, Nagata S, Miyatake K. Rapidity of progression of aortic stenosis in patients with congenital bicuspid aortic valves. *Am J Cardiol.* 1993;71:322–327.

14. Aboulhosn J, Child JS. Left ventricular outflow obstruction: subaortic stenosis, bicuspid aortic valve, supravalvar aortic stenosis, and coarctation of the aorta. *Circulation.* 2006;114:2412–2422.

15. Gatzoulis MA, Balaji S, Webber SA, et al. Risk factors for arrhythmia and sudden cardiac death late after repair of tetralogy of Fallot: a multicentre study. *Lancet.* 2000;356:975–981.

16. Khairy P, Landzberg MJ, Gatzoulis MA, et al. Value of programmed ventricular stimulation after tetralogy of fallot repair: a multicenter study. *Circulation.* 2004;109:1994–2000.

17. Therrien J, Siu SC, Harris L, et al. Impact of pulmonary valve replacement on arrhythmia propensity late after repair of tetralogy of Fallot. *Circulation.* 2001;103:2489–2494.

18. Mertens L, Hagler DJ, Sauer U, Somerville J, Gewillig M. Protein-losing enteropathy after the Fontan operation: an international multicenter study. PLE study group. *J Thorac Cardiovasc Surg.* 1998;115:1063–1073.

19. Ghai A, Harris L, Harrison DA, Webb GD, Siu SC. Outcomes of late atrial tachyarrhythmias in adults after the Fontan operation. *J Am Coll Cardiol.* 2001;37:585–592.

20. Digilio M, Marino B. Clinical manifestations of Noonan syndrome. *Images Paediatr Cardiol.* 2001;3:19–30.

21. Burch M, Sharland M, Shinebourne E, Smith G, Patton M, McKenna W. Cardiologic abnormalities in Noonan syndrome: phenotypic diagnosis and echocardiographic assessment of 118 patients. *J Am Coll Cardiol.* 1993;22:1189–1192.

22. Loeys BL, Schwarze U, Holm T, et al. Aneurysm syndromes caused by mutations in the TGF-beta receptor. *N Engl J Med.* 2006;355: 788–798.

23. Williams JA, Loeys BL, Nwakanma LU, et al. Early surgical experience with Loeys-Dietz: a new syndrome of aggressive thoracic aortic aneurysm disease. *Ann Thorac Surg.* 2007;83:S757–S763; discussion S785–S790.

24. Williams JC, Barratt-Boyes BG, Lowe JB. Supravalvular aortic stenosis. *Circulation.* 1961;24:1311–1318.

25. Schubert C. The genomic basis of the Williams-Beuren syndrome. *Cell Mol Life Sci.* 2009;66:1178–1197.

26. Shone JD, Sellers RD, Anderson RC, Adams P Jr, Lillehei CW, Edwards JE. The developmental complex of "parachute mitral valve," supravalvular ring of left atrium, subaortic stenosis, and coarctation of aorta. *Am J Cardiol.* 1963;11:714–725.

27. Freij BJ, South MA, Sever JL. Maternal rubella and the congenital rubella syndrome. *Clin Perinatol.* 1988;15:247–257.

28. Digilio MC, Sarkozy A, de Zorzi A, et al. LEOPARD syndrome: clinical diagnosis in the first year of life. *Am J Med Genet A.* 2006;140: 740–746.

chapter 10

Physiology/Biochemistry

Amar Krishnaswamy

QUESTIONS ● ● ●

1. At the level of the endothelium, nitric oxide (NO) causes the following:

   a. Promotes smooth muscle relaxation
   b. Reduced leukocyte adhesion
   c. Increased smooth muscle proliferation
   d. Downregulation of oxidative enzymes

2. The following cells are considered most important to the process of atherosclerosis:

   a. Monocyte/macrophage lineage
   b. Platelets
   c. Red blood cells
   d. B cells

3. The following are characteristics of a vulnerable plaque *except*

   a. high concentration of macrophages.
   b. high concentration of collagen.
   c. neovascularization.
   d. large necrotic core.

4. Arterial thrombosis after plaque rupture is initiated by

   a. tissue plasminogen activator.
   b. factor XIII.
   c. protein C.
   d. activated protein C.
   e. tissue factor.

5. Low levels of gene expression can be detected by

   a. Northern blot.
   b. Western blot.
   c. reverse transcriptase-polymerase chain reaction (RT-PCR).
   d. Southern blot.
   e. gene transfer.

6. The final common pathway of platelet aggregation is mediated through

   a. adenosine diphosphate (ADP) binding.
   b. collagen.
   c. thrombin.
   d. $\alpha_v\beta_3$ receptor.
   e. glycoprotein (GP) IIb/IIIa receptor.

7. Inducers of smooth muscle cell proliferation include the following *except*

   a. platelet-derived growth factor-β.
   b. basic fibroblast growth factor (bFGF).
   c. transforming growth factor-β (TGF-β).
   d. thrombin.
   e. oxidized low-density lipoprotein (LDL).

8. Inhibitors of cardiac myocyte apoptosis include

   a. insulin-like growth factor-1β.
   b. dobutamine.
   c. ischemia.
   d. caspase 3.
   e. Bid cleavage.

9. The following are endothelium-independent vasodilators *except*

   a. nitroglycerin.
   b. papaverine.
   c. adenosine.
   d. acetylcholine (ACh).
   e. verapamil.

ANSWERS ● ● ●

1. **c.** Increased smooth muscle proliferation. NO has important effects on the endothelium to produce vasodilation, reduced leukocyte adhesion and platelet reactivity, and downregulation of oxidative enzymes. Consistent with these beneficial effects, NO results in a reduction in smooth muscle proliferation, not an increase.

2. **b.** Monocyte/macrophage lineage. These cells bind oxidized LDL to form foam cells, which then release proinflammatory cytokines to perpetuate the atherosclerotic process.

3. **b.** High concentration of collagen. It is in fact the low concentration of collagen (due to low levels of smooth muscle cells) that results in the collagen-poor thin cap of vulnerable plaques. These plaques display high concentrations of macrophages (foam cells) and T-lymphocytes (producing interferon-γ), as well as significant neovascularization and a large necrotic core that is vulnerable to rupture and propagate thrombosis. In fact, saphenous vein graft (SVG) lesions tend to have a larger necrotic core than native coronary lesions, which is one factor that contributes to greater plaque friability and worse outcomes with SVG stenting.

4. **e.** Tissue factor. Tissue factor binding to factor VII is the initiating event for the extrinsic blood coagulation cascade. The complex can also cleave factor IX and contribute to activation of the intrinsic cascade as well. Tissue factor is normally not expressed in the vasculature, but, in atherosclerotic vessels, tissue factor is expressed by macrophages and smooth muscle cells. Tissue factor expression is increased in the lesions of patients who present with unstable angina. On plaque rupture, the exposure of tissue factor to blood-borne coagulation factors leads to thrombus formation.

5. **c.** Reverse transcriptase-polymerase chain reaction (RT-PCR). RT-PCR is capable of finding a single copy of RNA. Northern blot analysis requires at least 5 to 10 µg of total RNA. Western blot analysis is for determining protein levels. Southern blot analysis is for genotyping and requires multiple copies of DNA. Gene transfer is not a detection method.

6. **e.** Glycoprotein (GP) IIb/IIIa receptor. ADP, collagen, and thrombin bind independently, leading to platelet activation and, ultimately, to expression of the GP IIb/IIIa receptor. GP IIb/IIIa receptor expression leads to platelet clumping by binding to surrounding activated platelets. The $\alpha_v\beta_3$ receptor does not lead to platelet aggregation.

7. **c.** Transforming growth factor-β (TGF-β). Platelet-derived growth factor-β, bFGF, and thrombin are all smooth muscle mitogens. Oxidized LDL causes smooth muscle cell proliferation through the autocrine release of bFGF. TGF-β alters the smooth muscle cell phenotype from a proliferative to a synthetic state and, thus, is antiproliferative.

8. **a.** Insulin-like growth factor-1β. Insulin-like growth factor-1β overexpression has been shown to be cardioprotective because of decreased apoptosis in the setting of myocardial ischemia. Dobutamine has been shown to induce cardiomyocyte apoptosis. Caspase 3 and Bid cleavage are cytoplasmic markers of apoptosis, but do not directly influence apoptosis itself.

9. **d.** Acetylcholine (ACh). ACh, acting through muscarinic receptors, exerts its effect on the endothelium by promoting the conversion of L-arginine to NO. This in turn produces smooth muscle cell relaxation and consequent vasodilation. ACh is therefore an endothelium-dependent vasodilator. In patients with endothelial dysfunction, this effect is lost, and the direct action of ACh on smooth muscle cells producing vasoconstriction is more pronounced. The other agents listed are all endothelium-independent vasodilators.

SUGGESTED READINGS

Annex BH. Differential expression of TF protein in directional atherectomy specimens from patients with stable and unstable coronary syndromes. *Circulation.* 1995;91:619–622.

Bristow MR, Ginsburg R, Minobe W, et al. Decreased catecholamine sensitivity and beta-adrenergic-receptor density in failing human hearts. *N Engl J Med.* 1982;307(4):205–211.

Chai YC, Howe PH, DiCorleto PE, et al. Oxidized low density lipoprotein and lysophosphatidylcholine stimulate cell cycle entry in vascular smooth muscle cells. Evidence for release of fibroblast growth factor-2. *J Biol Chem.* 1996;27:17791–17797.

Chisolm GM 3rd, Hazen SL, Fox PL, et al. The oxidation of lipoproteins by monocytes/macrophages. Biochemical and biological mechanisms. *J Biol Chem.* 1999;274:25959–25962.

Hessler JR, Morel DW, Lewis LJ, et al. Lipoprotein oxidation and lipoprotein-induced cytotoxicity. *Arteriosclerosis.* 1983;3(3):215–222.

Li Q, Li B, Wang X, et al. Overexpression of insulin-like growth factor-1 in mice protects from myocyte death after infarction, attenuating ventricular dilation, wall stress, and cardiac hypertrophy. *J Clin Invest.* 1997;100:1991–1999.

Lowes BD, Gilbert EM, Abraham WT, et al. Myocardial gene expression in dilated cardiomyopathy treated with beta-blocking agents. *N Engl J Med.* 2002;346(18):1357–1365.

Morel DW, Hessler JR, Chisolm GM. Low density lipoprotein cytotoxicity induced by free radical peroxidation of lipid. *J Lipid Res.* 1983;24:1070–1076.

Moreno PR, Bernardi VH, Lopez-Cuellar J, et al. Macrophages, smooth muscle cells, and tissue factor in unstable angina. Implications for cell-mediated thrombogenicity in acute coronary syndromes. *Circulation.* 1996;94:3090–3097.

Nilsson J. Cytokines and smooth muscle cells in atherosclerosis. *Cardiovasc Res.* 1993;27: 1184–1190.

Reidy MA, Fingerle J, Lindner V. Factors controlling the development of arterial lesions after injury. *Circulation.* 1992;86(Suppl 6): III43–III46.

Rifai N, Ridker PM. Inflammatory markers and coronary heart disease. *Curr Opin Lipidol.* 2002;13(4):383–389.

Robbins M, Topol EJ. Inflammation in acute coronary syndromes. *Cleve Clin J Med.* 2002; 69(Suppl 2):SII130–SII142.

Rosenberg RD, Aird WC. Vascular-bed-specific hemostasis and hyper-coagulable states. *N Engl J Med.* 1999;340(20):1555–1564.

Topol EJ, Byzova TV, Plow EF. Platelet GPIIb–IIIa blockers. *Lancet.* 1999;353:227–231.

Toschi V, Gallo R, Lettino M, et al. Tissue factor modulates the thrombogenicity of human atherosclerotic plaques. *Circulation.* 1997;95: 594–599.

Zhang R, Brennan ML, Fu X, et al. Association between myeloperoxidase levels and risk of coronary artery disease. *JAMA.* 2001;286(17): 2136–2142.

chapter 11

Hypertension

Amanda R. Vest • Leslie S. Cho

QUESTIONS

1. A 35-year-old woman at 24 weeks of pregnancy is found to have several blood pressure readings in the range of 145 to 158 mmHg systolic, 80 to 92 mmHg diastolic. This is her first pregnancy and she has no prior history of hypertension. She reports bilateral mild ankle swelling and nausea, but no right upper quadrant pain, visual changes, headaches, or dyspnea. A 24-hour urine collection shows 360 g protein. The hemoglobin is 8.0 g/dL and the platelet count is 43,000 cells/mm³. Which of the following is the correct diagnosis?

   a. Chronic hypertension
   b. Gestational hypertension
   c. Preeclampsia
   d. Eclampsia

2. A 42-year-old woman presents for post hospitalization follow-up. She was recently admitted to hospital for 3 days due to sudden-onset dyspnea. Her blood pressure on presentation was 164/98 mmHg. Her examination and chest radiograph were consistent with pulmonary edema. She responded well to intravenous diuretics and was discharged on lisinopril. She has no family history of hypertension. On examination during the clinic visit, her blood pressure is 158/90 mmHg. She is normal in weight and has a normal cardiovascular examination except for a right-sided carotid bruit. Her blood tests are notable for a rise in creatinine from 0.9 to 1.8 mg/dL since hospital discharge. What is the most appropriate follow-up investigation?

   a. Coronary angiogram
   b. Duplex ultrasonography of the renal arteries
   c. Urinary catecholamines
   d. 24-Hour urinary-free cortisol

3. An 83-year-old woman presents to cardiology clinic for follow-up of her hypertension and coronary artery disease. Her only current symptom is dizziness on standing from a sitting position. The dizziness caused her to lose balance and fall on two occasions. Her current resting blood pressure is 144/90 mmHg with pulse 60 beats per minute (bpm). Her medications include hydrochlorothiazide 25 mg daily, doxazosin 2 mg daily, metoprolol XL 50 mg daily, simvastatin 40 mg daily, and aspirin 81 mg daily. What changes in medication therapy would you recommend?

a. Discontinue hydrochlorothiazide and start lisinopril 20 mg daily.

b. Discontinue atenolol and increase hydrochlorothiazide to 50 mg daily.

c. Discontinue doxazosin and initiate clonidine 0.4 mg twice daily.

d. Discontinue doxazosin and start lisinopril 5 mg daily.

e. Discontinue doxazosin and increase metoprolol to 100 mg daily.

4. A 64-year-old woman with hypertension, stage III chronic kidney disease (CKD), and diabetes is not yet at blood pressure goal on the following antihypertensives: lisinopril 40 mg, hydrochlorothiazide 25 mg, and metoprolol XL150 mg. Which of the following additional agents is contraindicated?

a. Aliskiren

b. Hydrochlorothiazide

c. Amlodipine

d. Methyldopa

5. A 57-year-old woman with multidrug-resistant hypertension presents to her primary care doctor with multiple complaints. Her antihypertensive regimen consists of valsartan, hydralazine, amlodipine, captopril, and hydrochlorothiazide. Which of the following pairings of medication and side effect are most likely to be correct?

a. Valsartan and cough

b. Hydralazine and ankle edema

c. Amlodipine and insomnia

d. Captopril and constipation

6. A 19-year-old young man presents with an aortic root diameter of 4.4 cm and a strong family history of aortic dissection. His father died of a type A dissection at age 42, and his older brother recently underwent aortic root repair for an aneurysm measuring 5.6 cm in diameter. Both brothers have the fibrillin-1 gene mutation. The patient currently receives metoprolol 50 mg daily, with a pulse of 55 bpm and blood pressure measurements in the range of 115 to 125/65 to 75 mmHg. Which additional medication should be added?

a. No additional medications

b. Amlodipine

c. Ramipril

d. Losartan

7. A 62-year-old man with type 1 diabetes mellitus receives intermittent hemodialysis for his end-stage renal disease. His blood pressure has become elevated over the past year and has not reached goal levels despite initiation of three antihypertensive medications. He takes several medications for comorbid conditions, several of which may be exacerbating his elevated blood pressure. Medications for which of the following conditions would not be expected to have a side effect of hypertension?

a. Diabetes

b. Anemia

c. Hyperparathyroidism

d. Glaucoma

e. Osteoarthritis

8. A 58-year-old man with resistant hypertension returns for outpatient follow-up. His blood pressure is 168/79 mmHg and pulse 70 bpm, despite 25 mg hydrochlorothiazide daily, 200 mg metoprolol XL daily, 320 mg valsartan daily,

10 mg amlodipine daily, and a 0.1 mg/24 hour clonidine patch. He is considering entering a sympathetic denervation trial and has some questions about the procedure. Which of the following is the most accurate brief description of the denervation procedure?

a. Access through a femoral vein, cryoablation of a unilateral renal artery

b. Access through a femoral artery, radiofrequency ablation of a unilateral renal artery

c. Access through a femoral vein, radiofrequency ablation of bilateral renal arteries

d. Access through a femoral artery, alcohol ablation of bilateral renal arteries

e. Access through a femoral artery, radiofrequency ablation of bilateral renal arteries

f. At this time renal denervation cannot be recommended for this patient population

9. Which of the following patient characteristics is a risk factor for development of angiotensin-converting enzyme inhibitor (ACEI)-induced angioedema?

a. Diabetes

b. Female gender

c. Age <45 years

d. Age >65 years

10. A 76-year-old man with hypertension has inadequate blood pressure control on chlorthalidone 25 mg daily. His primary care doctor is choosing a second antihypertensive agent. Which of the following comorbidities would be an evidence-based indication for choosing ramipril over amlodipine as the second agent?

a. Heart failure with preserved ejection fraction (HFPEF)

b. Peripheral arterial disease

c. Sleep apnea

d. Aortic aneurysm

11. A 30-year-old man with no past medical history presents to his primary care physician complaining of new-onset morning headaches that have been ongoing for the past few weeks. His blood pressure is noted to be 220/100 mmHg with a gradient between his brachial and popliteal arteries. On auscultation, there is a II/VI systolic crescendo–decrescendo murmur heard across the precordium. His electrocardiogram is significant for left ventricular hypertrophy. A chest X-ray shows cardiomegaly with evidence of rib notching. The patient most likely has what valvular abnormality?

a. Bicuspid aortic valve

b. Mitral regurgitation

c. Tricuspid regurgitation

d. Pulmonary stenosis

12. A 55-year-old man with diabetes mellitus presents to his cardiologist with a blood pressure of 165/95 mmHg. According to the JNC (Joint National Committee) 8 guidelines, what is his target blood pressure measurement?

a. Prehypertension, 140/90 mmHg

b. Stage 2, 130/80 mmHg

c. Stage 1, 140/90 mmHg

d. Stage 2, 110/70 mmHg

13. What is the mechanism of action of the antihypertensive medication aliskiren?

   a. ACEI

   b. Nonselective β-blockade

   c. Angiotensin receptor blocker (ARB)

   d. Direct renin inhibitor

14. A 35-year-old woman with no past medical history, not receiving oral contraceptives, and with a family history of hypertension presents with a gradual increase in blood pressure over the past few years. Today in clinic her blood pressure is 155/95 mmHg. What is the most appropriate next step?

   a. Patient has essential hypertension; start thiazide diuretic

   b. She is asymptomatic; therefore, observe patient and have her follow-up in 1 year

   c. Have her follow-up in a few weeks for repeat blood pressure measurements

   d. Renal magnetic resonance imaging (MRI)

15. A 68-year-old man with coronary artery disease, hypertension, diabetes mellitus, and stage II hypertension presents for routine follow-up in the cardiology clinic. His blood pressure is 180/100 mmHg. He is compliant with all his medications and is currently on hydrochlorothiazide, lisinopril, metoprolol, amlodipine, and isosorbide mononitrate. He recently has had two episodes of noncardiogenic pulmonary edema in the setting of an ejection fraction of 55% with no evidence of diastolic dysfunction. What is the most appropriate next step in the management of his hypertension?

   a. Addition of minoxidil

   b. Renal MRI

   c. Discussion of medical adherence

   d. Addition of hydralazine

16. A 44-year-old woman had a blood pressure of 115/75 mmHg a few years ago. She now has a blood pressure of 155/75 mmHg, which was confirmed on a repeat visit. How much has her risk for cardiovascular disease increased?

   a. No change

   b. Twofold

   c. Fourfold

   d. Tenfold

17. Which of the following antihypertensive agents is a known cause of autoimmune hemolytic anemia?

   a. Metoprolol

   b. Methyldopa

   c. Captopril

   d. Losartan

18. A patient is initiated on an ACEI. What is the recommended cutoff for rise in creatinine before stopping the medication?

   a. 10% increase in creatinine

   b. 20% increase in creatinine

   c. 35% increase in creatinine

   d. 50% increase in creatinine

19. A 68-year-old man with hypertension and history of a stroke presents for further management of his hypertension. He is currently prescribed a thiazide diuretic;

however, his blood pressure remains elevated. From the standpoint of decreasing his future risk of stroke, which of the following drug classes would be most beneficial?

a. Calcium channel blocker

b. ACEI

c. ARB

d. β-Blocker

20. A 56-year-old woman presents to your clinic for physical examination. She has no significant past medical history and is asymptomatic. Her vital signs are significant for a blood pressure of 145/95 mmHg. What are the next steps in her evaluation for hypertension?

a. She should return in 1 year for her yearly physical examination.

b. She should have a repeat blood pressure measurement at a later time point during her visit and return in a few weeks to obtain repeat testing if that measurement is elevated.

c. Start patient on thiazide diuretic at the initial clinic visit.

d. Begin evaluation for secondary causes of hypertension.

21. A 45-year-old woman with no significant past medical history is noted to have a blood pressure of 145/90 mmHg in the outpatient clinic. This is confirmed on repeat visits. Which of the following tests would not be indicated at this time?

a. Electrocardiogram

b. Urinalysis

c. Creatinine

d. Urine metanephrines

22. A 26-year-old man with no significant history presents to his primary care physician with complaints of episodic palpitations, morning headaches, and diaphoresis. He denies any illicit drug use. His physical examination is notable for a blood pressure of 230/120 mmHg. His ophthalmologic examination is significant for AV nicking. What is the most appropriate next step?

a. Toxicology screen

b. Urine metanephrines

c. MRI thorax

d. Start thiazide diuretic with follow-up in 1 month

23. A 65-year-old man with a history of hypertension and dyslipidemia is admitted to the coronary care unit with a diagnosis of a myocardial infarction. He undergoes an emergent cardiac catheterization with insertion of a drug-eluting stent to his left circumflex coronary artery. His vital signs show a blood pressure of 170/90 mmHg with a heart rate of 85 bpm and no evidence of heart failure on examination. Which of the following medications would be most appropriate to treat this patient's hypertension?

a. Amlodipine

b. Verapamil

c. Metoprolol

d. Nitroprusside

24. Which of the following antihypertensive drug classes is most effective at reducing carotid intimal thickness?

a. Calcium channel blocker

b. β-Blocker

c. ACEI

d. Thiazide diuretic

25. What is the long-term antihypertensive mechanism of action for thiazide diuretics?

    a. Decreased plasma volume
    b. Natriuresis
    c. Decreased cardiac output
    d. Decreased peripheral resistance

26. A 46-year-old woman, status post orthotopic heart transplantation, is currently taking mycophenolate, prednisone, and tacrolimus as an immunosuppressive regimen. On routine laboratory evaluation, she is found to have leukopenia. Mycophenolate levels have not been elevated in the past few months. Which of the following antihypertensive agents is the most likely culprit?

    a. Hydrochlorothiazide
    b. Metoprolol
    c. Captopril
    d. Clonidine

27. A 34-year-old man with isolated essential hypertension presents to clinic and is found to have a blood pressure of 180/100 mmHg after intensive lifestyle modifications. What is the most appropriate next step?

    a. Start hydrochlorothiazide.
    b. Start hydrochlorothiazide and lisinopril.
    c. Repeat blood pressure in 4 weeks.
    d. Start amlodipine.

28. A 62-year-old man with isolated essential hypertension, currently taking hydrochlorothiazide 25 mg PO daily, comes to you for his first clinic visit. He notes that his blood pressure at home is always less than 140/80 mmHg, but in clinic it is always at least 155/95 mmHg. What is the next step?

    a. Increase dose of thiazide
    b. Addition of second antihypertensive medication
    c. Do nothing as he has white coat hypertension
    d. Evaluate for secondary causes of hypertension

29. A 48-year-old man with diabetes mellitus, hypertension, and hyperlipidemia presents to the emergency room with hypertensive emergency. His mean arterial pressure is 150 mmHg, pulse 58 bpm. The electrocardiogram is notable for sinus bradycardia with PR prolongation (260 milliseconds) and no ST deviations or T-wave abnormalities. Which medications would be the most appropriate therapy for this patient?

    a. Intravenous nitroprusside
    b. Sublingual nifedipine
    c. Intravenous labetalol
    d. Intravenous nitroglycerin

30. A 48-year-old obese man with hypertension, dyslipidemia, and diabetes mellitus presents to the outpatient clinic for his yearly physical. He has refused medications in the past, but now is willing to consider treatment. His blood pressure is 145/95 mmHg with a heart rate of 80 bpm. His laboratory data are significant for a creatinine of 1.3 mg/dL with the presence of microalbuminuria. Which of the following mediations would be most appropriate?

    a. Carvedilol
    b. Lisinopril

    c. Chlorthalidone

    d. Terazosin

31. A 34-year-old woman with essential hypertension is considering becoming pregnant. Which of the following medications would be absolutely contraindicated to control her blood pressure during pregnancy?

    a. Methyldopa

    b. Labetolol

    c. Captopril

    d. Nifedipine

32. A 48-year-old Caucasian man with impaired fasting glucose presents to his physician for a follow-up visit after he was noted to have a blood pressure of 150/95 mmHg. On repeat evaluation his blood pressure is 155/95 mmHg. Which of the following medications would be the least favored?

    a. Hydrochlorothiazide 25 mg PO daily

    b. Lisinopril 10 mg PO daily

    c. Atenolol 25 mg PO daily

    d. Chlorthalidone 25 mg PO daily

33. A 65-year-old African American man with isolated hypertension presents to clinic for his yearly physical examination. He is noted to have a blood pressure of 170/95 mmHg. He is currently prescribed lisinopril and metoprolol. Which of the following medication changes would be most appropriate?

    a. Continue current medications at increased doses

    b. Conversion of patient to a calcium channel blocker and thiazide diuretic

    c. Addition of clonidine

    d. Stopping lisinopril because of concern for renal artery stenosis

34. A 42-year-old woman with a new diagnosis of diabetes mellitus presents for management of hypertension. She was previously an avid athlete, but over the past few years has noted increased weight gain, a radial fracture after a minor fall, and increasing hirsutism. She is currently on hydrochlorothiazide, amlodipine, and lisinopril. What is the most appropriate next step in the management of this patient's hypertension?

    a. Referral to nutrition specialist to assist her with weight loss

    b. Addition of clonidine

    c. 24-Hour urine cortisol test

    d. MRI of the brain

35. A 69-year-old woman with diabetes mellitus and hyperlipidemia and no history of hypertension is noted at her yearly clinic visit to have new-onset hypertension with a blood pressure of 180/110 mmHg. She undergoes screening for secondary causes of hypertension and is found to have a pheochromocytoma. What of the following medications is contraindicated as monotherapy?

    a. Metoprolol

    b. Lisinopril

    c. Phentolamine

    d. Hydrochlorothiazide

36. A 42-year-old man presents for a routine physical examination. He is noted to have a body mass index of 30 kg/m^2, impaired fasting glucose, and a blood pressure of 135/85 mmHg. What is the best treatment plan for this individual?

a. Aggressive lifestyle modification

b. Institute thiazide diuretic regimen

c. No treatment at this time

d. Initiate ACEI

37. A 50-year-old man with CKD and hypertension has a blood pressure of 165/110 mmHg. What is this patient's target blood pressure according to the JNC 8 guidelines?

a. 140/90 mmHg

b. 130/80 mmHg

c. 120/80 mmHg

d. 110/70 mmHg

38. A 36-year-old patient, status post heart transplantation, is found to have hypertension. He is currently taking prednisone, mycophenolate, and cyclosporine. Which of the following antihypertensive medications would increase cyclosporine levels?

a. Lisinopril

b. Hydrochlorothiazide

c. Diltiazem

d. Metoprolol

39. A 56-year-old man with resistant hypertension begins to take a new antihypertensive agent. Within the next few weeks he is diagnosed with pericarditis. Which of the following agents is most likely responsible?

a. Carvedilol

b. Minoxidil

c. Amlodipine

d. Captopril

40. A 27-year-old woman presents to the cardiology clinic for evaluation of uncontrolled hypertension. She was diagnosed 2 years ago and is currently taking hydrochlorothiazide, lisinopril, and amlodipine. She denies nonadherence and has a blood pressure of 170/100 mmHg that is equal in both arms. On routine laboratory examination, she has a potassium level of 2.9 mEq/L with a sodium level of 148 mEq/L. What is the most appropriate diagnostic test?

a. Renal MRI/magnetic resonance angiography

b. Morning renin and aldosterone concentrations

c. Adrenal vein sampling

d. 24-Hour urine cortisol concentration

41. A 58-year-old obese man with hypertension, diabetes mellitus, hyperlipidemia, and recent myocardial infarction presents for his annual physical examination. He is currently prescribed atenolol, hydrochlorothiazide, amlodipine, and quinapril. His blood pressure is at target values. His HbA1c is at goal. However, he has noted increasing lower extremity edema over the past few months and had a near-fatal car accident after falling asleep while driving. His echocardiogram reveals an ejection fraction of 65% with no evidence of diastolic dysfunction. Which of the following management decisions would be most appropriate at this time?

a. Discontinue calcium channel blocker

b. Polysomnography

    c. Addition of loop diuretic

    d. Maintain current regimen with advisement that his symptoms are typical with aging

42. A 56-year-old man on hydralazine, hydrochlorothiazide, lisinopril, and metoprolol begins to develop a malar rash and arthralgias. Which of the above antihypertensive agents is known to cause drug-induced lupus?

    a. Hydralazine

    b. Hydrochlorothiazide

    c. Lisinopril

    d. Metoprolol

43. A 47-year-old man with coronary artery disease, diabetes mellitus, and hypertension is currently taking clonidine. He is found to have a blood pressure of 170/90 mmHg after forgetting to take his medication for 48 hours. What is the best strategy to control his blood pressure?

    a. Restart clonidine.

    b. Start nitroprusside.

    c. Start esmolol.

    d. Add thiazide diuretic.

ANSWERS

1. **c.** Preeclampsia. Chronic hypertension is characterized by blood pressure ≥140/90 mmHg present before pregnancy, before the 20th week of gestation, or persisting beyond the 42nd postpartum day. Conversely, gestational hypertension develops beyond 20 weeks of gestation and usually resolves within 42 days postpartum. Preeclampsia is characterized by hypertension presenting beyond 20 weeks of gestation with >300 mg protein in a 24-hour urine collection or >30 mg/mmol in a spot urine sample, although in rare cases hypertension or proteinuria can be absent. Thrombocytopenia in this patient is very concerning for HELLP syndrome (hemolysis, elevated liver enzymes, and low platelets), a life-threatening condition showing significant overlap with preeclampsia. Eclampsia is the occurrence of seizures in a pregnant woman with preeclampsia. Edema is no longer considered to be part of the diagnostic criteria for preeclampsia because it occurs in more than half of normal pregnancies.

2. **b.** Duplex ultrasonography of the renal arteries. This young woman likely has hypertension secondary to fibromuscular dysplasia (FMD). FMD is a non-inflammatory, nonatherosclerotic vascular condition typically affecting young women. It most frequently presents with hypertension, transient ischemic attack, stroke, or an asymptomatic cervical bruit. Sudden onset of pulmonary edema and a significant rise in creatinine after ACEI/ARB initiation are also common manifestations and reflect the presence of renal artery stenosis. About 60% to 75% of cases of FMD involve the renal arteries. Duplex ultrasonography is a noninvasive investigation that is highly specific and sensitive for renal artery stenosis, whether the stenosis is caused by atherosclerosis or FMD, and therefore is often the first test for diagnosis of this condition. Duplex ultrasonography of the carotids would also have been a good choice in this patient given the presence of a carotid bruit. The classic "string-of-beads" appearance of the arteries may be seen on angiography. The clinical history is not suggestive of pheochromocytoma (Answer c) or Cushing syndrome (Answer d).

3. **d.** Discontinue doxazosin and start lisinopril 5 mg daily. The likely culprit of this patient's postural dizziness and falls is doxazosin. Elderly patients are more susceptible to drug side effects and management of hypertension should take into account such symptoms. Doxazosin demonstrated less effective blood pressure lowering than a thiazide in the antihypertensive and lipid lowering treatment to prevent heart attack trial (ALLHAT) study and was associated with excess cardiovascular events and incident heart failure. It would therefore be appropriate to discontinue doxazosin. There is minimal additional efficacy increasing from 25 to 50 mg of hydrochlorothiazide. The β-blocker should be continued due to the coronary artery disease history, but increasing to 100 mg metoprolol risks bradycardia. Clonidine 0.4 mg twice daily would also lower the heart rate and would be an excessive dose for initiation in an elderly patient who is already near blood pressure goal. The JNC recommendation of a "start low, go slow" approach in the elderly is intended to limit drug side effects, including hypotension. The discontinuation of doxazosin and initiation of 5 mg lisinopril is therefore the most appropriate option.

4. **a.** Aliskiren. The U.S. Food and Drug Administration issued a black box warning in 2012 that aliskiren should not be used with ACEIs or ARBs in patients with diabetes, because of the risk of renal impairment. There is also a warning to avoid the use of aliskiren with ACEIs or ARBs in patients with a glomerular filtration rate <60 mL/min. Conversely, methyldopa usually does not reduce glomerular filtration rate, renal blood flow, or filtration fraction. Normal or elevated plasma renin activity may decrease during methyldopa therapy. Hydrochlorothiazide may be a useful addition in stage III CKD but is unlikely to be effective in patients with a glomerular filtration rate <30 mL/min. Amlodipine is also a reasonable add-on medication to consider in this scenario.

5. b. Hydralazine and ankle edema. Vasodilatory lower extremity edema is most commonly seen with direct arteriolar dilators such as hydralazine and minoxidil. Dihydropyridine calcium antagonists, such as amlodipine, and α-adrenergic antagonists, such as doxazosin, are also associated with extremity edema. ACEIs are associated with an approximate 20% incidence of cough, which is purported to be bradykinin mediated. Angiotensin receptor antagonists, such as valsartan, do not directly inhibit angiotensin-converting enzyme activity or inhibit the breakdown of bradykinin. However, there are reports of angiotensin receptor antagonist-associated cough, but the incidence, severity, and frequency of dry cough in patients receiving valsartan or losartan are equivalent to those receiving placebo. Sleep disturbance is a side effect of β-blockers, especially those that cross the blood-brain barrier (e.g., propranolol and metoprolol). Constipation is a frequent side effect of verapamil.

6. d. Losartan. Both brothers carry the gene mutation for Marfan syndrome; presumably their father's fatal aortic dissection was also a result of this connective tissue disease. Recent data suggest that the ARB losartan may slow the progression of aortic root dilatation in Marfan syndrome. Initially promising animal model studies demonstrating the benefits of transforming growth factor-beta pathway blockade by losartan have now translated into human clinical trials demonstrating benefit for patients with Marfan syndrome. In a randomized controlled trial of 233 Marfan patients, aortic root dilatation rate per MRI was significantly lower in the losartan group, when compared with controls, at a mean of 3-year follow-up.

7. a. Diabetes. There are no established links between hypertension and oral or subcutaneous therapies for diabetes. However, all four other conditions can be treated with medications that may be iatrogenic causes or contributors to hypertension. Approximately 20% to 30% of patients who receive erythropoietin intravenously for anemia of CKD develop an elevation in diastolic pressure of 10 mmHg or more. Secondary hyperparathyroidism is common in CKD patients, and cinacalcet can lower parathyroid hormone levels by increasing the sensitivity of the calcium-sensing receptor to extracellular calcium. However, hypertension is an adverse effect in approximately 7% of patients. Systemic absorption of ophthalmic drops is limited, but α-adrenergic agonists such as brimonidine may raise the pulse and blood pressure. Nonsteroidal anti-inflammatory medications such as ibuprofen are a common cause of fluid retention and hypertension exacerbation, especially for patients with renal dysfunction.

8. e. Access through a femoral artery, radiofrequency ablation of bilateral renal arteries. Current renal denervation catheters are introduced via standard femoral artery access. These catheters have a radiofrequency energy electrode tip that delivers a series of 2-minute ablations along the lumen of each renal artery to disrupt the sympathetic nerve fibers. Symplicity HTN-2 was a randomized, controlled trial comparing 54 patients receiving standard medical therapy for resistant hypertension with 52 patients who underwent percutaneous renal sympathetic denervation. The denervation group demonstrated a mean 32/12 mmHg blood pressure reduction at 6 months, compared with a 1/0 mmHg reduction in controls. However, the larger Symplicity 2 study did not show any difference. Thus, at this time, renal denervation cannot be recommended as therapy.

9. b. Female gender. ACEIs are the leading cause of drug-induced angioedema in the United States because they are so widely prescribed, accounting for 20% to 40% of all emergency room visits for angioedema. ACEIs induce angioedema in approximately 0.2% of recipients and the risk appears equivalent between the different ACEI medications. Severe reactions can be observed many months or even years after initiation of ACEI therapy. One large Veteran's Affairs study by Miller et al. documented an almost fourfold higher rate of ACEI angioedema in blacks compared with whites, a 50% higher rate in women and a 12% lower rate in patients with diabetes. Patient age quartiles were unassociated with angio-edema risk.

10. b. Peripheral arterial disease. There is now evidence to support the specific use of ramipril in patients with peripheral arterial disease and intermittent claudication. Ramipril has been associated with a significant increase in pain-free and maximum treadmill walking times at 6 months, as compared with placebo. Relative to placebo, ramipril also significantly improved the physical functioning component of a quality of life score. Although blood pressure control is an important management component for hypertensive patients with HFPEF, there is no compelling evidence for superiority of one medication over another in this setting. There is also no strong evidence to guide a specific antihypertensive choice for a patient with sleep apnea, although the presence of increased sympathetic nerve activity and a nocturnal diuresis in sleep apnea patients may explain reports that β-blockers tend to lower blood pressure more than thiazide diuretics in this setting. β-Blockers and ACEIs or ARBs are commonly used for blood pressure control in patients with aortic aneurysms.

11. a. Bicuspid aortic valve. This young man has a classic presentation of coarctation of the aorta. This secondary cause of hypertension is the result of stenosis of the aorta, usually at the embryonic site of the ligamentum arteriosum and is typically distal to the origin of the left subclavian artery. The presentation in adulthood is varied and is twice as common in men. Symptoms of hypertension or congestive heart failure are common. The electrocardiogram is characterized by left ventricular hypertrophy. Right ventricular hypertrophy is common if a concomitant ventricular septal defect is present. The most common associated valvular abnormality is a bicuspid aortic valve seen in 22% to 42% of cases. Intracranial aneurysms are seen in up to 10% of cases. Patients will often have a characteristic systolic precordial murmur secondary to the development of collateral arteries. Long-term management involves surgical or transcatheter correction. Patients will often continue to have systemic hypertension after repair and should be treated accordingly.

12. b. Stage 2, 130/80 mmHg. The most recent JNC 8 guidelines recommend that patients with diabetes have blood pressure goal of less than 140/90 mmHg based on the large ACCORD-BP (Action to Control Cardiovascular Risk in Diabetes — Blood–Pressure-lowering arm) study. The new guideline makes no distinction between patients with CKD or diabetes mellitus with no or with otherwise uncomplicated hypertension in patients less than 60 years of age. The most controversial aspect of the new guideline involves patients >60 years whose treatment goal is now <150/90 mmHg if they have no CKD or diabetes mellitus.

13. d. Direct renin inhibitor. Aliskiren is a direct renin inhibitor. The renin enzyme controls the rate-limiting step in the generation of angiotensin II. Aliskiren reaches peak concentration in 2 to 4 hours with a half-life of 24 to 36 hours. It is 50% protein bound. Diarrhea is the most common side effect occurring in up to 9.5% of patients. A dose of 150 mg daily will decrease systolic blood pressure on average 12.5 mmHg with a further 2.7 mmHg decrease when the dose is increased to 300 mg PO daily as compared with placebo. Aliskiren has been shown to have similar blood pressure-lowering effects when compared with thiazide diuretics as well as ACEIs. However, to date there are limited data on the effect of aliskiren on hypertension-induced end-organ damage and clinical outcomes.

14. a. Patient has essential hypertension; start thiazide diuretic. The patient likely has essential hypertension. The age of onset is typically between the early 20s to the late 50s. The presence of a family history of hypertension, the mild elevation in blood pressure, and the gradual onset make the diagnosis of essential hypertension more likely. First-line therapy in this individual, assuming she is not trying to become pregnant, is the use of a thiazide diuretic. Reevaluation in 1 year would not be appropriate, given the long-term complications associated with uncontrolled hypertension. A repeat evaluation in a few weeks is not necessary, given the documented hypertension over the past few years. The presence of unilateral renal artery stenosis from vascular hyperplasia is a possibility; however, the clinical history is most consistent with essential hypertension.

15. **b.**   Renal MRI. The distinction between essential hypertension and secondary causes is critical in the management of a patient with long-standing hypertension that is difficult to control. In this scenario, the inability to control the patient's blood pressure with multiple medications increases the pretest probability of a secondary etiology. In this individual, the presence of multiple cardiac risk factors, along with repeat episodes of noncardiogenic pulmonary edema, suggests the diagnosis of bilateral renal artery stenosis. Addition of further antihypertensive medications would be indicated, but not prior to initiating a workup for renal artery stenosis. A renal MRI would be the most appropriate of the mentioned answers.

16. **b.**   Twofold. Increasing blood pressure beginning at 115/75 mmHg is noted to be a risk factor for stroke, heart failure, and myocardial infarction. For every 20 mmHg increase in systolic blood pressure and for every 10 mmHg in diastolic blood pressure, there is a twofold increase in the risk of cardiovascular disease. For the above patient, her risk of cardiovascular disease has increased by twofold.

17. **b.**   Methyldopa. The central α-agonist methyldopa is known to cause an autoimmune hemolytic anemia in up to 20% of patients taking the medication. Other common side effects include sedation, insulin resistance, and galactorrhea. Methyldopa is not a first-line agent for treatment of hypertension and is usually reserved for pregnant patients and those with resistant hypertension.

18. **c.**   35% increase in creatinine. According to the JNC 7 guidelines, patients initiated on an ACEI should be continued on that medication unless the creatinine increases by more than 35% or another indication for discontinuation presents itself.

19. **a.**   Calcium channel blocker. The Blood Pressure Lowering Treatment Trialist Collaboration Study found that calcium channel blockers provided a greater benefit in the reduction of stroke when compared with other antihypertensive agents. However, there was no difference in cardiovascular mortality or overall cardiovascular events.

20. **b.**   She should have a repeat blood pressure measurement at a later time point during her visit and return in a few weeks to obtain repeat testing if that measurement is elevated. The JNC 7 guidelines suggest that the diagnosis of hypertension requires at least two separate blood pressure measurements during a clinic visit. The patient should be resting in a chair for at least 5 minutes and should have her arm supported at heart level when the blood pressure is measured. Blood pressure measurements should be evaluated in the contralateral arm and while standing as well. Elevations in blood pressure should be confirmed in a timely manner on a repeat visit, the timing of which is dependent on the level of hypertension and the presence of comorbid conditions. The patient in this vignette has mild isolated hypertension and should return in a few weeks (6 to 8 weeks). Those with more elevated blood pressure should return sooner. Antihypertensive medications should not be initiated on this initial visit as diurnal variations in blood pressure are common and she may not have hypertension. Ambulatory monitoring of blood pressure should be attempted. An evaluation for secondary cause is premature as the diagnosis of hypertension is not confirmed. Waiting

to reevaluate the patient in 1-year time is unacceptable, as hypertension, if left untreated, increases the risk of stroke, myocardial infarction, heart failure, and renal insufficiency.

21. **d.**   Urine metanephrines. The initial assessment of any patient with a new diagnosis of hypertension requires evaluation for evidence of hypertension-induced end-organ damage. All patients with a new diagnosis of hypertension should have the following testing: serum hematocrit, blood urea nitrogen, serum creatinine, serum potassium, serum calcium, blood glucose, an electrocardiogram, an ophthalmologic examination, a fasting lipid panel, and a urinalysis. Evaluation for secondary causes of hypertension should be limited to those with uncontrolled hypertension after treatment.

22. **b.**   Urine metanephrines. This patient's medical history is consistent with a diagnosis of pheochromocytoma. Pheochromocytomas arise from chromaffin cells. These tumors are most commonly found in the adrenal glands, but may be present anywhere there are sympathetic nerves. Classic symptoms are episodic palpitations, headaches, and diaphoresis. Rarely, patients may present with orthostatic hypotension. Initial diagnostic testing would involve the evaluation of a urine specimen for urine metanephrines. A toxicology screen is not indicated given his clinical history. An MRI of the abdomen would be helpful to evaluate for intra-abdominal masses, but an MRI of the thorax would be of limited benefit. Starting a thiazide diuretic would be beneficial, but ultimately the patient requires surgical therapy for correction of his hypertension.

23. **c.**   Metoprolol. The initial choice of antihypertensive medication in this patient should be a β-blocker. Multiple studies have shown the benefit of β-blockers in the post-myocardial infarction period. The morphine in acute myocardial infarction (MIAMI-1) and International Study of Infarct Survival (ISIS-1) trials in the fibrinolytic era both showed trends toward a decrease in mortality with the use of intravenous β-blockers. The clopidogrel and metoprolol in myocardial infarction (COMMIT) trial found decreases in the rate of reinfarction and ventricular fibrillation with intravenous metoprolol followed by oral metoprolol; however, there was a 30% increase in the risk of cardiogenic shock. A meta-analysis of the post-myocardial infarction use of β-blockers has shown up to a 40% decrease in cardiovascular mortality. The American Heart Association 2013 ST-segment elevation myocardial infarction (STEMI) guidelines recommend initiation of oral β-blockers in the first 24 hours, providing that heart failure signs, evidence of a low-output state, risk factors for cardiogenic shock, or other contraindications to β-blockers are absent. However, intravenous β-blockers carry a class IIa indication in STEMI, given the concern for possible complications.

24. **a.**   Calcium channel blocker. Calcium channel blockers are the most effective of the antihypertensive regimens at reducing carotid atherosclerosis. Studies comparing various calcium channel blockers with thiazide diuretics, ACEIs, and β-blockers have shown that calcium channel blockers have greater ability to decrease carotid intimal thickness.

25. **d.**   Decreased peripheral resistance. The initial mechanism of action for lowering blood pressure is a decrease in plasma volume secondary to natriuresis. This triggers an increase in the activity of the rennin-angiotensin system, resulting in a return of plasma volume to normal. However, there is a long-term decrease in peripheral resistance that produces the chronic antihypertensive effects of thiazide diuretics.

26. **c.**   Captopril. Aside from mycophenolate, the ACEI captopril is the most likely cause of this patient's leukopenia. When immunosuppressive therapy is combined with ACEIs, there are reports of the development of anemia, neutropenia,

leukopenia, and agranulocytosis. The best treatment strategy in this patient would be to use an alternative antihypertensive agent and monitor blood counts closely.

27. **b.** Start hydrochlorothiazide and lisinopril. The most appropriate initial step in the management of the patient in this clinical vignette is the initiation of two antihypertensive medications as recommended in the JNC 7 guidelines. In general, if patients have a blood pressure of greater than 20/10 mmHg above goal, they should be initiated on two antihypertensive agents because monotherapy will typically be ineffective in achieving target blood pressure. Most patients should be started on a thiazide diuretic when commencing treatment of hypertension, as confirmed by the results of the Antihypertensive and Lipid Lowering Treatment to Prevent Heart Attack trial. Care should be taken in patients at risk for hypotension, specifically elderly patients, those with diabetes, and those with autonomic dysfunction.

28. **c.** Do nothing as he has white coat hypertension. The patient in the above clinical vignette has a diagnosis of white coat hypertension. It is defined as a clinic blood pressure of >140/80 mmHg in at least three clinic settings, with blood pressure measurements of <140/80 mmHg in at least two nonclinic settings, and with absence of end-organ damage. Multiple studies have been undertaken to evaluate if isolated elevations in blood pressure in the medical setting are associated with increased cardiovascular events. A 10-year follow-up study comparing cardiovascular events between patients with white coat hypertension and those with sustained hypertension found worse outcomes in those with sustained hypertension. The risk of myocardial infarction was two times greater and the risk of a cerebral vascular event was four times greater in the sustained hypertension group. Comparison of normotensive patients with those with white coat hypertension has noted a greater prevalence of left ventricular hypertrophy in the white coat hypertension group. However, there are no clear data that white coat hypertension increases long-term cardiovascular events. Treatment of white coat hypertension is associated with decreases in clinic blood pressure with no significant decrease in ambulatory blood pressure. Patients with white coat hypertension should be monitored closely for development of sustained hypertension, but do not need to be initiated on antihypertensive therapy.

29. **a.** Intravenous nitroprusside. Treatment of hypertensive emergency requires the use of intravenous medications to decrease the mean arterial blood pressure by 25% in the first few hours. Lower target blood pressure goals increase the risk of inducing a cerebral vascular event from decreased cerebral perfusion. Sublingual nifedipine is no longer used for hypertensive emergencies due to its dramatic and unpredictable blood pressure–lowering effects and the associated adverse clinical outcomes. Nitroprusside, labetalol, and nitroglycerin are all reasonable options. However, given the rapid onset and offset of nitroprusside, and the evidence of conduction delay that may limit labetalol use, nitroprusside would be the most appropriate medication for rapid and safe titration of blood pressure.

30. **b.** Lisinopril. The patient in the vignette has a target blood pressure of 130/80 mmHg according to the JNC 7 guidelines. The correct choice of initial blood pressure medication in this patient would be an ACEI. The ALLHAT study suggested that patients with diabetes mellitus have better long-term outcomes when using a thiazide diuretic compared with an ACEI. However, the patient in this vignette has evidence of protein in his urine. JNC 7 recommends that a thiazide diuretic should be first-line therapy, unless there is a specific indication. In this patient, the presence of proteinuria and diabetes mellitus makes the choice of an ACEI a better option than the thiazide. α-Blockers are not considered first-line therapy in hypertensive patients. In the ALLHAT study, there was

an increased incidence of heart failure when comparing the α-blocker group (doxazosin) with the thiazide group.

31. c. Captopril. ACEIs and ARBs are contraindicated during pregnancy, because of the increased risk of congenital malformations. Methyldopa is the medication most commonly used to control blood pressure in pregnancy. There is significant evidence that it does not produce any harmful outcomes to the fetus. β-Blockers have been used in pregnancy with what appear to be safe results. However, the data are contradictory. There is some evidence that β-blockers, especially when used early in pregnancy, may increase the risk of fetal bradycardia, hypoglycemia, small placental weight, and a small-for-gestational-age fetus. Calcium channel blockers have been used in pregnancy without deleterious results, but the number of published cases is small. In general, methyldopa is the safest antihypertensive during pregnancy. β-Blockers and calcium channel blockers may be used with caution. ACEIs and ARBs are absolutely contraindicated due to teratogenic effects including renal dysplasia and intrauterine growth restriction.

32. c. Atenolol 25 mg PO daily. The least effective option is atenolol. The ALLHAT study showed that the use of thiazide diuretics as first-line therapy for treatment of uncomplicated hypertension was as effective as, if not superior to, amlodipine and lisinopril in preventing fatal coronary artery disease and nonfatal myocardial infarction. The choice of an ACEI would be reasonable, given the presence of glucose intolerance. β-Blockers would not be indicated as first-line therapy in this patient. Multiple meta-analysis comparing β-blockers with placebo or other antihypertensive agents have shown no statistically significant decreases in mortality, myocardial infarction, and stroke. The Anglo Scandinavian Cardiac Outcomes Trial (ASCOT) trial comparing atenolol with amlodipine found a 23% greater risk of stroke in the atenolol group versus the amlodipine-based regimen.

33. b. Conversion of patient to a calcium channel blocker and thiazide diuretic. Analysis of the clinical trials in hypertension has noted that there are differences in the effectiveness of antihypertensive medications between different ethnic groups. African Americans are more responsive to calcium channel blockers and thiazide diuretics than other antihypertensive agents. This patient is on an ACEI and a β-blocker. Altering his regimen to include more effective antihypertensive agents would be indicated rather than increasing his medications, adding additional medications, or evaluating him for secondary causes of hypertension. The new JNC 8 guidelines make recommendation of medication based on the race of the patient.

34. c. 24-Hour urine cortisol test. This patient's medical history is consistent with a secondary cause of hypertension, in particular, Cushing syndrome. This syndrome is characterized by an excess of cortisol. It may be secondary to a pituitary tumor/hyperplasia (Cushing disease), an adrenal tumor, or ectopic adrenocorticotropic production. Clinical manifestations include diabetes mellitus, hypertension, obesity, hypokalemia, osteoporosis, and fungal infections. The initial step in diagnosis is a 24-hour urine free cortisol test. Treatment is surgical.

35. a. Metoprolol. Pheochromocytoma is a rare cause of hypertension. Treatment ultimately requires surgical removal. The use of β-blocker monotherapy is contraindicated as part of the medical management of pheochromocytomas. The catecholamines secreted by these tumors activate both peripheral α- and β-receptors. Blockage of these peripheral β-receptors results in unopposed α-activation. This can result in severe hypertension. Typical medical management of pheochromocytomas involves the use of antihypertensives with α-blocking capability. For example, prazosin or phenoxybenzamine may be used. Only once α-blockade is established should the use of a β-blocker be entertained.

36. a. Aggressive lifestyle modification. Patients with prehypertension are at increased risk for cardiovascular events compared with normotensive individuals; therefore, care of these patients should be focused on aggressive control of all cardiovascular risk factors. Analysis of the Women's Health Initiative compared cardiovascular outcomes in prehypertension patients with normotensive patients and found that the prehypertension patients had hazard ratios indicating a 1.58 (95% confidence interval [CI], 1.12 to 2.21) greater risk for cardiovascular death; 1.76 (95% CI, 1.40 to 2.22) greater risk for myocardial infarction; 1.93 (95% CI, 1.49 to 2.50) greater risk for stroke; 1.36 (95% CI, 1.05 to 1.77) greater risk for hospitalized heart failure; and a 1.66 (95% CI, 1.44 to 1.92) greater risk for any cardiovascular event. Not only are these patients at increased risk for cardiovascular events, but they also have a high incidence of hypertension development. In the Trial of Preventing Hypertension (TROPHY) trial, patients with prehypertension were randomized to candesartan or placebo. Over a period of 4 years, 67% of the untreated group developed hypertension as defined by the JNC 7 guidelines. These data suggest that patients with prehypertension are a high-risk population and should be treated aggressively. According to the JNC 7 guidelines, these individuals should increase their activity level, modify their diet, avoid excessive alcohol, and attempt weight loss. Initiation of antihypertensive medications should be reserved for those who progress to evident hypertension.

37. a. 140/90 mmHg. JNC 8 guidelines recommend that in patients with CKD or diabetes mellitus, the target blood pressure should be <140/90 mmHg.

38. c. Diltiazem. Patients who have undergone heart transplantation often have preexisting hypertension or develop hypertension subsequent to the heart transplant. This is a unique patient population as many of the immunosuppressive medications used after transplantation have multiple drug interactions. With respect to antihypertensive agents, most if not all calcium channel blockers have been shown to increase cyclosporine levels. Diltiazem and verapamil, in particular, are potent inhibitors of protein P-glycoprotein and CYP3A4. These enzymes are critical for the metabolism of diltiazem, and their inhibition can increase cyclosporine levels up to sixfold. It is recommended that patients who require diltiazem and are on cyclosporine have their cyclosporine dose decreased by 25% to 50%. Diltiazem can also increase tacrolimus levels.

39. b. Minoxidil. Pericarditis is a known complication of the direct vasodilator minoxidil often accompanied by a pericardial effusion. Its other major side effect is hirsutism. Prompt withdrawal of the medication once the diagnosis of a pericardial effusion or pericarditis is made is recommended. Minoxidil is a potent peripheral vasodilator and is typically reserved for patients with severe or difficult-to-control hypertension.

40. b. Morning renin and aldosterone concentrations. The patient in this vignette has secondary hypertension from Conn syndrome. This is primary hyperaldosteronism from uncontrolled secretion of aldosterone. Classic laboratory findings include hypokalemia and mild hypernatremia. The initial diagnostic test of choice is an aldosterone-renin ratio. A ratio of >20 is considered diagnostic. In this patient, the presence of lisinopril complicates the testing. ACEIs are known to decrease renin levels, and ideally the test should be done in the early morning after withdrawal of ACEI therapy. Adrenal vein sampling would be helpful in the diagnosis of primary hyperaldosteronism; however, it is not the initial test of choice. A 24-hour urine test would be more appropriate if Cushing syndrome were suspected. The patient's clinical description is not consistent with this diagnosis. The presence of FMD should be suspected in any young woman with suspected secondary hypertension. However, the laboratory abnormalities are more suggestive of Conn syndrome than renal artery stenosis.

41. b. Polysomnography. The patient's clinical history is consistent with the presence of obstructive sleep apnea; therefore, polysomnography (an overnight sleep study) would be the best option. Multiple studies have found evidence for increased risk of hypertension in patients with obstructive sleep apnea. There is no definitive evidence that treating patients with sleep apnea can lower blood pressure; however, there is an increasing hypertension risk as the number of overnight apneic episodes increases. Patients with >30 apnea or hypopnea episodes per hour have an odds ratio of 1.37 of developing hypertension versus those patients with <1.5 apnea or hypopnea episodes per hour.

42. a. Hydralazine. Hydralazine is known to cause a lupus-like syndrome in 5% to 20% of patients taking the medication. This syndrome is characterized by arthralgias, myalgias, pericarditis, fever, and rash. Lisinopril, metoprolol, and hydrochlorothiazide are not known to induce lupus. Other side effects of hydralazine include nausea, vomiting, tachycardia, anorexia, flushing, and diarrhea. Treatment of hydralazine-induced lupus involves withdrawal of the medication.

43. a. Restart clonidine. Rebound hypertension is a known complication of clonidine. Immediate treatment of clonidine withdrawal involves reinstitution of therapy with a slow taper. The mechanism of action is thought to be an increase in sympathetic nervous system activity.

SUGGESTED READINGS

Ahimastos AA, Walker PJ, Askew C, et al. Ramipril for PAD effect of ramipril on walking times and quality of life among patients with peripheral artery disease and intermittent claudication. *JAMA*. 2013;309(5):453–460.

ALLHAT Officers and the Coordinators for the ALLHAT Collaborative Research Group. Major outcomes in high risk hypertensive patients randomized to angiotensin converting enzyme inhibitors or calcium channel blockers vs. diuretic. *JAMA*. 2002;288:2981–2997.

Bertogn SC, Sobotka PA, Sievert H. Renal denervation for hypertension. *J Am Coll Cardiol Intv*. 2012;5(3):249–258.

Blood Pressure Lowering Treatment Trialists' Collaboration. Blood pressure dependent and independent effects of agents that affect the renin angiotensin system. *J Hypertens*. 2007;25:951–958.

Blood Pressure Lowering Treatment Trialists' Collaboration. Effects of ACE inhibitors, calcium antagonists, and other blood-pressure-lowering drugs: results of prospectively designed overviews of randomized trials. *Lancet*. 2000;356:1955–1964.

Blood Pressure Lowering Treatment Trialists' Collaboration. Effects of different blood pressure regimens on cardiovascular events: results of prospectively designed overview of randomized trials. *Lancet*. 2003;362:1527–1535.

Chobanian AV. Isolated systolic hypertension in elderly. *N Engl J Med*. 2007;357:789–796.

Chobanian AV, Bakris GJ, Black HR, et al. The Seventh Report of the Joint National Committee on prevention, detection, evaluation, and treatment of high blood pressure: the JNC 7 report. *JAMA*. 2003;289:2560–2572.

Clement DC, Buyzere MD, Bacquer DA, et al. Prognostic value of ambulatory blood pressure recordings in patients with treated hypertension. *N Engl J Med*. 2003;348:2407–2415.

Dahlof B, Sever PS, Poulter NR, et al. Prevention of cardiovascular events with an antihypertensive regimen of amlodipine adding perindopril as required versus atenolol adding bendroflumethiazide as required, in the Anglo Scandinavian Cardiac Outcomes Trial-Blood Pressure Lowering Arm (ASCOT-BLA). *Lancet*. 2005;366:895–906.

Devereux RB, Dahlof B, Gerdts E, et al. Regression of hypertensive left ventricular hypertrophy by losartan compared to atenolol: the Losartan Intervention for End Point Reduction in Hypertension (LIFE) study. *Circulation*. 2004;110:1456–1462.

Devereux RB, Palmieri V, Sharpe N, et al. Effects of once daily angiotensin converting enzyme inhibition and calcium channel blockade based antihypertensive treatment regimens on left ventricular hypertrophy and diastolic filling in hypertension. *Circulation*. 2001;19:303–309.

Esler MD, Krum H, Sobotka PA, et al. Renal sympathetic denervation in patients with treatment-resistant hypertension (the Symplicity HTN-2 trial): a randomised controlled trial. *Lancet*. 2010;376(9756):1903–1909.

Gradman AH, Kad R. Renin inhibition in hypertension. *J Am Coll Cardiol*. 2008;51:519–528.

Groenink M, den Hartog AW, Franken R, et al. Losartan reduces aortic dilatation rate in adults with Marfan syndrome. *Eur Heart J*. 2013 Sep 2 [Epub ahead of print].

Hsia J, Margolis KL, Eaton CB, et al. Prehypertension and cardiovascular disease risk in the Women's Health Initiative. *Circulation*. 2007; 115:855–860.

Julius S, Nesbitt S, Egan BM, et al. Feasibility of treating prehypertension with an angiotensin receptor blocker. *N Engl J Med*. 2006;354:1685–1697.

Khattar RS, Senior R, Lahiri A. Cardiovascular outcome in white-coat versus sustained mild hypertension: a 10-year follow-up study. *Circulation*. 1998;98:1892–1897.

Krapf R, Hulter HN. Arterial hypertension induced by erythropoietin and erythropoiesis-stimulating agents (ESA). *Clin J Am Soc Nephrol*. 2009;4(2):470.

Lidenfield J, Page RL, Zolty R, et al. Drug therapy in the heart transplant recipient part III: common medical problems. *Circulation*. 2005;113:113–117.

Lindholm LH, Carlberg B, Samuelsson O. Should beta-blockers remain first choice in the treatment of primary hypertension? A meta-analysis. *Lancet*. 2005;366(9496):1545–1553.

Miller DR, Oliveria SA, Berlowitz DR, et al. Angioedema incidence in US veterans initiating angiotensin-converting enzyme inhibitors. *Hypertension*. 2008;51:1624–1630.

Nieto FJ, Young TB, Lind BK, et al. Association of sleep disordered breathing, sleep apnea and hypertension in a large community based study. *JAMA*. 2000;283:1829–1836.

Olin JW. Recognizing and managing fibromuscular dysplasia. *Cleve Clin J Med*. 2007;74(4):273–274, 277–282.

Page RL, Miller GG, Lidenfield J. Drug therapy in the heart transplant recipient part IV: drug-drug interactions. *Circulation*. 2005;111:230–239.

Prospective Studies Collaboration. Age-specific relevance of usual blood pressure to vascular mortality: a meta-analysis of individual data for one million adults in 61 prospective studies. *Lancet*. 2002;360:1903–1913.

Salpeter S, Ormiston T, Salpeter E. Cardioselective beta-blockers for chronic obstructive pulmonary disease. *Cochrane Libr*. 2006;3:1–25.

Salpeter S, Ormiston T, Salpeter E. Cardioselective beta-blockers in reactive airway disease. *Cochrane Libr*. 2006;3:1–45.

Sega R, Trocino S, Lanzarotti A, et al. Alterations in cardiac structure in patients with isolated office, ambulatory or home hypertension: data from the general population Pressione Arteriose Monitorate E Loro Associazioni [PAMELA] Study. *Circulation*. 2001;104(12): 1385–1392.

Simon A, Gariepy J, Moyse D, et al. Differential effects of nifedipine and co-amilozide on the progression of early carotid wall changes. *Circulation*. 2001;103:2949–2954.

Terpesta WF, May JF, Smit AJ, et al. Effect of amlodipine and lisinopril on intima media thickness in previously untreated elderly hypertensive patients (the ELVERA Trial). *J Hypertens*. 2004;22:1309–1316.

Wachtell K, Lehto N, Gerdts E, et al. Angiotensin II receptor blockade reduces new onset atrial fibrillation and subsequent stroke compared to atenolol: the Losartan Intervention for End Point Reduction in Hypertension (LIFE) Study. *J Am Coll Cardiol*. 2005;45:712–719.

chapter 12

Hyperlipidemia

Michael B. Rocco

QUESTIONS ● ● ●

1. Familial hypercholesterolemia (FH) is a common autosomal dominant disorder resulting from mutations leading to impaired hepatic clearance of low-density lipoprotein (LDL) from the circulation. All of the following statements are true regarding heterozygous FH except that

   a. it occurs in 1 in 5,000 persons.

   b. it is associated with serum low-density lipoprotein cholesterol (LDL-C) two to three times above the average.

   c. it is associated with four- to sixfold increased risk of premature coronary heart disease (CHD).

   d. without treatment, the average age for development of symptomatic CHD is 45 years in men and 55 years in women.

   e. ninety percent of FH heterozygotes exhibit detectable xanthomas on the extensor tendons of the hands or on the Achilles tendons by the age of 39.

2. Phenotypic presentation of FH has been demonstrated to be caused by various mutations associated with all but one of the following:

   a. Defects in the hepatic LDL receptor (LDL-R)

   b. Defects in apolipoprotein B (apoB)

   c. Loss-of-function mutation of PCSK9

   d. Loss-of-function mutation of LDLRAP1

3. A 31-year-old man is referred to you for hyperlipidemia assessment. He has no previous cardiovascular history himself and denies any first-degree relatives with a history of CHD although his father and paternal uncle are treated for elevated cholesterol and triglycerides (TGs). He reports that two uncles and a cousin have had heart attacks at young ages. His physical examination reveals a body mass index (BMI) of 32, arcus cornea and xanthelasmas but no xanthomas, and a blood pressure (BP) of 150/80 mmHg. His fasting lipid profile is as follows: total cholesterol (TC) 300 mg/dL, TGs 430 mg/dL, high-density lipoprotein cholesterol (HDL-C) 50 mg/dL, direct LDL-C 202 mg/dL. Fasting blood glucose is 112 mg/dL. Which primary dyslipidemia is this patient most likely to have?

   a. Polygenic hypercholesterolemia

   b. Heterozygous FH

   c. Familial combined hyperlipidemia

    d. Hyperapobetalipoproteinemia

    e. Familial endogenous hypertriglyceridemia

4. Which of the following statements regarding FH is NOT true?

    a. The Food and Drug Administration (FDA) indications for LDL apheresis after maximal tolerated pharmacologic therapy include (a) homozygous FH patients and (b) heterozygous FH in the absence of CHD when LDL-C $\geq$300 mg/dL and in the presence of CHD when LDL-C $\geq$200 mg/dL.

    b. Mipomersen (which inhibits the translation of apoB100 mRNA, thus blocking the production of apoB100 and formation of very low-density lipoprotein [VLDL] and LDL particles) lowers LDL-C by 28% to 36% in individuals with homozygous and heterozygous FH.

    c. TC levels are generally >600 mg/dL with LDL-C levels 6- to eightfold higher than average in individuals with homozygous FH.

    d. Lomitapide has been approved to treat homozygous and heterozygous FH.

    e. Simon Broome Register Group criteria for definite FH requires (a) TC >290 mg/dL in adults or TC >260 mg/dL in children under 16 years OR LDL-C >190 mg/dL in adults or >155 mg/dL in children PLUS (b) tendon xanthomas in the patient, or first- or second-degree relative OR DNA-based evidence of mutations such as LDL-R mutation or familial defective apoB100.

5. Recent statistics from the American Heart Association (AHA) Statistical Update in 2014 report that all of the following regarding dyslipidemia in the United States are true EXCEPT that

    a. 98,900,000 U.S. adults over 20 years of age have elevated TC >200 mg/dL (43.4%).

    b. 35.8% of adults have LDL >130 mg/dL (71 million adults).

    c. 48.7 million adults (21.8%) have HDL <40 mg/dL.

    d. National Health and Nutrition Examination Survey (NHANES) data through 2006 reported that 10.3% of adolescents (12 to 19 years) have abnormal lipid levels.

    e. inadequate control of dyslipidemia is responsible for 4 million yearly deaths worldwide and 350,000 in the United States.

    f. 68.2% of adults and 31.8% of children/adolescents are overweight or obese.

6. Many randomized clinical trials (RCTs) and meta-analyses have contributed to the lipid management guidelines over the past two decades. Which of the following statements is NOT correct?

    a. PROVE-IT/TIMI-22 showed that individuals post myocardial infarction (MI) treated with the more potent statin atorvastatin versus pravastatin had a 16% relative risk reduction.

    b. The JUPITER trial demonstrated that in individuals without documented cardiovascular disease (CVD) and median LDL-C of 108 mg/dL, aggressive statin therapy with rosuvastatin offered greater benefit in individuals with ultrasensitive C-reactive protein (usCRP) >2 versus <2 mg/L.

    c. Primary prevention hypertensive patients in the ASCOT-LLA trial showed reductions in nonfatal MI, CHD death but not all-cause mortality when patients with average lipids and hypertension were treated with atorvastatin 10 mg daily for an average of 3.3 years.

    d. WOSCOPS and AFCAPS/TexCAPS were both primary CHD prevention studies, which showed significant clinical benefits for statin therapy, with similar percentage reductions in LDL-C. The main difference between these trials was that subjects in AFCAPS/TexCAPS had considerably lower baseline LDL-C levels than those in WOSCOPS.

   e. Scandinavian Simvastatin Survival Study (4S), Cholesterol and Recurrent Events (CARE), and Long-Term Intervention with Pravastatin in Ischemic Disease (LIPID) all involved secondary prevention of CHD.

   f. Meta-analyses have demonstrated a >20% reduction in CHD events for every 1 mmol/L reduction in LDL-C with similar proportional reductions in diabetics versus nondiabetics. Similar percent reductions were seen even in lower-risk groups with <5% 5-year risk for CVD.

7. The Framingham Risk Score (FRS) was popularized in the National Cholesterol Education Project: Adult Treatment Panel (NCEP ATP) III guidelines. Potential limitations of the FRS include the following:

   1. Does not take family history into account

   2. May overestimate lifetime risk in individuals ≤50 years of age with ≥1 NCEP risk factor

   3. May not accurately calculate risk in certain ethnic groups because original Framingham population was almost entirely of European origin

   4. Incorporates risk due to insulin-resistant conditions such as metabolic syndrome

   5. Does not include emerging risk factors such as CRP, lipoprotein(a), and apoB

      a. All of the above

      b. 1, 3, and 5

      c. 1, 3, 4, and 5

      d. None of the above

8. Based on the definition proposed by the NCEP ATP III guidelines, metabolic syndrome would be present if three or more of five criteria were present. Which of the following is NOT one of the criteria?

   a. BP ≥130/≥85 or on treatment for hypertension

   b. TGs ≥150 mg/dL

   c. HDL-C of <40 mg/dL in men and women

   d. Fasting glucose =100 mg/dL

   e. Waist circumference of >40 inches in men and >35 inches in women

9. NCEP ATP III was published in 2001. Modifications to NCEP ATP III published in 2004 include all of the following except that

   a. LDL-C goal <70 mg/dL is a therapeutic option for very high-risk patients.

   b. LDL-C goal <70 mg/dL extends to patients at very high risk even with baseline LDL-C <100 mg/dL.

   c. factors that favor the optional goal of <70 mg/dL include CVD plus multiple major risk factors (especially diabetes), severe and poorly controlled risk factors (especially smoking), metabolic syndrome, and acute coronary syndromes.

   d. for moderately high-risk patients, LDL-C <100 mg/dL is an option with consideration of initiation of therapy with statins for LDL-C between 100 and 130 mg/dL.

   e. both higher-dose statins and addition of fibrates and niacin to achieve non–HDL-C goals should be considered to achieve secondary targets and to further reduce cardiovascular event rate.

10. A 53-year-old obese, sedentary woman undergoes lipid screening, revealing TC of 310, TG of 720, HDL-C of 41. LDL-C was not calculated due to elevated TG. HbA1c is 5.9 and thyroid-stimulating hormone (TSH) is normal. NCEP ATP III guideline recommendations for TGs and HDL-C management include all but which of the following:

a. If TGs are ≥500 mg/dL, then TG is the primary target with use of therapeutic options to prevent pancreatitis including fibrates or niacin before LDL-lowering therapy, than treat LDL-C to goal.

b. In patients attaining LDL-C goals, those with TG ≥200 mg/dL have an increased cholesterol content of TG-rich, atherogenic lipoprotein particles. Non–HDL-C takes into account cholesterol in these and LDL particles and is a secondary target for therapy.

c. Therapeutic goal for TG is <150 mg/dL and for HDL-C is >40 in men and >50 in women.

d. HDL-C <40 mg/dL is defined as low and is a risk factor for CVD.

e. Non–HDL-C goal equals the LDL-C goal +30 mg/dL.

f. Combining a fibrate or nicotinic acid with an LDL-C-lowering drug can be considered.

11. Guidelines for management of dyslipidemia emphasize the importance of weight management, dietary choices, and exercise. TLC or Therapeutic Life Style Therapies for primary prevention of CVD include all of the following except

a. diet to reduce intake of saturated fats and dietary cholesterol with total fat range of 25% to 30% of total calories, saturated fat <7% of calories, and low intake of transfatty acids and <200 mg/day of cholesterol.

b. increased intake of plant stanols/sterols up to 2 g/day as a therapeutic option to reduce LDL-C.

c. increased intake of viscous (soluble) fiber to at least 5 to 10 g/day.

d. omega-3 polyunsaturated fatty acid supplements of 800 to 1,000 mg a day.

e. regular physical activity: >30 minutes five to seven times per week or enough moderate activity to expend at least 200 kcal/day.

f. weight loss to maintain BMI <25 kg/m².

12. Secondary causes of dyslipidemia include all EXCEPT which of the following?

a. Hyperthyroidism

b. Obstructive liver disease/biliary cirrhosis

c. Renal disorders including nephrotic syndrome and chronic renal failure

d. Drugs including estrogen/progestins, protease inhibitors, anabolic steroids, corticosteroids, isotretinoin (Accutane®), and cyclosporine

e. Metabolic syndrome or diabetes mellitus (DM)

f. Pregnancy

13. According to NCEP ATP III, CHD risk equivalent defines high-risk individuals who would benefit from more intensive lipid-modifying therapies and include individuals with all of the following except

a. diabetes and additional cardiovascular risk factors.

b. FRS indicating a 10-year risk of MI or coronary death of >10%.

c. claudication with an ankle brachial index of 0.78.

d. individual status post aortic aneurysm endograft.

e. history of transient ischemic attack (TIA) followed by carotid endarterectomy.

Questions 14 to 16

You see a 52-year-old man with a history of type 2 DM on metformin. He has a history of hypertension controlled on amlodipine and an angiotensin-converting enzyme inhibitor. His BMI is 31.7 and waste circumference is 41 inches. His father had a coronary stent at the age of 54. He has the following fasting laboratory values:

Total C: 212 mg/dL

LDL-C: 120 mg/dL

HDL-C: 36 mg/dL

TG: 278 mg/dL

Non–HDL-C: 176 mg/dL

Glucose: 156 mg/dL

HbA1c: 7.6%

TSH: 1.2 mU/L

LFTs (liver function tests): WNL (within normal limits)

14. Based on NCEP ATP III and American Diabetes Association (ADA) guidelines, the most appropriate lipid goals for therapy in this patient are

   a. LDL <70 mg/dL and non-HDL <100.
   b. LDL <100 mg/dL and non-HDL <130.
   c. LDL <70 mg/dL and non-HDL <130.
   d. LDL <130 mg/dL and non-HDL <160.

15. Additional secondary goals for therapy in this patient based on these guidelines include

   a. apoB <80 mg/dL.
   b. apoB <90 mg/dL.
   c. LDL particle number (LDL-P) <1,200.
   d. LDL-P <1,000.
   e. usCRP <2.
   f. Answers a and d.
   g. Answers a and e.

16. The best initial treatment for this patient's dyslipidemia would be

   a. atorvastatin 40 mg/day.
   b. fenofibrate 148 mg/day.
   c. extended release niacin 2,000 mg/day.
   d. simvastatin 20 mg/day.
   e. ezetimibe 10 mg/day.
   f. omega-3 fish oil 4,000 mg/day.

17. The patient above was started on rosuvastatin 20 mg/day, metformin dose was increased, an aerobic exercise program was recommended, and he was referred for dietary advice. Repeat laboratory values in 4 months are as follows:

	Baseline	4 Months
Total C	212	150 mg/dL
LDL-C	120	66 mg/dL
HDL-C	36	38 mg/dL
TG	278	229 mg/dL
Non–HDL-C	176	126 mg/dL
Glucose	156	112 mg/dL
A1C	7.6	6.8%
LFT	WNL	WNL

The most appropriate additional therapies recommended by NCEP ATP II at this time would include all but

    a. nicotinic acid.

    b. fenofibrate.

    c. ezetimibe.

    d. intensification of diet, exercise, and weight loss program.

    e. intensification of statin therapy, increase rosuvastatin to 40 mg/day.

    f. all of the above.

    g. none of the above.

18. Patients such as the one above with diabetes are considered at high risk for CVD events. Which of the following statements is not true in regard to patients with diabetes?

    a. Atherosclerosis accounts for approximately 65% to 75% of all diabetic mortality with 75% of these deaths due to coronary atherosclerosis.

    b. A diabetic patient without a clinical history of prior MI or coronary artery disease (CHD) has a mortality rate from CHD and MI rate equal to a nondiabetic who has had a previous MI.

    c. NHANES data from 2010 indicate that although goals of HbA1c <7 mg/dL, systolic BP <130 mmHg, and LDL-C <100 mg/dL are recommended for diabetics, only 32% of diabetics in the survey currently achieve all three of these goals.

    d. Risk for atherosclerotic events is two- to fourfold greater in diabetics than in nondiabetics.

    e. Atherosclerosis begins years to decades prior to diagnosis of type DM2 and >50% already have clinical CHD at the time of the diagnosis of DM.

19. Additional markers beyond standard risk factors have been shown to help reclassify risk assessment particularly in individuals in an intermediate-risk category (e.g., FRS of 10% to 20% or American College of Cardiology [ACC]/AHA guideline risk score of 5% to 7.5%). All but one of the following may be useful in hyperlipidemia treatment decisions:

    a. usCRP

    b. LDL-P

    c. Coronary artery calcification score (CACS)

    d. HDL particle size and number

    e. Lipoprotein(a)

20. Major differences in the ACC/AHA hyperlipidemia treatment guidelines of 2013 compared with NCEP ATP III recommendations include all of the following except

    1. elimination of LDL-C and non–HDL-C targets for therapy.

    2. a focus on risk reduction targeting therapy to four major groups demonstrated to benefit from statin therapy based on RCT data rather than targeted to risk category and LDL-C level.

    3. replacing the FRS with a newly developed risk calculator that includes ethnicity and family history and broadens the outcome events to include stroke.

    4. that since the absolute benefit in CVD risk reduction is proportional to the baseline risk of the individual and to the intensity of statin therapy, treatment is focused on intensity of statin treatment and does not recommend use of low-dose statin therapies.

    5. that decreasing statin dose is reasonable if LDL-C on therapy is <40 mg/dL.

        a. None, all are true

        b. 1, 3, and 5

    c. 3 and 5

    d. All are not true

    e. 3, 4, and 5

21. The ACC/AHA hyperlipidemia guidelines of 2013 identify four groups shown to benefit from high-intensity and moderate-intensity statin therapy for use in secondary and primary prevention of CVD. High-risk individuals who would be a candidate for high-intensity statin therapy for LDL-C lowering would include all except

    a. those with clinical atherosclerotic cardiovascular disease (ASCVD).

    b. primary elevations of LDL-C $\geq$160 mg/dL.

    c. individuals with diabetes aged 40 to 75 years with LDL-C 70 to 189 mg/dL without clinical ASCVD and with ASCVD risk $\geq$7.5%.

    d. without clinical ASCVD or diabetes with LDL-C 70 to 189 mg/dL and estimated 10-year ASCVD risk $\geq$7.5%.

22. The American Academy of Pediatrics (AAP) 2008 lipid management recommendations for children and teenagers include all of the following except

    a. screening as early as 2 years of age in setting of family history of CVD or hyperlipidemia.

    b. lower LDL cut points for initiation of treatment dependent on risk level.

    c. bile acid sequestrants as initial therapy in younger patients under 16 years of age.

    d. considering initiation of therapy as early as 8 years of age in high-risk children.

    e. emphasis on overweight, high TG, and low HDL managed with lifestyle interventions and weight management.

    f. fiber up to 20 g/day and use of dietary plant stanols/sterols.

23. In decisions regarding screening for and treating hyperlipidemia in children and adolescents, it is important to remember that all of the following are true except that

    1. cholesterol is lowest intrauterine and at birth.

    2. concentrations are similar to young adult levels by 2 years of age with strongest relation to adult levels at 5 to 10 years and 17 to 19 years.

    3. cholesterol levels decrease from 10% to 20% during pre-pubertal and pubertal development.

    4. low-fat diets should not be implemented until after age 5 years.

    5. statins have not been shown to have an adverse effect on sexual or physical maturation.

    6. impact on the atherosclerotic process and clinical outcomes has been demonstrated with statin treatment in children and adolescents.

        a. None of the above

        b. 2, 4, and 6

        c. 4 and 6

        d. 3, 5, and 6

        e. All of the above

24. Although statin therapy and LDL-C reduction is the main thrust of pharmacologic therapies, there has been an interest in treating beyond LDL-C with other therapies directed toward HDL-C and TG to further reduce CVD events. This concept is supported by the following observations except that

    a. cardiovascular events occur in individuals with treated LDL-C even after aggressive LDL lowering with statins.

b. patients with diabetes studied in clinical trials on statins have CVD event rates higher than the CVD event rates of those patients without diabetes on placebo.

c. intravascular ultrasound (IVUS) studies have shown LDL-C <70 to 80 mg/dL to be associated with plaque regression but the 20% of individuals that progress on therapy often have DM, less increase in HDL, and less decrease in apoB on treatment.

d. the action to control cardiovascular risk in diabetes clinical trial (ACCORD) trial demonstrated a benefit of fenofibrate when added to baseline simvastatin therapy in diabetic patients.

e. observational studies have noted an impact of low/abnormally functioning HDL, VLDL remnants, elevated TG small dense LDL, LDL-P, and apoB/apoA ratios on adverse outcomes.

f. epidemic of obesity, diabetes, and metabolic syndrome associated with dyslipidemia is marked by only modest elevations in LDL-C but increases in HDL-C and TG.

25. In the setting of strong observational and epidemiologic data supporting HDL-C's relationship to CVD risk, the limitations of current therapies, and the increase in incidence of diabetes/metabolic syndrome, there remains a strong interest in focusing on other therapeutic interventions in addition to LDL-C lowering, particularly HDL modulation. HDL is more than a simple carrier of cholesterol. Which of the following statements regarding HDL-C metabolism and function is not true?

a. In addition to reverse cholesterol transport, HDL may have beneficial effects due to antioxidant and anti-inflammatory effects.

b. ATP-binding cassette transporter 1 (ABCA1) and ABCG1 both facilitate free cholesterol efflux to lipid-poor pre-β1-HDL.

c. Cholesteryl ester transfer protein (CETP) enables exchange of cholesterol esters for TGs between HDL and apoB-containing lipoproteins (LDL and VLDL).

d. HDL can deliver cholesterol to the liver via both direct and indirect reverse cholesterol transport.

26. Since most lipid-lowering guidelines emphasize the use of statin therapy and at potent doses in the highest-risk individuals, it is important to recognize side effects. Clinically significant adverse effects of statins include all of the following except

a. muscle-related adverse events.

b. liver-related adverse events.

c. renal insufficiency.

d. headaches.

e. dyspepsia.

27. You see a 68-year-old woman recently started on a statin for a calculated FRS of 18% 10-year risk and elevated usCRP. She returns in 6 weeks complaining of left lower extremity aching, which she had not experienced before. Regarding muscle-related side effects with statin drugs, all of the following statements are true except that

a. myopathy occurs in approximately 0.1% to 0.5% of patients on statin monotherapy and is dose dependent.

b. the incidence of statin-associated rhabdomyolysis across large, randomized, controlled statin trials is <0.1% and the reported incidence of fatal rhabdomyolysis with statins is extremely rare with 0.15 death per 1 million prescriptions.

c. a review of five large-scale controlled clinical trials of statin safety reported a rate of myopathy ranged from 0.1% to 0.6% and rate of rhabdomyolysis ranged from 0.03% to 0.05%.

d. myalgia symptoms reported in prescribing information range from 5% to 10%.

e. identifying factors that may contribute to myopathy should lead to statin dose reduction.

28. For the patient in Question 27, you obtain a creatine phosphokinase (CPK) which is 282 (upper normal in laboratory of 220 U/L). No baseline CPK is available for comparison. She has no reproducible pain or weakness on examination. She denies darkening of the urine. Should you stop the statin?

a. Yes

b. No

29. You see a 49-year-old obese, sedentary woman with type 2 DM, hypertension, and family history of coronary stent in her father at age 53. LDL-C was 173 mg/dL. Based on NCEP ATP III and 2013 ACC/AHA guidelines she is a candidate for intensive statin therapy. Laboratory values obtained 3 months after treatment with 40 mg of atorvastatin revealed alanine transaminase (ALT)/aspartate transaminase (AST) of 102/96 (upper normal in laboratory of 50/42 U/L). Which of the following regarding liver abnormalities with statin use is not true?

a. Reversal of transaminase elevation is frequently noted with continuation of statins or a reduction in statin dose.

b. Elevations do not often recur with either readministration or selection of another statin.

c. Statins have been shown to worsen the outcome in persons with chronic transaminase elevations due to hepatitis B or C.

d. In this patient review other drugs and supplements, continue the current dose, and repeat in 6 to 12 weeks.

e. Baseline measurement of ALT should be performed before starting therapy.

30. Later that afternoon you are referred a 58-year-old man with waist circumference of 42 inches, fasting glucose of 112 mg/dL, hypertension, current smoker with brother with MI at age 54. LDL-C is 163 mg/dL, TG 275 mg/dL, and HDL-C 47 mg/dL. When first seen prior to initiation of any therapy, he had LFTs similar to those reported for the patient in the previous question (approximately two times upper limit of normal [ULN]). The patient is very worried about taking statins due to concerns of liver failure. Which of the following can you tell him? 10 year risk by Framingham Risk Score is >30% and ACC/AHA calculator score is 21.2.

a. Statin use has not been investigated in patients with baseline LFT abnormalities but should be used due to his high risk.

b. Statins have been studied in patients with baseline elevations and have been shown to further increase the LFTs.

c. Elevations of LFTs greater than two times ULN is a contraindication to starting statins.

d. Statin therapy may lower the LFTs in patients with fatty liver infiltration.

e. Progression to liver failure has never been reported.

31. In 2012, the FDA issued an alert reporting a relationship between statin use and increase in blood glucose and new incidence of diabetes. Which of the following statements is TRUE?

1. A large meta-analysis has reported an approximate 18% increase in relative risk of developing diabetes on statin therapy.

2. This observation appears to be dose dependent with a meta-analysis of high-versus moderate-dose trials reporting an absolute increase in rate of 0.4%.

3. Increase in blood glucose with statins does not attenuate the CVD reduction benefit of statins.

4. Development of diabetes on statin therapy is independent of risk factors for diabetes.

5. Reducing the dose of statin should be utilized to avoid diabetes development in those at risk, for example, metabolic syndrome, obesity, and impaired fasting glucose.
   a. All of the above
   b. 1, 3, and 5
   c. 2 and 3
   d. 2, 3, and 5
   e. None of the above

32. Your patient is a 51-year-old man with heterozygous FH with predrug therapy LDL-C of 202 mg/dL who had been tried on atorvastatin, simvastatin, and lovastatin in the past but stopped all three due to complaints of muscle aching, had gastrointestinal complaints with resins, and refused further treatment. He recently had an ST-segment elevation MI treated with direct stenting. He was given a prescription to start atorvastatin again but was hesitant to have it filled and comes to you for advice. He has increased his frequency of aerobic exercise and has been following a low-saturated fat diet. LDL-C measured 2 months after the MI was 188 mg/dL. Appropriate options to consider in managing this patient include

1. trial of rosuvastatin beginning at 5 mg two to three times a week followed by slow titration.

2. pretreatment with coenzyme Q10 followed by rechallenge with a different statin or lower dose of previously used statin.

3. niacin titrated to highest tolerated dose in combination with ezetimibe.

4. LDL-C apheresis.

5. emphasis on aggressive lifestyle intervention including very low saturated fat to vegetarian diet, plant sterols/stanols, and high dietary and supplementary fiber.

6. mipomersen.
   a. All of the above
   b. 1, 2, 3, and 5
   c. 1, 2, 3, 4, and 5
   d. 1, 3, and 5
   e. None of the above

33. Statements regarding fibrates include all of the following except that
   a. side effects include gastrointestinal complaints, gallstones, and increase in need for cholecystectomy and elevated hepatic transaminase levels.
   b. monotherapy trials have not uniformly demonstrated reductions in CVD risk but subanalysis of groups with a metabolic pattern (elevated TG and low HDL) have been more strongly associated with CVD event reduction.
   c. although difficult to demonstrate in individual studies, meta-analysis of fibrate trials has demonstrated reduction in cardiovascular mortality on therapy.
   d. myopathy has been reported with both monotherapy and combination therapy with statin.
   e. increase in creatinine is more common with gemfibrozil compared with fenofibrate.

34. The following statements regarding use of niacin are true except that

   a. possible concerns with niacin use include risk of gout, worsening glucose control, and flushing.

   b. combination therapy of statins with niacin has been shown to exert favorable effect on some surrogate markers for CVD outcomes.

   c. the Coronary Drug Project in the pre-statin era demonstrated a beneficial effect on MI and mortality in secondary prevention patients with coronary disease treated with high-dose niacin.

   d. niacin can raise HDL-C from 20% to 25% and lower TGs from 30% to 50% depending on dose and pretreatment TG levels but has little effect on LDL-C.

   e. to reduce adverse event severity, start niacin at low dose and titrate over weeks, take with a light snack, and take aspirin 30 minutes prior.

ANSWERS   ● ● ●

1. **a.** It occurs in 1 in 5,000 persons. Homozygous FH occurs in 1 in 1 million individuals while heterozygous FH in 1 in 500 individuals. The other statements are true.

2. **d.** LDLRAP1 mediates internalization of LDL-C via clathrin-coated pits, and loss-of-function mutations would decrease LDL-C clearance. Defects in apolipoprotein B (apoB). The LDL-R on the hepatocyte binds to apoB (acts as ligand, binding LDL particle to receptor) on the LDL particle inducing internalization via clathrin-coated pits (mediated by LDLRAP1) and endocytosis of the complex. Defects in the receptor itself or the apoB molecule may reduce LDL-C clearance. The protein PCSK9 can bind to the LDL/LDL-R complex and when internalized prevents recycling of the LDL-R to the hepatocyte surface. A gain in function mutation of PCSK9 (by further reducing recycling of LDL-Rs) has been shown to be associated with increase in LDL-C and CVD.

3. **c.** Familial combined hyperlipidemia. Familial combined hyperlipidemia is a common dyslipidemia (1 in 33 to 1 in 100 individuals) characterized by complex inheritance. Xanthomas are rarely present (unlike in heterozygous FH), but xanthelasmas and arcus cornea can be seen. They are generally overweight, are hypertensive, and have insulin resistance or diabetes. Affected individuals generally exhibit a TC of 250 to 350 mg/dL, LDL-C of 200 to 300 mg/dL, and TG of >140 mg/dL (two-thirds of patients have TG of 200 to 500 mg/dL). Patients with polygenic hypercholesterolemia (1 in 20 to 1 in 100 individuals) have alterations in the function or expression of several key proteins involved in LDL metabolism including defective LDL-R and apoB100, and the presence of the apoE4 allele (which has a higher affinity for the LDL-R than the other apoE isoforms leading to downregulation of LDL-R). They have similar elevations in LDL-C as familial combined hyperlipidemia except they do not generally have elevated TG. Hyperapobetalipoproteinemia is associated with increased apoB synthesis. TG may be normal or elevated and arcus cornea and xanthelasmas may be present. However, LDL-C is typical below 160 mg/dL. Familial endogenous hypertriglyceridemia is associated with increased hepatic VLDL formation and TG of 200 to 500 mg/dL but without significant elevations in LDL-C and is not consistently linked with increased CVD risk.

4. **d.** Lomitapide has been approved to treat homozygous and heterozygous FH. Homozygous FH occurs in 1 in 1 million individuals. TC levels are generally >600 mg/dL, with LDL-C levels six- to eightfold higher than average. Without treatment, death from MI occurs in the first or second decades of life. In addition to the xanthomas observed in heterozygotes, FH homozygotes are commonly affected by interdigital xanthomas; tuberous xanthomas on the hands, elbows, buttocks, and feet; and planar xanthomas on the posterior thighs, buttocks, and knees. The mainstay of therapy for FH homozygotes is LDL apheresis and has been associated with stabilization or regression of atherosclerotic lesions and improvement in symptoms. Since immediate reductions in LDL-C of 50% to 80% rebound quickly, the process is performed every 2 to 4 weeks to keep intrapheresis LDL-C ≤120 mg/dL.

Both mipomersen and lomitapide were FDA approved in 2013 as orphan drugs for management of patients with homozygous FH only. Mipomersen is a subcutaneously injectable RNA antisense oligonucleotide. Lomitapide blocks microsomal TG transport protein (a key protein in assembly and secretion of apoB-containing lipoproteins in the liver and intestines) reducing hepatic secretion of VLDL. These therapies have a small target population, require risk evaluation and mitigation strategy limiting use to specialized centers, and have concerns with liver toxicity and hepatic steatosis due to accumulation of TGs not secreted into VLDL.

Several clinical diagnostic criteria for FH exist, with the 15-year Simon Broome Register Group being the most commonly used. Definite FH is as defined above. Possible FH by this criteria is defined as (a) above PLUS and (b) MI before age 50 in second-degree relative, or before 60 in first-degree relative or elevated cholesterol in first-degree relative, or >290 mg/dL in second-degree relative.

5. **d.** National Health and Nutrition Examination Survey (NHANES) data through 2006 reported that 10.3% of adolescents (12 to 19 years) have abnormal lipid levels. In adolescents between the ages of 12 and 19, the number of individuals with one or more abnormal lipid level is higher at 20.3% and increases further to 42.9% in association with obesity. All the other facts noted are true. The AHA has established TC <170 mg/dL in children and <200 mg/dL in adults as one of seven goals for ideal cardiovascular health. In one survey in 2010, 38.1% of children and 52.7% of adults did not meet these criteria. Although average adult TC levels have been dropping over the past two decades from 208 to 197 mg/dL, obesity and lack of physical activity (two factors associated with dyslipidemia and diabetes risk) have been on the rise. From 2011 to 2012 only 20.7% of adults and 49.5% of adolescents, respectively, achieved recommended activity levels. These facts and more can be found in the most recent Heart Disease and Stroke Statistics-2014 Update from the AHA published in *Circulation*.

6. **b.** The JUPITER trial demonstrated that in individuals without documented cardiovascular disease (CVD) and median LDL-C of 108 mg/dL, aggressive statin therapy with rosuvastatin offered greater benefit in individuals with ultrasensitive C-reactive protein (usCRP) >2 versus <2 mg/L. JUPITER demonstrated that primary prevention patients with only modest elevations in LDL-C but elevated usCRP above 2 mg/L benefited from treatment with statins. However, the trial only enrolled individuals with usCRP >2 mg/L. There was no comparison arm to individuals with low LDL-C and low usCRP. While ASCOT-LLA showed reductions in nonfatal MI and CHD death, coronary events or procedures, stroke, and chronic stable angina, but did not show a reduction in total mortality. However, this trial did demonstrate that initiation of moderate intensity statin therapy in higher-risk individuals without clinical CVD and without significant elevations in LDL-C significantly reduced CVD events. The study with average LDL-C at entry of 130 mg/dL was stopped early by the safety monitoring board. Primary prevention trials WOSCOPS and AFCAPS/TexCAPS and secondary prevention trials including 4S, CARE, PIPID, and Heart Protection Study (HPS) across a wide range of pretreatment LDL-C and using various statins demonstrated approximately 1% reduction in CVD events for every 1% reduction in LDL-C.

7. **b.** 1, 3, and 5. In making treatment decisions regarding initiation and intensity of treatment for dyslipidemia in patients without documented CVD or diabetes, assessment of future risk of CVD development is important. In individuals with two or more standard cardiovascular risk factors (hypertension, family history, low HDL-C, and smoking), the FRS can be used to calculate 10-year risk of MI or coronary disease mortality. The calculator is based on assessment of TC (or LDL-C), HDL-C, hypertension history, age, and smoking stratified by gender. It does not incorporate family history, assessment of metabolic syndrome, or other nontraditional risk markers such as usCRP, lipoprotein(a), and CACS. Risk may be underestimated in younger individuals and data may not be transferable to ethnic groups not well represented in the cohort. Other risk assessment tools include some of these additional risk markers such as the Reynolds Risk Score (usCRP and family history), PROCAM (prospective cardiovascular Münster heart study) Score (TG and family history), and SHAPE (Screening for heart attack prevention and education) guidelines (carotid intimal medial thickness [CIMT] and CACS). The recent 2013 ACC/AHA guideline on the treatment of blood cholesterol to reduce atherosclerotic cardiovascular risk in adults has promoted a new Pooled Cohort Equations risk calculator that incorporates race into the calculation and stroke as an outcome event.

8. **c.** HDL-C of <40 mg/dL in men and women. Metabolic syndrome is characterized by abdominal obesity, an atherogenic dyslipidemia with elevated TG, increased number of small LDL particles, low HDL-C, elevated BP, insulin resistance (glucose intolerance), a prothrombotic state, and a proinflammatory state. There is an increased risk of CVD development of two- to fourfold in individuals with metabolic syndrome. Focus of treatment should be on intensive lifestyle intervention. In the NCEP ATP III recommendations for diagnosis of metabolic syndrome, cutoffs for HDL-C are <40 mg/dL in men but <50 mg/dL in women. The other criteria listed are correct. Modifications since initial publication include lowering the fasting glucose cutoff to 100 mg/dL and population-specific waist circumferences such as ≥90 cm in men and ≥80 cm in women of South Asian ancestry. Metabolic syndrome is present if three or more of these criteria are identified.

9. **e.** Both higher-dose statins and addition of fibrates and niacin to achieve non-HDL-C goals should be considered to achieve secondary targets and to further reduce cardiovascular event rate. Between NCEP ATP III in 2001 and the update in 2004, multiple randomized controlled clinical trials offered new information supporting more aggressive treatment of hyperlipidemia and led to lowering the treatment goals and pretreatment LDL-C cutoffs for treatment in high- and intermediate-risk individuals (Table 12.1). The HPS demonstrated statin benefit in high-risk patients even with low pretreatment LDL-C. The ASCOTT LLA and Collaborative Atorvastatin Diabetes Study (CARDS) trials showed benefit when treating high-risk primary prevention patients with

TABLE 12-1	Treatment Goals and Low-Density Lipoprotein Cholesterol Levels for Initiation of Pharmacologic Therapies Based on Modifications of the National Cholesterol Education Project: Adult Treatment Panel III Guidelines in 2004

Risk Category	LDL-C (mg/dL)	Non–HDL-C (mg/dL)	Consider Drug Therapy for LDL-C
CHD/CHD risk equivalents (10-y risk >20%)	<100 Optional <70	<130 Optional <100	≥100 Optional <100
≥2 risk factors (10-y risk 10–20%)	<130 Optional <100	<160 Optional <130	>130 Optional 100–129
≥2 risk factors (10-y risk <10%)	<130	<160	>160
0–1 risk factor	<160	<190	>190 Optional 160–190

CHD, coronary heart disease; HDL-C, high-density lipoprotein cholesterol; LDL-C, low-density lipoprotein cholesterol.

hypertension or DM even if LDL-C was not significantly elevated. Studies such as Treat to New Targets (TNT) and PROVE-IT TIMI-22 demonstrated that increasing the intensity of LDL-C lowering using higher doses or more potent statins in secondary prevention populations was associated with incremental cardiovascular risk reduction. The guidelines recommend that in treating individuals with hyperlipidemia the first priority of treatment is to lower LDL-C; the first line of drug therapy to manage LDL-C is statin therapy and intensity of therapy should be selected to achieve at least a 30% to 40% LDL reduction. Intensity of therapy and LDL-C goals should be based on level of CVD risk. Although NCEP ATP III recommended non-HDL-C (TC minus HDL-C) as a secondary therapeutic goal after achieving LDL-C goals and considering addition of niacin and fibrates to achieve this goal, this has not yet been definitively shown in clinical trials to reduce adverse cardiovascular events when added to adequate statin therapy.

10. e. Non–HDL-C goal equals the LDL-C goal +30 mg/dL. Although the ADA, the American Association of Clinical Endocrinologists (AACE), and the AHA/ACC women's preventive guidelines set specific goals for TG below 150 mg/dL and HDL-C >50/40 mg/dL in women/men, NCEP ATP III guidelines do not and instead focus on non–HDL-C targets. The primary target for therapy is LDL-C reduction and statins remain the primary therapy for reducing LDL-C. However, in individuals with TGs >500 mg/dL initial therapy with aggressive diet and lifestyle intervention and medications should be first addressed. Non–HDL-C is recommended as a secondary target after achieving LDL-C goals if TG are greater than 200 mg/dL with therapeutic options to lower non–HDL-C including more intense LDL-C lowering or addition of niacin, fibrates, or high-dose omega-3 fish oils. Bile acid sequestrants should be avoided in individuals with TG over 300 mg/dL. NCEP ATP III recognizes a role for HDL-C as an important determinant of risk and if low a reason to achieve LDL-C and non–HDL-C goals as well as cause to emphasize diet and exercise. Although specific treatment to raise HDL-C may be considered in very high-risk individuals, the best therapies to accomplish this are not known and clinical trials documenting CVD risk reduction with HDL-C–directed therapies are lacking. An appropriate approach to HDL-C management is lifestyle. Dietary changes are associated with a 3% to 15% increase in HDL-C with an average 0.35 mg/dL increase in HDL for each 1 kg of weight loss. About 120 to 180 minutes of aerobic exercise a week and discontinuation of smoking can each raise HDL-C by 5% to 10%.

11. d. Omega-3 polyunsaturated fatty acid supplements of 800 to 1,000 mg a day. Diets high in omega-3 saturated fat are recommended but universal use of supplements is not. The AHA recommends 800 to 1,000 mg/day in dietary consumption and to consider supplements in secondary prevention patients without an adequate dietary source. Omega-3 fatty acids have a role in managing high TGs (>500 mg/day) by using high doses of prescription or supplement forms at 2,000 to 4,000 mg/day. Long-term outcome data supporting definitive reduction in CVD events with omega-3 supplementation in primary prevention populations are lacking. All of the other recommendations listed are supported by the guidelines.

12. a. Hyperthyroidism. Identifying and treatment of or modifying secondary causes of dyslipidemia is an important component in the management of dyslipidemia. Treating hypothyroidism and better control of diabetes may have significant impact on correcting lipid abnormalities. If possible, identification of medications associated with dyslipidemia and substitution of alternate medications when possible may help. Cholesterol and TGs rise progressively throughout pregnancy. Drugs such as statins, niacin, and ezetimibe are contraindicated during pregnancy and lactation.

13. b. FRS indicating a 10-year risk of MI or coronary death of >10%. Any clinically significant non-coronary vascular diseases such as peripheral artery disease, carotid artery disease, and aortic disease would qualify. Diabetics also fall into this category, particularly those >40 years of age and with at least one additional CVD risk factor. CHD risk equivalent status is present in individuals without clinically evident CHD, other CVD, or diabetes but with two or more CVD risk factors and FRS associated with a 10-year risk of a fatal or nonfatal MI of >20% not >10%. All of these individuals would be candidates for aggressive lipid management. The NCEP ATP III guidelines recommend LDL-C goals <100 mg/dL and optional LDL-C goals <70 mg/dL in this group. The ACC/AHA 2013 hyperlipidemia guidelines have eliminated LDL-C goals for therapy and recommend high-intensity statin therapy to achieve LDL-C lowering of >50% in high-risk groups <75 years old. This includes individuals with coronary and non-coronary disease, diabetics with new Pooled Cohort Equation calculator risk of >7.5% 10-year risk.

14. a. LDL <70 mg/dL and non-HDL <100.

15. f. Answers a and d.

16. a. Atorvastatin 40 mg/day. Patients with diabetes are CHD risk equivalent patients and therefore at high cardiovascular risk and candidates for aggressive lipid-lowering therapy. The NCEP ATP III update in 2004, ACC/ADA consensus statement in 2008, and the ADA and AAACE (American Association of Clinical Endocrinologists) guidelines in 2013 all support a primary LDL-C goal of <70 mg/dL and secondary non–HDL-C goal of <100 mg/dL. In addition, the consensus statement and recent ADA/AACE guidelines recommend considering apoB of <80 mg/dL and LDL-P of <1,000 as secondary targets for therapy. usCRP is a marker for CVD risk and reduced by many therapies including statins and lifestyle interventions but is not a recognized specific target or therapeutic goal (Tables 12.2 and 12.3).

The first-line therapy is statins, at a dose needed to achieve LDL-C reductions of at least 30% to 40%. Only atorvastatin 40 mg/day would achieve recommended treatment goals. Simvastatin at this dose is unlikely to result in sufficient LDL-C reduction to achieve goals and since the FDA alert in 2011, doses higher than 20 mg are not recommended in combination with amlodipine. Monotherapy with ezetimibe generally lowers LDL-C <20% and outcome benefit has not

TABLE 12-2	Treatment Goals: American Diabetes Association/American College of Cardiology Consensus Statement 2008		
	LDL-C (mg/dL)	Non–HDL-C (mg/dL)	apoB (mg/dL)
Highest-risk patients			
Known CVD or diabetes plus one or more additional CVD risk factors	<70	<100	<80
High-risk patients			
No diabetes or known CVD but two or more major CVD risk factors or diabetes but no other CVD risk factors	<100	<130	<90

CVD, cerebrovascular disease; HDL-C, high-density lipoprotein cholesterol; LDL-C, low-density lipoprotein cholesterol.

TABLE 12-3 American Association of Clinical Endocrinologists Lipid Targets for Patients with Type 2 Diabetes

	Moderate-Risk Patients	High-Risk Patients
LDL-C (mg/dL)	<100	<70
Non–HDL-C (mg/dL)	<130	<100
Triglycerides (mg/dL)	<150	<150
TC/HDL-C	<3.5	<3.0
ApoB (mg/dL)	<90	<80
LDL particle number (nmol/L)	<1,200	<100

ApoB, apolipoprotein B; HDL-C, high-density lipoprotein cholesterol; LDL-C, low-density lipoprotein cholesterol; TC, total cholesterol.

been demonstrated. Although LDL-C is not significantly elevated and the TG and HDL-C abnormalities may be improved by the other listed therapies, statins remain the primary treatment choice, supported by beneficial outcome data in trials such as CARDS and diabetic subsets in other large prospective trials and meta-analyses. Outcome data regarding cardiovascular risk reduction with these other listed therapies are lacking or less robust. New lipid treatment guidelines from the ACC/AHA published in November 2013 recommend a different approach to the management of lipids. These new guidelines support therapy initiation and intensity dependent on the level of risk and they recognize that most patients with diabetes are candidates for high-intensity statin therapy (defined as a statin able to achieve >50% reduction in LDL-C, e.g., 40 to 80 mg of atorvastatin or 20 to 40 mg of rosuvastatin).

17. **f.** All of the above. On statin therapy, the LDL-C goal of <70 mg/dL has been achieved but non–HDL-C remains above an ideal goal of <100 mg/dL. Any of these therapies would help to achieve the secondary non–HDL-C goals. NCEP ATP III recommends intensification of statins, further LDL-C lowering with non-statin therapies, niacin, or fibrates to achieve secondary non–HDL-C goal. There are clinical trial data to support further risk reduction with intensification of statin therapy although outcome data are absent when niacin, fibrates, fish oil, or ezetimibe is added to adequate statin therapy. Intensification of lifestyle interventions should be a part of any pharmacologic intervention in this patient. The patient is on a high-intensity statin with <50% reduction in LDL-C. Based on new ACC/AHA 2013 guidelines for management of hyperlipidemia, there is insufficient RTC evidence that adding additional therapies will further reduce cardiovascular events. Intensification of statin therapy does appear to offer benefit. In individuals receiving maximum tolerated intensity of statin with less than anticipated therapeutic response and in high-risk groups, the addition of non-statin therapy may be considered if the CVD risk reduction benefits outweigh the adverse effects.

18. **c.** NHANES data from 2010 indicate that although goals of HbA1c <7 mg/dL, systolic BP <130 mmHg, and LDL-C <100 mg/dL are recommended for diabetics, only 32% of diabetics in the survey currently achieve all three of these goals. The NHANES survey in 2010 demonstrated that although greater than 50% of diabetic patients achieved LDL <100 mg/dL, systolic BP <130 mmHg, or HbA1c <7 mg/dL, only <20% achieved all three goals. Studies such as the

East-West study in 1998 demonstrated that a diabetic without CHD history had a similar approximate 20% incidence of MI over 7 years compared with a non-diabetic with known previous MI. Diabetics have a two- to fourfold increased risk of CVD events and the majority of deaths in patients with diabetes are due to CVD, accounting for up to 75% of deaths. These observations emphasize the concept of diabetes as a CHD equivalent and a rationale for intensive therapy of hyperlipidemia.

19. **d.** HDL particle size and number. usCRP has been shown in studies such as the Women's Health Study (WHS) to reclassify risk when added to the FRS and in the JUPITER trial to be a factor in determining benefit of early statin therapy for primary prevention of CVD. Similar reclassification of risk has been demonstrated with anatomic measurements for preclinical atherosclerosis such as CACS and CIMT. Post hoc analyses of studies such as the WHS and MESA (multi-ethnic study of atherosclerosis) have demonstrated LDL-P to be a better predictor of future cardiovascular risk, and the National Lipid Association has recommended it as a tool for further risk assessment. However, data supporting the benefit and use of HDL particle size and number in assessing risk and guiding treatment are absent. NCEP ATP III recommends that intermediate-risk patients (FRS 10% to 20% estimated 10-year risk) with these additional risk markers should be considered for more intensive therapies. The ACC/AHA hyperlipidemia guidelines in 2013 suggest that in selected individuals, particularly those with a 10-year CVD risk of 5% to 7.5% not falling into defined treatment groups for high- or moderate-intensity statin therapy, factors including LDL-C >160 mg/dL, family history of premature CVD, usCRP >2 mg/dL, CACS >300 Agatston units or >75th percentile for age/sex/ethnicity, and ankle brachial index <0.9 may be used to consider initiation or intensification of pharmacologic therapy.

20. **a.** None, all are true. The ACC/AHA 2013 guidelines have attempted to offer recommendations based on a balance of benefit and therapeutic risk of treatment strategies as supported whenever possible by RTCs. The guidelines are based on observations including the absolute benefit in CVD risk reduction is proportional to baseline risk; cholesterol-lowering medications used in clinical trials (particularly statins) reduce risk of cardiovascular events proportional to the intensity of stain therapy rather than LDL-C achieved and therefore more intensive statin therapy could reduce risk more than moderate- or lower-intensity statin therapy; and statins are associated with similar relative risk reductions for CVD events across the majority of patient groups studied, and little clinical trial evidence to support use of other non-statin therapies particularly when added to treatment with statins. Therefore, in these guidelines a greater degree of emphasis is placed on level of treatment with statins and less on other lipid-lowering therapies either alone or in combination with statins. Patients or groups at higher baseline absolute risk will derive greater absolute benefit from initiation of statin therapy over a period of 5 to 10 years as studied in clinical trials. Like the NCEP ATP III recommendations, intensity of therapy is based on a measure of level of CVD risk but defined as dose or potency of statin therapy to be used rather than titration to specific LDL-C and non–HDL-C goals. Both sets of guidelines recommend statin therapy as primary and most beneficial therapy for CVD risk reduction although the ACC/AHA recommendations deemphasize the use of add-on non-statin therapies in the absence of RCT data and balance the risk of pharmacologic therapies in lower-risk populations. The ACC/AHA guidelines position treatment of TGs and use of non–HDL-C in treatment decision making as future clinical questions to be addressed and updated after future clinical trials. It should be mentioned that since these guidelines have appeared many have offered criticism of the document, including the elimination of LDL-C targets and concern with use of a new risk assessment tool that has not been prospectively validated, may overexpand treatment of lower-risk

populations, and delay treatment in other high-risk populations. It should be remembered that these are guidelines and not doctrine and individual treatment plans should be tailored to the individual patient's risk and needs after carefully assessing side effects and risk of treatment and discussion with the patient.

21. **b.** Primary elevations of LDL-C ≥160 mg/dL. In these recommendations, LDL-C would need to be above 190 mg/dL to be considered for high-intensity statin therapy (Table 12.4). Clinical ASCVD is defined as acute coronary syndromes, a history of MI, stable or unstable angina, coronary or other arterial revascularization, stroke, TIA, or peripheral arterial disease of atherosclerotic origin. It is recommended that the absolute 10-year ASCVD risk (defined as nonfatal MI, CHD death, and including nonfatal and fatal stroke) should be used to guide the initiation and intensity of statin therapy and should be estimated using the Pooled Cohort Equations for the primary prevention of ASCVD in individuals without clinical ASCVD and LDL-C 70 to 189 mg/dL and to determine intensity of therapy in diabetics (DM types 1 and 2). For those with clinical ASCVD or with LDL-C ≥190 mg/dL who are already in a statin benefit group, it is not appropriate to estimate 10-year ASCVD risk. In individuals over 75 years of age falling into these groups or diabetics with 10-year risk <7.5%, consider moderate-intensity therapy to reduce possible side effects.

22. **c.** Bile acid sequestrants as initial therapy in younger patients under 16 years of age. The AAP recommends screening beginning as early as 2 years of age and before age 10 in children with family history of hyperlipidemia or premature

---

TABLE 12-4   American College of Cardiology/American Heart Association 2013 Guidelines: Four Treatment Groups and Intensity of Statin Therapy

High-Intensity Statin Therapy (average LDL-C lowering >50%)	Moderate-Intensity Statin Therapy (average LDL-C Lowering 30–50%)
Indicated for	**Indicated for**
1. Clinical ASCVD age <75	1. Clinical ASCVD age ≥75
2. LDL-C ≥190 mg/dL	2. LDL-C ≥190 mg/dL (unable to tolerate high-intensity statin)
3. Diabetics aged 40–75 with LDL-C 70–189 mg/dL with 10-y ASCVD risk ≥7.5%	3. Diabetics aged 40–75 with LDL-C 70–189 mg/dL with 10-y ASCVD risk <7.5%
4. Others aged 40–75, LDL-C 70–189 mg/dL and ASCVD risk ≥7.5%	4. Others aged 40–75 with LDL-C 70–189 mg/dL with 10-y ASCVD risk ≥7.5%
Considered high-intensity statins	**Considered moderate-intensity statins**
Atorvastatin (40)–80 mg	Atorvastatin 10 (20) mg
Rosuvastatin 20 (40) mg	Rosuvastatin (5) 10 mg
	Simvastatin 20–40 mg
	Pravastatin 40 (80) mg
	Lovastatin 40 mg
	Fluvastatin XL 80 mg
	Fluvastatin 40 mg bid
	Pitavastatin 2–4 mg

ASCVD, atherosclerotic cardiovascular disease; HDL-C, high-density lipoprotein cholesterol; LDL-C, low-density lipoprotein cholesterol.

CVD in parents and grandparents or if family history is not known and other risk factors (overweight, obese, hypertension, smoking, and DM) are present. They now recommend considering pharmacologic treatment with statins as the first choice drug rather than resins and consider beginning pharmacologic therapy as early as 8 years of age if after lifestyle intervention LDL-C remains >190 mg/dL, >160 mg/dL with one or more other cardiovascular risk factors (including obesity), or >130 mg/dL if diabetes is present.

23. **c.**   4 and 6. Child and Adolescent Trial for CV Health reported that 13.3% of fourth graders had TC >200. NHANES 2010 notes that approximately 8% of adolescents have TC >200. A population approach including weight mainte-nance, healthy diet, and exercise is recommended for all children. An individ-ual approach to therapy is reserved for those at higher risk for CVD and with elevated LDL-C levels as summarized in the previous question. Other high-risk children and adolescents for whom earlier pharmacologic therapy may be con-sidered include post transplantation, human immunodeficiency virus (HIV), chronic inflammatory disease such as lupus and rheumatoid arthritis, renal dis-ease (nephrotic syndrome), Kawasaki disease, overweight/obese with metabolic syndrome, and childhood cancer survivors. Statins have not been shown to delay or adversely affect physical and sexual development. Cholesterol levels may drop significantly during pubertal development. Therefore, screening before or after is most representative. Studies in ages 7 months to adolescents have shown safety of low total fat, saturated fat, and cholesterol diets and initiation of low-fat diet is recommended after age 2 years. Benefits of statin treatment on the atherosclerotic process have been demonstrated in children using surrogate markers such as flow-mediated dilatation and CIMT. However, the impact on clinical outcomes has not been studied in large prospective trials. Since there are little outcome data to show that treatment in childhood decreases adult CVD, treatment recommendations are based on extrapolations from adult studies.

24. **d.**   The ACCORD trial demonstrated a benefit of fenofibrate when added to baseline simvastatin therapy in diabetic patients. Observational studies support that for every 1 mg/dL increase in HDL-C, there is a 2% to 3% decrease in CVD risk. The Framingham Heart Study recognized that the lower the level of HDL-C, the greater the risk of a coronary event, regardless of LDL-C level. In fact, a per-son with a "desirable" LDL-C of 100 mg/dL but a low HDL-C of 25 mg/dL had the same risk of a cardiac event as a person with an LDL-C of 220 mg/dL and an HDL-C of 45 mg/dL. Further strengthening the link between HDL-C and TG and poor CVD outcomes is the observation that patients presenting with a new diag-nosis of CHD have higher TGs and lower HDL-C than those without CHD. In the TNT trial, this relationship continued to exist even following aggressive statin therapy. When a subgroup of individuals all achieving LDL-C below 70 mg/dL was examined, CVD events increased significantly when HDL-C was below 42 mg/dL even in this group with very low LDL-C levels. A meta-analysis in 2010 of multiple statin trials reported that the inverse relationship of HDL-C to CVD events was not altered by statin therapy. Meta-analyses have shown a relationship between elevations of TG and CVD risk even when controlling for confounding factors and HDL-C. In the treatment arms of statin placebo-controlled studies and even when including those in which very low LDL-C levels are achieved, a significant residual CVD risk persists. NHANES reports that of the 48% of U.S. adults with dyslipidemia approximately a third have elevations in TGs and/or HDL-C. With the growing prevalence of obesity, diabetes, inactivity, and meta-bolic syndrome more individuals are presenting with a combined dyslipidemia characterized by only moderate elevation of LDL-C but increased numbers of small dense LDL and other atherogenic apoB particles, elevated TGs, and low high density HDL-C. Particularly in these groups it is reasonable to hypothesize that therapies beyond LDL-C lowering may be beneficial. Evidence supports

titration of statin to higher doses or use of more potent statins to achieve greater risk reduction. However, data from long-term outcome studies demonstrating incremental benefit when therapy directed toward low HDL-C and TG is added to statins have been disappointing. The AIM-HIGH (Atherothrombosis Intervention in Metabolic Syndrome with Low HDL/High Triglycerides: Impact on Global Health) trial and HPS-THRIVE (Treatment of HDL to Reduce the Incidence of Vascular Events) did not demonstrate improved outcomes when niacin preparations were added to individuals with well-controlled LDL-C on statin ± ezetimibe (LDL-C prerandomization of 74 and 63, respectively). The ACCORD trial did not demonstrate benefit when fenofibrate was added to baseline statin therapy in the total population of diabetics studied. A prospectively defined but subanalysis noted a borderline statistically significant 31% CVD event reduction in a subgroup with TG above 204 mg/dL and HDL-C below 34 mg/dL. However, until further studies are available there still may remain a role for niacin, fibrates, or ezetimibe in the management of elevated non-HDL after maximally tolerated statin therapy, those not at LDL-C goal after maximally tolerated statin therapy, or those intolerant to statins. The NCEP ATP III, ADA, and ACCE guidelines do recommend considering therapies including niacin and fibrates to achieve non–HDL-C goals after treating LDL-C. The AHA/ACC 2013 guidelines are less enthusiastic regarding the addition of non-statin therapies. Also note that other recommendations still recommend treatment targets and utilization of non-statin therapies in certain populations.

25. b. ATP-binding cassette transporter 1 (ABCA1) and ABCG1 both facilitate free cholesterol efflux to lipid-poor pre-β1-HDL. There are many proposed mechanisms offered to explain the beneficial anti-atherosclerotic activity of HDL-C including increase in nitric oxide production and enhanced endothelial function, inhibition of LDL-C oxidation, reduction of cytokine-induced endothelial vascular cell adhesion molecule induction and macrophage infiltration, as well as anti-inflammatory, antithrombotic (including reduction of platelet activation/aggregation, activation of protein C–mediated anticoagulant effects, and stimulation of fibrinolysis), and antioxidant effects. However, reverse cholesterol transport, the transfer of cholesterol from the peripheral tissues to the liver for excretion in the feces or bile, appears to offer the greatest cardioprotective role. The mature α-HDL particles are generated from lipid-free apolipoprotein A1 (apoA1) or lipid-poor pre–β1-HDL as the precursors are produced by the liver or intestine, released from lipolyzed VLDL and chylomicrons or released by interconversion of mature HDL particles. ABCA1 facilitates efflux of cholesterol from cells and initial lipidation of these precursors. Lipid efflux to more mature HDL particles also occur via ABCG1-mediated transfer. Enzymatic modification with lecithin cholesterol acyltransferase (LCAT) enables esterification of cholesterol and generates spherical particles that continue to grow with ongoing cholesterol esterification. The larger mature HDL particles are converted into smaller HDL particles via CETP-enabled exchange of cholesterol esters for TGs between HDL and apoB-containing lipoproteins (LDL and VLDL) and scavenger receptor class-B type 1 (SR-B1) selective uptake of cholesteryl esters into liver and steroidogenic organs. HDL can deliver cholesterol to the liver via the SR-B1 receptor or by holoparticle uptake (direct reverse cholesterol transport). It may also dispose of cholesterol via CETP-mediated transfer of cholesterol esters to LDL and VLDL and removal through normal clearance by hepatic LDL-Rs (indirect reverse cholesterol transport).

Studies in atherogenic animals show that raising HDL-C via genetic modification, infusion of HDL has favorable effects on experimental plague size and structure and reports of the ability of apoA1 Milano infusion therapy to reduce IVUS measured atherosclerotic plaque volume over a short period of 6 weeks in individuals following MI rekindled the interest in newer HDL-directed therapies. This raised hopes that synthetic forms of HDL, HDL mimetics, reconstituted

HDL, reinfusion of delipidated HDL, and other therapies designed to increase HDL-C would be potential therapeutic approaches to reduce CVD. Upregulation of liver X receptor (LXR), the nuclear receptor that protects cells from cholesterol toxicity, may be of benefit by resulting in the cellular transduction of the ATP-binding cassette sterol transporters that efflux free cholesterol into either nascent HDL or mature HDL. Enhancing LCAT activity increases the esterification of cholesterol in HDL, resulting in HDL maturation. Modifying the holo-particle uptake of HDL (a possible mechanism of niacin) may delay catabolism by allowing the HDL particle to continue circulating and potentially increase reverse cholesterol transport. Genetic and pharmacologic studies in mice suggest that overexpression of apoA1 and SR-B1 or LXR agonists may be beneficial. Unfortunately methodology, delivery concerns, and off-target adverse effects have so far limited the use of these therapeutic approaches in humans. Despite many new possible therapeutic strategies only inhibiting CETP which increases HDL particle size and delays catabolism of HDL is currently under active clinical phase 3 trial investigations. Two previous studies with CETP inhibitors (which raise HDL-C anywhere from 30% to 140%) were stopped early for adverse events with torcetrapib or lack of benefit/futility with dalcetrapib, but ongoing outcome trials with the more potent anacetrapib and evacetrapib continue.

26. **c.** Renal insufficiency. Statins have not been shown to worsen renal function. There was concern raised when proteinuria was noted in clinical trials with rosuvastatin. However, in analyses of RCTs, creatinine has not been shown to worsen and may improve. The other adverse effects listed above have all been noted with statins. In a meta-analysis by Naci et al. in 2013 comparing statins to placebo, the odds ratio for elevation in LFTs was 1.51, diabetes development 1.09, myalgia 1.07, CPK abnormality 1.13, and cancer 0.96, statistically significant only for liver test abnormalities and diabetes. Concerns have been raised about memory loss but there is a lack of large prospective trials designed to address this question and limited. A recent report in fact suggests a reduction in dementia with statin therapy.

27. **d.** Myalgia symptoms reported in prescribing information range from 5% to 10%. Definitions specified by the ACC/AHA NHLBI (National Heart, Lung, and Blood Institute) 2002 Clinical Advisory offer the following terminology to describe muscle injury: myalgias (muscle ache/weakness without CPK elevation), myopathy (muscle symptoms with CPK levels more than 10 times ULN), rhabdomyolysis (muscle symptoms with marked CPK elevation typically more than 10 times ULN with creatinine elevation and often with urinary myoglobin). Myalgia is reported in prescribing information at 1.2% to 3.2% but up to 11% in registries. Myopathy occurs in 0.1% to 0.5% of patients in a dose-dependent fashion. Fortunately, the risk of rhabdomyolysis is quite rare and reported <0.1%. Meta-analysis has reported rates of 0.03% to 0.05%. Muscle symptoms are more likely to occur at higher doses and doses should not exceed those recommended to achieve treatment goals. Attention should be paid to factors that may increase risk for myopathy. Concomitant medications such as fibrates, nicotinic acid (rarely), cyclosporine, azole antifungals, itraconazole, ketoconazole, macrolide antibiotics, erythromycin, clarithromycin, HIV protease inhibitors, nefazodone (antidepressant), verapamil, amiodarone, large quantities of grapefruit juice (>1 qt/day), and alcohol abuse may increase drug exposure and increase myopathy risk. This may be particularly true for simvastatin (metabolized via CYP3A) prompting an FDA advisory not to exceed 40 mg dose in general and reduce dose to 10 to 20 mg with concomitant use of drugs such as high-dose niacin, verapamil, ranolazine, and amiodarone. Other factors contributing to a higher likelihood of muscle symptoms include advanced age (especially >80 years; women more than men), small body frame, frailty, multisystem disease (e.g., chronic renal insufficiency, especially due to diabetes), and perioperative periods.

28. b.   No. Routine measurement of CPK on statin therapy is not recommended but it is reasonable to obtain at baseline prior to therapy in individuals at higher risk for myopathy and if new symptoms develop on treatment. When a patient presents with complaints of pain, tenderness, stiffness, cramping, weakness, or fatigue the first approach should be to document the severity of the symptoms, obtain CPK, creatinine, and urinalysis to exclude rhabdomyolysis, and search for other causes (such as hypothyroidism, rheumatologic disorders, vitamin D deficiency, and steroid use). If there are clinical signs of severe pain, new muscle weakness, CPK greater than 10 times ULN, or myoglobinuria the statin should be stopped. If symptoms are mild to moderate and CPK is less than three times ULN it is reasonable to hold the statin until symptoms can be evaluated. If symptoms resolve rechallenge with the same or lower dose of the statin to establish whether a causal relationship exists. If so starting a low dose of a different statin is reasonable followed by slow titration. If an asymptomatic individual on statin therapy has an elevated CPK, complete a thorough muscular examination and if unremarkable check for other causes. If greater than 10 times ULN, hold statin and evaluate for other primary or secondary myopathies. If a baseline CPK is known to be elevated prior to therapy, it is not an absolute contraindication to initiate statin therapy if less than three times ULN and asymptomatic. If higher, a search for other causes such as hypothyroidism, recent injury, and other myopathies would be prudent before initiating therapy with a statin and consideration of referral to a rheumatologist for further evaluation.

29. c.   Statins have been shown to worsen the outcome in persons with chronic transaminase elevations due to hepatitis B or C. Dose-related elevation in AST or ALT has been reported between 0.1% and 2%. Statins have not been shown to worsen the outcome in persons with chronic transaminase elevations due to hepatitis B or C. A search for other causes of LFT elevations is essential including review of prescription and over-the-counter drugs and supplements, recent infections, and alcohol use. In this patient with LFT less than three times ULN, it is reasonable to repeat in 6 to 12 weeks on the same or a lower dose. If LFTs greater than three times ULN repeat in 2 weeks and if continued elevation stop statin, recheck in 2 to 4 weeks and if improving consider rechallenge with a lower-dose or different statin. Reversal of transaminase elevation is frequently noted with a reduction in statin dose, and elevations do not often recur with either readministration or selection of another statins.

30. d.   Statin therapy may lower LFTs in patients with fatty liver infiltration. Prior to initiation of statin therapy it is reasonable to exclude other causes for LFT elevation. However, there are small studies supporting the safety of use in appropriate patients. Kiyici et al. examined 44 patients with biopsy-proven NASH (nonacoholic steatosis) and found that on atorvastatin 10 mg for 6 months there was a decrease in cholesterol, AST, ALT, AP (alkaline phosphatase), and GGT (gammaglutaryl transferase). Chalasani et al. examined the effect of statins over 6 months in patients with baseline moderate elevations in LFTs. In patients with normal LFTs placed on statin, the incidence of mild/moderate or severe elevation in LFTs was 1.9% and 0.2%, respectively, in those with baseline elevations placed on statin (4.7% and 0.6%) compared with those not placed on statin (6.4% and 0.4%). Progression to liver failure due to statins is not zero but exceedingly rare reported at 0.02 to 0.07 per million treated. In this patient, an ultrasound of the liver confirmed fatty infiltration. Manufacturer's prescribing information lists unexplained ALT greater than three times ULN as a contraindication to statin therapy. The best approach is to counsel on a diet program low in sugar and carbohydrates, weight loss, and exercise, and start statin therapy following the LFTs more closely.

31. c.   2 and 3. Sattar in a meta-analysis of 13 statin trials in 91,140 patients noted that 4,278 developed DM (4.89% on statins versus 4.5% on placebo; 0.39%

absolute increased difference and 9% relative risk of incident diabetes). This represented 1 additional case of DM per 1,000 patient-years. Preiss published a meta-analysis of 5 trials in 32,772 patients comparing high- versus moderate-dose statins and reported 2,749 developed DM (8.8% versus 8.4% or an absolute increase of 0.4%). There were two additional cases of DM (18.9 versus 16.9) per 1,000 patient-years of follow-up. The development of diabetes did not appear to reduce the benefits of treatment. Sattar found 5.4 less cardiac events for 255 patients treated over 4 years for each 1 mmol/L reduction in LDL-C compared with 1 extra case of diabetes for the same time period. Preiss noted 1 additional case of diabetes for every 498 patients over 1 year compared with 1 fewer CVD event for every 155 patients over 1 year. In a separate analysis of three high-dose atorvastatin trials, Waters et al. reported no difference in CVD events occurring in 11.3% with new DM and 10.8% without new DM. This compared with those with diabetes at baseline (10.1% versus 17.5%). The FDA reported this association in February 2012 but added that it does not appear to reduce the benefits of statin therapy in appropriately selected patients. Therefore, statin therapy should not be denied or appropriate doses reduced to avoid diabetes. However, since the individuals that developed diabetes are those at risk for diabetes it is prudent to measure for glycemic control more frequently and emphasize lifestyle interventions to reduce diabetes risk. This approach has been supported in the ACC/AHA 2013 guidelines.

32. b. 1, 2, 3, and 5. This patient is at very high risk for recurrent events. Since the greatest reduction in CVD events has been demonstrated with statins, further attempts to rechallenge with statins are appropriate. Small clinical trials and observational studies have shown that tolerance may be improved by trying multiple alternate statins, often using a potent statin beginning at low and intermittent rather than daily dosing with slow titration. Small investigations of coenzyme Q10 appear to lower the incidence of muscle complaints when added to statins. An analysis of patients referred to the Cleveland Clinic for intolerance to statins (the majority due to muscle complaints) revealed that over two-thirds of patients were able to tolerate some statin regimen with average LDL-C reduction of ~28% in those able to tolerate daily dosing. Niacin in high doses has been shown in the Coronary Drug Project to reduce recurrent MI and mortality after MI and is a reasonable component of a combination therapy program in patients resistant to all statins. Both LDL-C apheresis and mipomersen can lower LDL-C but with LDL-C levels in this range he would not meet the FDA recommendation for apheresis and although trials with mipomersen have been shown to be effective in both homozygous and heterozygous FH patients it is only currently approved for homozygotes.

33. c. Although difficult to demonstrate in individual studies, meta-analysis of fibrate trials has demonstrated reduction in cardiovascular mortality on therapy. An increase in myopathy has been reported with both gemfibrozil and fenofibrate as monotherapy but to a greater extent when added to statins (5.5-fold increased risk of myopathy when combined with statins) and more so with gemfibrozil compared with fenofibrate. A meta-analysis of monotherapy fibrate trials published in 2007 in the *American Heart Journal* reported a reduction in nonfatal MI but no reduction in fatal MI or total/cardiovascular mortality. Subanalyses of individuals with a metabolic dyslipidemia in fibrate trials such as BIP (bezafibrate infarction prevention), FIELD (fenofibrate intervention and event lowering in diabetes), and ACCORD trials demonstrated significant reduction in the primary endpoint of combined cardiovascular events, although not in the overall populations studied. Renal status should be evaluated within 3 months of initiation of therapy and every 6 months thereafter. Plasma half-life of fenofibric acid is prolonged in renal insufficiency and requires lower dose with glomerular filtration rate (GFR) 30 to 59 and avoidance if GFR <30. An increase in creatinine of 12% was reported in the FIELD study using fenofibrate, usually reversible with discontinuation of therapy.

34. d. Niacin can raise HDL-C from 20% to 25% and lower TGs from 30% to 50% depending on the dose and pretreatment TG levels but has little effect on LDL-C. Flushing and skin reactions are the most common reasons limiting niacin use. Gout episodes are more common in individuals with a prior history of gout. A small increase in blood glucose levels and HbA1c has been reported but is generally not of clinical significance and manageable with adjustments in glucose-lowering therapies. Baseline LFTs, fasting glucose, or HBA1c and uric acid should be obtained prior to therapy. While studies have suggested a benefit on surrogate markers for CVD events such as CIMT in the Arterial Biology for the Investigation of the Treatment Effects of Reducing Cholesterol (ARBITER) trials, there are currently no large longitudinal controlled trials demonstrating incremental benefit on clinical events when niacin is added to adequate statin therapy. Results of the AIM-HIGH and HPS-THRIVE were reviewed in Question 25. Niacin has a beneficial effect on multiple components of the lipid panel including a 20% to 35% increase in HDL-C, up to 20% lowering of LDL-C, and up to 30% to 50% reduction in TG. The Coronary Drug Project, initiated in the late 1960s, was a large secondary prevention study among men with several treatment arms, one of which utilized up to 3 g/day of niacin (Table 12.5). Compared with placebo, niacin lowered TC by 10% and TG by 26% (although HDL-C data not available) and after 6 years, significantly reduced nonfatal MI by 27%. A 15-year follow-up analysis (9 years after the interventions had ended) revealed a significant 11% decrease ($p < 0.004$) in total mortality. Further analysis has demonstrated equivalent reductions in CVD risk regardless of entry fasting glucose level, presence or absence of diabetes at entry, or change in fasting glucose while on therapy.

TABLE 12-5	Pharmacologic Therapies for Lipid Management				
Drug	**% Decrease LDL**	**% Increase HDL**	**% Decrease TG**	**Side Effects**	**Contraindications**
Statins	18–55	5–15	7–30	Myopathy, increased LFTs, diabetes	Liver disease
Bile acid sequestrants	15–30	3–5	May increase	GI distress, constipation, decreased drug absorption	Very elevated TG
Cholesterol absorption inhibitor	15–25	1–3	5–14	GI distress, increased LFTs, myopathy	Liver disease
Nicotinic acid	5–25	15–35	20–50	Flushing, GI distress, increased LFTs, increased glucose and uric acid	Liver disease, severe gout, peptic ulcer disease
Fibric acids	5–20, may increase	10–20	20–50	GI distress, gallstones, myopathy	Severe renal disease or liver disease
Omega-3 fish oil	May increase	10–20	20–50	GI distress	Fish allergy

GI, gastrointestinal; HDL, high-density lipoprotein; LDL, low-density lipoprotein; LFTs, liver function tests; TG, triglyceride.

SUGGESTED READINGS

ACCORD Study Group. Effects of combination lipid therapy in type 2 diabetes mellitus. *N Engl J Med*. 2010;362:1563–1574.

The AIM-HIGH Investigators. The role of niacin in raising HDL-C to reduce cardiovascular events in patients with atherosclerotic cardiovascular disease and optimally treated LDL-C AIM-HIGH: rationale and study design. *Am Heart J*. 2011;161:471–477.

American Diabetes Association. Executive summary: standards of medical care in diabetes—2012. *Diabetes Care*. 2012;35(Suppl 1):S5–S10.

Baigent C, Blackwell L, Emberson J, et al. Cholesterol Treatment Trialists' (CTT) Collaboration. Efficacy and safety of more intensive lowering of LDL cholesterol: a meta-analysis of data from 170,000 participants in 26 randomised trials. *Lancet*. 2010;376:1670–1681.

Baigent C, Keech A, Kearney PM, et al. Cholesterol Treatment Trialists' (CTT) Collaborators. Efficacy and safety of cholesterol-lowering treatment: prospective meta-analysis of data from 90,056 participants in 14 randomised trials of statins. *Lancet*. 2005;366:1267–1278. Errata in *Lancet*. 2008;371:2084, *Lancet*. 2005;366:1358.

Brugts JJ, Yetgin T, Hoeks SE, et al. The benefits of statins in people without established cardiovascular disease but with cardiovascular risk factors: meta-analysis of randomised controlled trials. *BMJ*. 2009;338:b2376.

Brunzell JD, Davidson M, Furberg CD, et al.; American Diabetes Association; American College of Cardiology Foundation. Lipoprotein management in patients with cardiometabolic risk: consensus statement from the American Diabetes Association and the American College of Cardiology Foundation. *Diabetes Care*. 2008;31:811.

Canner, PL, Berge KG, Wenger NK, et al. Fifteen year mortality in Coronary Drug Project patients: long-term benefit with niacin. *JACC*. 19868:1245–1255.

Cholesterol Treatment Trialists' (CTT) Collaborators; Mihaylova B, Emberson J, Blackwell L, et al. The effects of lowering LDL cholesterol with statin therapy in people at low risk of vascular disease: meta-analysis of individual data from 27 randomised trials. *Lancet*. 2012;380:581–590.

Colhoun HM, Betteridge DJ, Durrington PN, et al. Primary prevention of cardiovascular disease with atorvastatin in type 2 diabetes in the Collaborative Atorvastatin Diabetes Study (CARDS): multicentre randomised placebo-controlled trial. *Lancet*. 2004;364:685–696.

Coronary Drug Project Research Group. Clofibrate and niacin in coronary heart disease. *JAMA*. 1975;231:360–381.

Downs JR, Clearfield M, Whitney E, et al. Primary prevention of acute coronary events with lovastatin in men and women with average cholesterol levels. *JAMA*. 1998;279:1615–1622.

FIELD Study Investigators. Effects of long-term fenofibrate therapy on cardiovascular events in 9795 patients with type 2 diabetes mellitus (the FIELD study): randomised controlled trial. *Lancet*. 2005;366:1849–1861.

Garber AJ, Abrahamson MJ, Barzilay JI, et al. American Association of Clinical Endocrinologists' Comprehensive Diabetes Management Algorithm 2013 Consensus Statement. *Endocr Pract*. 2013;19(3):536–557.

Go AS, Mozaffarian D, Roger VL, et al.; on behalf of the American Heart Association Statistics Committee and Stroke Statistics. Heart Disease and Stroke Statistics—2014 Update: A Report from the American Heart Association. *Circulation*. 2014;129:e28–e292.

Goff DC Jr, Lloyd-Jones DM, Bennett G, et al. 2013 ACC/AHA guideline on the assessment of cardiovascular risk: a report of the American College of Cardiology/American Heart Association Task Force on Practice Guidelines. *Circulation*. 2013 Nov 12 [Epub ahead of print].

Grasso A, Rocco MB. Dyslipidemias. In: Griffin BP, Kapadia SR, Rimmerman CM, eds. *The Cleveland Clinic Board Review*, 2n ed. Philadelphia, PA: Lippincott Williams & Wilkins; 2013 :781–805.

Grundy SM, Brewer HB, Cleeman JI, et al. Definition of metabolic syndrome: report of the National Heart, Lung, and Blood Institute/American Heart Association conference on scientific issues related to definition. *Circulation*. 2004;109:433–438.

Grundy SM, Cleeman JI, Bairey Merz CN, et al. Implications of recent clinical trials for the National Cholesterol Education Program Adult Treatment Panel III guidelines. *Circulation*. 2004;110:227–239.

Haffner SM, Lehto S, Ronnemaa T, Pyorala K, Laakso M. Mortality from coronary heart disease in subjects with type 2 diabetes and in nondiabetic subjects with and without prior myocardial infarction. *N Engl J Med*. 1998;339:229–234.

Kearney PM, Blackwell L, Collins R, Keech A, Simes Baigent C. Cholesterol Treatment Trialists' (CTT) Collaborators. Efficacy of cholesterol-lowering therapy in 18,686 people with diabetes in 14 randomised trials of statins: a meta-analysis. *Lancet*. 2008;371:117–125.

LaRosa JC, Grundy SM, Waters DD, et al. Intensive lipid lowering with atorvastatin in patients with stable coronary disease. *N Engl J Med*. 2005;352:1425–1435.

The Long-Term Intervention with Pravastatin in Ischaemic Disease (LIPID) Study Group. Prevention of cardiovascular events and death with pravastatin in patients with coronary heart disease and a broad range of initial cholesterol levels. *N Engl J Med*. 1998;339:1349–1357.

MRC/BHF Heart Protection Study of cholesterol lowering with simvastatin in 20,536 high-risk individuals: a randomised placebo-controlled trial. *Lancet*. 2002;360:7–22.

Naci H, Brugts J, Ades T. Meta-analysis of 246 955 participants from 135 randomized, controlled trials. comparative tolerability and harms of individual statins: a study-level network. *Circ Cardiovasc Qual Outcomes*. 2013;6:390.

Pasternak RC, Smith SC Jr, Bairey-Merz CN, et al. Statin advisory: clinical precautions when prescribing statin therapy. *Circulation*. 2002;106:1024.

Preiss D, Seshasai SR, Welsh P, et al. Risk of incident diabetes with intensive-dose compared with moderate-dose statin therapy: a meta-analysis. *JAMA*. 2011;305:2556–2564.

Ridker PM, Danielson E, Fonseca FAH, et al. Rosuvastatin to prevent vascular events in men and women with elevated C-reactive protein. *N Engl J Med*. 2008;359:2195–2207.

Rocco, MB. Statins and diabetes risk: fact, fiction and clinical implications. *Cleve Clin J Med*. 2012;79(12):883–893.

Rubins HB, Robins SJ, Collins D, et al. Gemfibrozil for the secondary prevention of coronary heart disease in men with low levels of high-density lipoprotein cholesterol. Veterans Affairs High-Density Lipoprotein Cholesterol Intervention Trial Study Group. *N Engl J Med*. 1999;341:410–418.

Sacks FM, Pfeffer MA, Moye LA, et al. The effect of pravastatin on coronary events after myocardial infarction in patients with average cholesterol levels. *N Engl J Med*. 1996;335:1001–1009.

Sattar N, Preiss D, Murray HM, et al. Statins and risk of incident diabetes: a collaborative meta-analysis of randomised statin trials. *Lancet*. 2010;375:735–742.

Scandinavian Simvastatin Survival Study Group. Randomised trial of cholesterol lowering in 4444 patients with coronary heart disease: the Scandinavian Simvastatin Survival Study (4S). *Lancet*. 1994;344:1383–1389.

Schwartz GG, Olsson AG, Abt M, et al.; dal-OUTCOMES Investigators. Effects of dalcetrapib in patients with a recent acute coronary syndrome. *N Engl J Med*. 2012;367:2089–2099.

Sever PS, Dahlof B, Poulter NR, et al. Prevention of coronary and stroke events with atorvastatin in hypertensive patients who have average or lower-than-average cholesterol concentrations, in the Anglo-Scandinavian Cardiac Outcomes Trial—Lipid Lowering Arm (ASCOT-LLA): a multicentre randomised controlled trial. *Lancet*. 2003;361:1149–1158.

Shepherd J, Barter P, Carmena R, et al. Effect of lowering LDL cholesterol substantially below currently recommended levels in patients with coronary heart disease and diabetes: the Treating to New Targets (TNT) study. *Diabetes Care.* 2006;29:1220–1226.

Stone NJ, Robinson J, Lichtenstein AH, et al. 2013 ACC/AHA guideline on the treatment of blood cholesterol to reduce atherosclerotic cardiovascular risk in adults: a report of the American College of Cardiology/American Heart Association Task Force on Practice Guidelines. *J Am Coll Cardiol.* 2013;S0735–1097(13):06028-2.

Taylor AJ, Sullenberger LE, Lee HJ, et al. Arterial Biology for the Investigation of the Treatment Effects of Reducing Cholesterol (ARBITER) 2: a double-blind, placebo-controlled study of extended-release niacin on atherosclerosis progression in secondary prevention patients treated with statins. *Circulation.* 2004;110:3512–3517.

Taylor F, Huffman MD, Macedo AF, et al. Statins for the primary prevention of cardiovascular disease. *Cochrane Database Syst Rev.* 2013;1:CD004816.

Third report of the National Cholesterol Education Program (NCEP) expert panel on detection, evaluation, and treatment of high blood cholesterol in adults (Adult Treatment Panel III). Final report. *Circulation.* 2002;106:3143–3421.

Waters DD, Ho JE, DeMicco DA, et al. Predictors of new-onset diabetes in patients treated with atorvastatin: results from 3 large randomized clinical trials. *J Am Coll Cardiol.* 2011;57:1535–1545.

Wiegman A, Hutten BA, de Groot E, et al. Efficacy and safety of statin therapy in children with familial hypercholesterolemia: a randomized controlled trial. *JAMA.* 2004;109:551–566.

chapter 13

Pericardial Disease

Wael A. Jaber • Parag R. Patel

QUESTIONS ● ● ●

1. A 62-year-old man is admitted with chronic obstructive pulmonary disease (COPD) and mild left ventricular (LV) dysfunction (ejection fraction [EF] 45%) as well as symptomatic, recurrent atrial fibrillation (heart rate [HR] 120s to 150s) despite antiarrhythmic drug therapy and direct current cardioversion in the past. After rate control with intravenous (IV) β-blockers, the HR improves and the patient feels better. Given his recurrent atrial fibrillation despite optimal medical therapy, the patient is referred for radiofrequency ablation of atrial fibrillation (pulmonary vein isolation) procedure. The procedure is performed on anticoagulation (international normalized ratio >2.0) and is deemed a success, with no inducible atrial fibrillation at the end of the case. A small atrial septal defect (ASD) was noted with intracardiac echocardiography at the end of the case, with no other remarkable findings. That evening in the post-anesthesia care-unit (PACU), the patient is noted to be hypotensive and tachycardic with increasing dyspnea. There is a concern for cardiac tamponade; however, the arterial line does not show a significant respiratory variation of the blood pressure (BP) waveform (pulsus paradoxus). An echocardiogram is performed, demonstrating a large circumferential effusion and the patient is referred for urgent pericardiocentesis. Which of the following explains why the patient did not develop a pulsus on the arterial line, despite a large, hemodynamically significant pericardial effusion?

   a. Presence of an ASD

   b. Administration of excess IV fluid during the ablation

   c. LV dysfunction

   d. COPD

2. A 38-year-old patient with no prior medical history presents to the emergency room with 4 days of chest discomfort. He denies any recent trauma, fever, or use of anticoagulants. The pain is positional and the patient reports mild upper respiratory infection (URI) symptoms in the preceding week. Laboratory work is notable for elevated white blood cell count (neutrophil predominance) as well as elevated erythrocyte sedimentation rate (ESR)/high-sensitivity C-reactive protein (hsCRP); his troponin and other laboratory work is otherwise negative/normal. Electrocardiogram (ECG) is consistent with pericarditis. There is a low suspicion for acute coronary syndrome, and acute pericarditis is diagnosed with small effusion on the echocardiogram; the pain improves with analgesics. Which of the following regimens is the most appropriate therapy for this patient to treat the acute episode and maintain remission?

a. Ibuprofen 600 TID for 2 weeks followed by taper and colchicine 0.5 mg BID for 3 months

b. Aspirin 325 daily and colchicine 0.5 mg BID for 2 weeks followed by taper

c. Ibuprofen 400 BID and colchicine 0.5 mg BID for 2 weeks followed by no taper

d. Prednisone 10 mg daily and ibuprofen 600 TID for 3 months followed by no taper

3. A 62-year-old man with cardiac risk factors of tobacco use, hypertension, and diabetes mellitus returns for follow-up after late-presenting mid-left anterior descending artery (LAD) ST-elevation myocardial infarction (MI). He had an occluded mid-LAD, which was successfully aspirated and stented with a single drug-eluting stent; no significant disease elsewhere is noted. The next day he reports progressive chest discomfort and mild fever and has developed a two-component pericardial friction rub on physical examination. His ECG is concerning for pericarditis (Dressler syndrome) and an echo is performed showing no interval change from discharge other than the presence of a small pericardial effusion. Which of the following regimens would be the most appropriate therapy in this patient?

a. Aspirin 650 TID for 2 weeks with taper to 81 mg daily + colchicine 0.5 mg BID for 3 months

b. Aspirin 325 daily for 2 weeks, then taper to 81 mg daily + ibuprofen 600 mg TID for 3 months

c. Ibuprofen 600 mg TID for 2 weeks with taper + colchicine 0.5 mg BID for 3 months

d. Indomethacin 50 mg TID for 3 months as well as aspirin 650 mg TID for 3 months with taper to 81 mg

4. A 45-year-old male patient with a history of acute pericarditis now returns for outpatient follow-up with increasing dyspnea and lower extremity edema. The patient was seen and started on high-dose aspirin and colchicine (no nonsteroidal anti-inflammatory drugs [NSAIDs] due to allergy) and has not been able to taper for the past 6 months due to persistent low-level symptoms. He has an elevated jugular venous pulse without inspiratory decline, 2+ pedal edema, and congested liver without ascites, as well as a soft pericardial knock. Laboratory values are notable for mild transaminitis as well as elevated ESR/hsCRP. ECG is unremarkable and echo shows a small persistent pericardial effusion with tubular-shaped LV with normal function, along with diastolic bounce and conical-shaped right ventricle (RV) as well as plethoric inferior vena cava and respirophasic transmitral and trans-tricuspid variation all consistent with constrictive pericarditis. Which of the following would be the next most appropriate step in management?

a. Initiate steroid therapy (0.25 to 0.5 mg/kg/day) along with colchicine, and initiate PO diuretic

b. Admit for IV diuresis and transition to PO diuretic regimen after cardiac catheterization for constriction evaluation

c. Repeat echo in 2 to 3 months aspirin and colchicine at current doses

d. Surgical evaluation for pericardiectomy/stripping

5. A 39-year-old patient with no prior medical visits presents with cardiac tamponade and undergoes urgent pericardiocentesis. He is from sub-Saharan Africa and has never been seen by a physician before—reports feeling progressively ill for the past month and brought to the hospital after syncopal episode today. Fluid analysis is performed and listed below:

Gram stain: no gram-positive/gram-negative bacteria noted

Peripheral cell count: normal (peripheral cell count <10 × 10^9 cells/L)

Pericardial fluid differential (lymphocyte/neutrophil): >1.0 (monocytes present as well)

Protein: elevated

hsCRP: markedly elevated

Lactate dehydrogenase (LDH): elevated (>2.0 times peripheral LDH level)

Adenosine deaminase (ADA): >40 U/L

Interferon gamma: >50 pg/mL

Glucose: low

Culture and cytology/acid fast staining: pending

The most likely etiology for the effusion would be

   a. tuberculous pericarditis.

   b. endemic malignancy (i.e., Epstein-Barr virus–associated Burkitt's) with metastatic spread.

   c. malarial (*Plasmodium vivax*).

   d. unable to determine—require pericardial biopsy to confirm.

6. A 47-year-old man with constrictive pericarditis is undergoing an echocardiogram for follow-up. The sonographer asks you to explain the difference between the annulus reversus and annulus paradoxus phenomena. Which of the following statements is correct?

   a. Annulus reversus refers to reversal of septal and lateral mitral tissue Doppler velocities (E′ septal > E′ lateral) and annulus paradoxus refers to inverse correlation of E/E′ and LV end-diastolic pressure.

   b. Annulus reversus refers to reversal of septal and lateral mitral tissue Doppler velocities (A′ septal > A′ lateral) and annulus paradoxus refers to inverse correlation of E/E′ and LV end-diastolic pressure.

   c. Annulus reversus refers to reversal of septal and lateral mitral tissue Doppler velocities (E′ septal < E′ lateral) and annulus paradoxus refers to positive correlation of E/E′ and LV end-diastolic pressure.

   d. Annulus reversus refers to reversal of septal and lateral mitral tissue Doppler velocities (A′ septal < A′ lateral) and annulus paradoxus refers to a positive correlation of E/E′ and LV end-diastolic pressure.

7. A 51-year-old male patient is admitted to the hospital with anasarca and progressive dyspnea and functional limitation. He has a prior history of coronary artery bypass grafting and post-pericardiotomy syndrome with relapsing pericarditis that has likely advanced to constrictive physiology (despite slow taper steroid therapy), given his presenting symptoms and physical examination findings. During the admission he is aggressively diuresed with IV diuretics with improvement in his renal and liver function, as well as symptom improvement (edema and dyspnea). He is unable to go for a magnetic resonance imaging (MRI) for further assessment (prior metallic implant in his spine for scoliosis) and his echocardiogram images are technically difficult due to his distorted spine and prior cardiac surgery.

He is referred for dual transducer cardiac catheterization for hemodynamic evaluation of right- and left-sided pressures as part of his diagnostic workup. The catheterization laboratory team begins the procedure and calls you to discuss the case. They note a sinus rhythm at 90 bpm with occasional premature ventricular contraction and a central venous pressure of 4 mmHg and nonelevated end-diastolic pressures at the beginning of the study (due to recent diuresis); they are unable to elucidate diastolic equalization of pressures, significant "dip and plateau," or respiratory discordance of the ventricular pressure waveforms.

A potential mechanism for the discordant catheterization findings would be

  a. lack of preload due to overdiuresis.
  b. borderline tachycardia and ectopy preventing accurate analysis.
  c. presence of only mild constrictive physiology.
  d. presence of restrictive cardiomyopathy and physiology.

8. A 32-year-old white man presented initially with low-grade fever, cough, and pleuritic chest pain. He was found on ECG to have diffuse ST-segment elevation. A transthoracic echocardiogram (TTE) revealed a large pericardial effusion, and serologies were positive for coxsackievirus B infection. He was diagnosed with acute viral pericarditis and treated with indomethacin. He returns 4 weeks later for follow-up and states that he no longer has any pain, but he notes some mild ankle swelling. His ECG is normal. A repeat TTE shows resolution of the effusion but new findings consistent with mild constriction. What is the next step in managing this patient?

  a. Obtain cardiac MRI to better assess the pericardium.
  b. Have a cardiothoracic surgical consultation for pericardiectomy.
  c. Reassure the patient and observe him over the next 3 months for worsening of symptoms.
  d. Start a course of steroids.

9. A 45-year-old woman with a history of treated carcinoma of the breast presents to the local emergency department with a few days of severe chest pain. In the emergency department, she appears ill and pale and in moderate discomfort. Her BP is 135/60 mmHg; her respiratory rate is 24 breaths per minute; her HR is 82 bpm; and her temperature is 100.8°F. The resident on call reads her chest X-ray (CXR) as unremarkable. Her ECG is shown in Figure 13.1. What is the most reasonable next step?

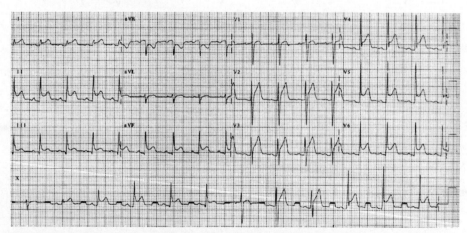

Figure 13.1 • (From Wagner GS, ed. *Marriott's Practical Electrocardiography*, 9th ed. Baltimore, MD: Williams & Wilkins; 1994, with permission.)

  a. Give aspirin and nitroglycerin and prepare to administer thrombolytics.
  b. Call the cardiac intervention team and rush the patient to the catheterization laboratory for emergency coronary intervention.
  c. Give a nonsteroidal anti-inflammatory medication.
  d. Discharge the patient and refer her for a gastroenterology follow-up as an outpatient.

10. A 59-year-old man with a history of coronary artery disease (CAD) and remote coronary bypass surgery presents with progressive dyspnea and vague chest pain. He had a stress echocardiogram for these symptoms that demonstrated normal

LV function with no stress-induced wall motion abnormalities. However, he returned to the emergency department a few days later with recurrent symptoms. This time the house officer examining the patient notes 3+ pedal edema. The patient is admitted and started on diuretics. His blood tests are as follows:

White blood cell count = 11,000

Hemoglobin = 14.2

Platelets = 172,000

Albumin = 4.6

Urea = 11

Creatinine = 0.9

Owing to the recurrent symptoms, his cardiologist decides to refer him for a right and left heart catheterization. The coronary grafts are all patent. The tracings from the study are shown in Figure 13.2. What is the most logical explanation for this patient's symptoms?

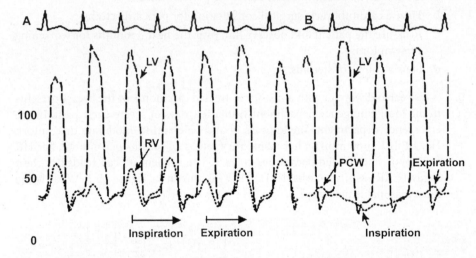

Figure 13.2 • PCW, pulmonary capillary wedge.

   a. Constrictive pericardial disease
   b. Small-vessel CAD
   c. Diastolic dysfunction related to his chronic CAD
   d. Cardiac amyloid
   e. Cardiac tamponade

11. A 73-year-old man with no cardiac history presents with chronic lower extremities edema. His primary care physician attributed his symptoms to old age. He was treated with hydrochlorothiazide. Initially, he reported a good response to the therapy, but, over the past few months, his edema recurred, and doubling the diuretic dose did not alleviate his symptoms. On his initial examination, you notice distended neck veins and a quiet precordium. He has mild hepatomegaly and 4+ pedal edema. A TTE is suboptimal because of the patient's inability to lie flat and obstructive lung disease. His blood work is as follows:

White blood cell count = 6,000

Hemoglobin = 12.7

Platelets = 225,000

Urea = 43

Creatinine = 2.4

Albumin = 3.6

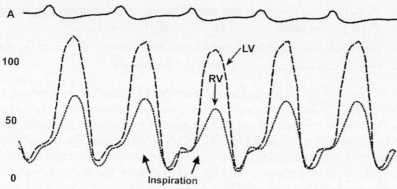

Figure 13.3 • Pressure tracings in the LV and RV.

A cardiac catheterization is performed. He has normal coronary arteries with mild impairment in LV systolic function. The tracings from the study are shown in Figure 13.3. What is your explanation of his symptoms?

   a. You agree with his primary care physician. You tell the patient that he probably has peripheral venous insufficiency.

   b. This patient has significant diastolic dysfunction, and his prognosis is guarded.

   c. This patient's symptoms are due to the LV systolic dysfunction and volume overload.

   d. This patient should be referred for surgical evaluation for possible pericardial stripping.

12. A 56-year-old male smoker with a family history significant for CAD is presenting with dyspnea on exertion and nonexertional vague chest pain. His physical examination and his initial ECG are unremarkable. His CXR demonstrates an increased cardiac silhouette. There is also a small nodule seen in his right upper lobe. The radiologist is not certain about its significance. Given his risk factors and symptoms, he is referred for a perfusion stress test. The images from the stress test are shown in Figure 13.4. Which of the following does the patient clearly have?

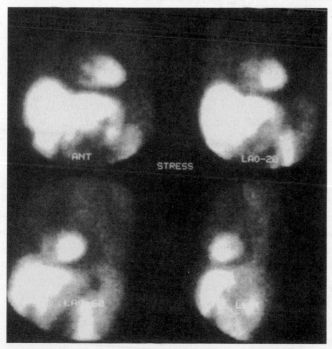

Figure 13.4 • (From Pohost GM, O'Rourke GA, Berman DS, et al., eds. *Imaging in Cardiovascular Disease.* Philadelphia, PA: Lippincott Williams & Wilkins; 2000, with permission.)

a. He has coronary ischemia and should be referred for coronary angiography.

b. There is no evidence of pathology to justify his symptoms.

c. His symptoms are related to impairment of RV filling and pericardial disease.

d. He has mild ischemia and can be treated medically.

13. A 58-year-old man, with cardiac risk factors of tobacco use, hypertension, and hypercholesterolemia, presented to the emergency department a few days ago with an acute onset of left-sided chest pain. His evaluation revealed a diaphoretic man in moderate discomfort. An ECG was performed and showed a pattern consistent with an inferior wall acute MI. The patient was treated with thrombolytics. Forty-five minutes after the initial dose of the thrombolytics, he felt better and had complete resolution of his symptoms and normalization of the ECG. On the third day after the event, he reports midsternal chest pain, vague in nature, with mild diaphoresis and shortness of breath. An ECG is performed, as shown in Figure 13.5. Which of the following should you tell the patient is the next step in managing his condition?

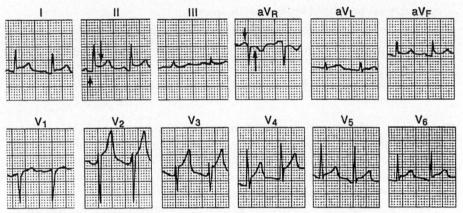

Figure 13.5 • (From Braunwald E, ed. *Heart Disease: A Textbook of Cardiovascular Medicine*, 5th ed. Philadelphia, PA: WB Saunders; 1997, with permission.)

a. There is evidence of reocclusion of the infarct-related artery, and a percutaneous intervention is needed.

b. There is evidence of reocclusion of the infarct-related artery, and rebolus with thrombolytics and heparin is indicated.

c. He is showing signs of early postinfarction pericarditis, and a nonsteroidal anti-inflammatory medication should be started.

d. An LV aneurysm has developed, and a TTE is needed to evaluate the extent of the aneurysm.

14. A 19-year-old male college student presents to his local physician for evaluation of a dry cough. His symptoms started 3 days ago but now appear to be resolving. He had planned a trip overseas but was concerned and is now seeking advice. His physical examination is unremarkable. A CXR is performed and is read as showing an enlarged right cardiac silhouette. A TTE is ordered, which is shown in Figure 13.6. The patient most likely has which of the following conditions?

a. He has a pericardial cyst that is benign; no further treatment should be offered.

b. He has cardiac tamponade requiring a pericardial tap.

c. He has a pleural effusion.

d. There is no pathology. The CXR was misread.

e. He has mesothelioma.

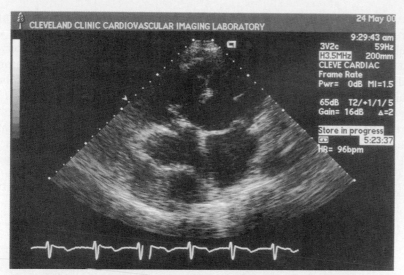

Figure 13.6

15. You are called to the emergency department to see a 74-year-old man. He has a history of heavy smoking and hypertension. The patient cannot remember his medications, but he reports not taking them on a routine basis. In the past few hours before presentation, he experienced a sudden onset of severe left-sided chest pain with radiation to the left scapula. Approximately half an hour later, he noted some difficulty breathing. In the emergency department, he is noted to be diaphoretic and in significant respiratory distress. His physical examination reveals a BP of 160/90 mmHg, elevated jugular venous pressures, and a quiet precordium. His ECG is reported as sinus tachycardia with no acute ST-T changes. After initial pain and BP management, a transesophageal echocardiography (TEE) is performed to rule out aortic dissection. The findings of the TTE are shown in Figure 13.7. What is your recommendation?

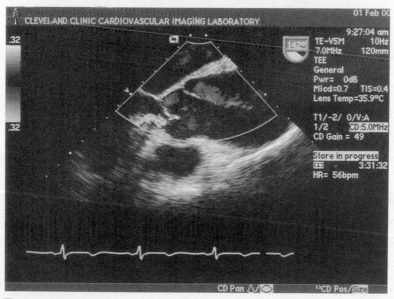

Figure 13.7

a. The patient should have immediate surgical intervention.

b. The patient needs BP control and surgical evaluation once he is medically stabilized.

c. The patient should have percutaneous pericardial drainage to manage the cardiac tamponade and then a surgical evaluation.

d. The diagnosis is unclear; a computed tomographic (CT) scan or an aortic angiogram is needed.

16. A 42-year-old man was referred for evaluation of symptomatic mitral regurgitation. He was diagnosed with mitral valve prolapse that was not suitable for repair. Given his family history of CAD and tobacco use, he underwent a coronary angiogram, which revealed no evidence of obstructive coronary disease. He underwent an uneventful mitral valve replacement. He was extubated and transferred from the intensive care unit 48 hours after the operation. On postoperation day 3, you note the patient to be pale and lethargic and in mild respiratory distress. His BP is 100/60 mmHg. His cardiac and lung examination is compromised by the presence of rapid breathing and chest tubes. His ECG reveals normal sinus rhythm (NSR) at 97 bpm with no acute ST-T changes. A TTE is performed. Selected views are shown in Figure 13.8A. As the patient continues to deteriorate and becomes hypotensive, a TEE is performed next, as shown in Figure 13.8B. What should you recommend?

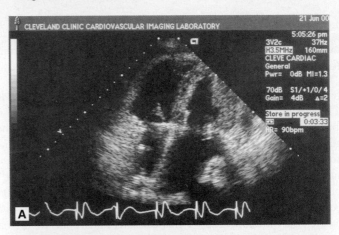

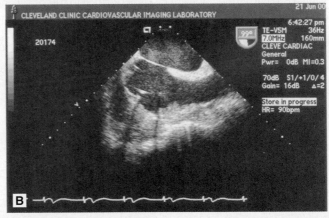

Figure 13.8

a. Immediate surgical exploration of the pericardium

b. Percutaneous aspiration of the fluid present in the pericardium

c. Immediate surgical intervention for malfunction of the prosthetic mitral valve

d. A 500-cc bolus of IV normal saline solution should be started because the patient is dehydrated, and no further intervention is needed

17. A 49-year-old black man with hypertension and chronic renal insufficiency presents with dyspnea and fluid overload with decreased urine output. He is treated in the hospital with diuretics, and his symptoms improve. However, his renal function continues to deteriorate with an increasing blood urea nitrogen of 90 and a creatinine of 5.4. In addition, the patient is noted to have several bruises on his arms from needlestick blood draws and IV lines. On hospital day 4, the patient is noted to be hypotensive and tachycardic: BP, 80/40 mm Hg; HR, 110 bpm.

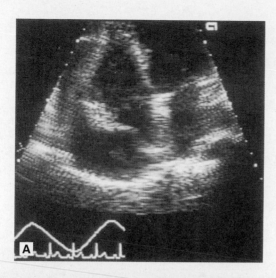

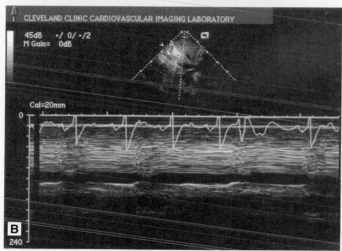

Figure 13.9 ∙ (From Otto CM, Pearlman AS. *Textbook of Clinical Echocardiography.* Philadelphia, PA: WB Saunders; 1995, with permission.)

No jugular venous distention is noted, but heart sounds are diminished, and a loud pericardial rub is heard. His TTE is shown in Figure 13.9. What is the next step in management?

a. Urgent pericardiocentesis

b. IV hydration

c. Immediate dialysis

d. The continuation of diuretics with serial TTE

18. A 42-year-old white male chef is brought into the emergency department after a motor vehicle accident in which he fell asleep at the wheel and ran into a tree. He is reporting anterior chest discomfort and shortness of breath. He relates no prior medical conditions and takes no medications. Vitals are stable with a BP of 120/60 mmHg and an HR of 90 bpm. His ECG is shown in Figure 13.10A. A TTE is performed. Diastolic images are shown in Figure 13.10B. Laboratory tests show modest elevation of creatinine phosphokinase at 240. Which of the following is the most reasonable next step in managing this patient?

a. Start the patient on a nonsteroidal anti-inflammatory agent with follow-up as an outpatient in 1 week.

b. Admit the patient for observation on telemetry with a follow-up TTE.

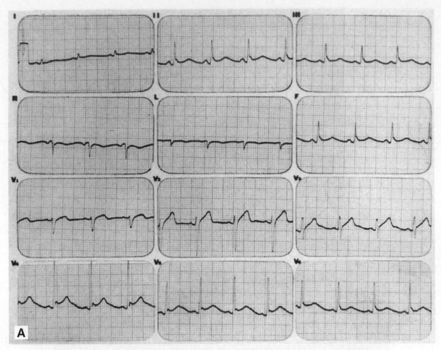

Figure 13.10A • (From Chou T-C. *Electrocardiography in Clinical Practice*, 4th ed. Philadelphia, PA: WB Saunders; 1996, with permission.)

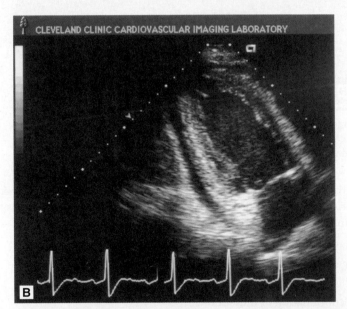

Figure 13.10B • (From Chou T-C. *Electrocardiography in Clinical Practice*, 4th ed. Philadelphia, PA: WB Saunders; 1996, with permission.)

    c. The patient needs immediate percutaneous revascularization.

    d. Send the patient for surgical treatment of pericardial rupture.

19. A 22-year-old white man is newly diagnosed with non-Hodgkin lymphoma. He undergoes a metastatic workup that includes an MRI of the chest and abdomen, which is shown in Figure 13.11. The plan is for chemotherapy, but you are consulted for cardiac assessment before beginning chemotherapy. Radionuclide ventriculography shows a normal LV EF of 65%. What should you recommend?

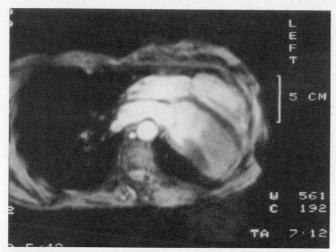

Figure 13.11 • (MRI image was provided by Dr. Richard White, Head, Section of Cardiovascular Imaging, Departments of Radiology and Cardiovascular Medicine, The Cleveland Clinic Foundation.)

a. Ordering a TTE to delineate the abnormality

b. Cardiothoracic surgical consultation before starting chemotherapy

c. Exercise stress testing

d. Proceeding with chemotherapy without further cardiac evaluation

20. A 44-year-old white man with rheumatoid arthritis is referred to your office for evaluation after his rheumatologist heard a loud heart sound. On questioning, the patient mainly reports joint pains in his fingers. He denies any chest discomfort or shortness of breath. He has been on methotrexate and prednisone for the past year. His examination is significant for mild erythema and swelling of his distal interphalangeal joints, rheumatoid nodules on his right forearm, clear lungs, distant heart sounds with a loud friction rub, and moderate peripheral edema. You order a TTE to further assess his heart. Selective images are shown in Figure 13.12. What is your recommendation?

a. Because he currently has no cardiac symptoms, no further treatment is needed except to continue methotrexate and prednisone.

b. You want the patient to start indomethacin, continue methotrexate and prednisone, and follow up in 4 weeks.

c. The best treatment at this time for his pericardial effusion is drainage with the instillation of steroids to prevent recurrence.

d. A surgical evaluation for pericardiectomy is necessary because the findings on his TTE indicate that he will develop problems in the future if this is not taken care of soon.

21. A 55-year-old white man presents for evaluation of chest pain. He has no prior medical problems, but he has noted burning epigastric and chest discomfort for the past few months for which he was taking antacids with some relief of his symptoms. However, because the symptoms persisted, he sought medical attention and was referred for an esophagogastroduodenoscopy, which was performed earlier today. He was found to have a fundal hiatal hernia with a gastric ulcer that was cauterized, and he was started on omeprazole. On returning home, he noted a new sharp anterior chest pain, somewhat positional related, that was not relieved with antacids or omeprazole. This pain progressively worsened over the next few hours, and he came to the emergency department. Examination in the emergency department revealed a temperature of 38.1°C, an HR of 110 bpm, and a BP of 120/70 mmHg. Lung sounds were clear. Heart sounds appeared normal with the patient sitting

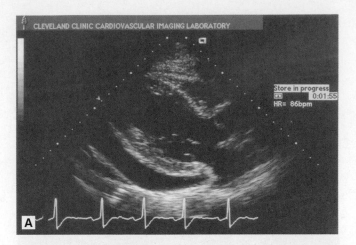

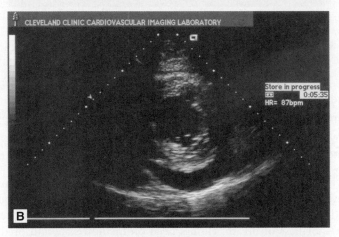

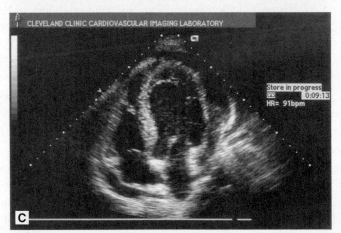

Figure 13.12

upright, but they were diminished with the patient lying in the supine position. An ECG did not show any acute ST-T wave abnormalities to suggest infarction. A CXR was performed, as shown in Figure 13.13. You are called to further assess the patient. After reviewing the available data, which of the following is your next step?

a. Immediate surgical consultation

b. Immediate pericardiocentesis

c. Start a nonsteroidal anti-inflammatory medication and admit him for observation

d. No further treatment is needed because his symptoms are caused by the hiatal hernia

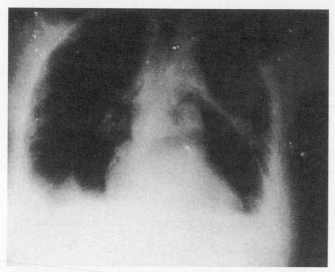

Figure 13.13 • (From Spodick DS. *The Pericardium: A Comprehensive Textbook.* New York: Marcel Dekker; 1997, with permission.)

22. A 71-year-old man presents to the hospital with palpitations of 2 to 3 days' duration. He has no known medical history, and he is not on any medications. Initial evaluation is unremarkable except for a BP of 160/90 mmHg and an ECG showing atrial fibrillation with a ventricular rate of 120 to 130 bpm. Given the duration of his symptoms, he is treated with β-blockers for rate control and heparin for anticoagulation. On hospital day 2, he is referred for early transesophageal-guided cardioversion. The TEE reveals normal LV and RV function. There are no echocardiographic contraindications for cardioversion. An uneventful cardioversion is performed, and the patient converts to NSR. On hospital day 3, the patient is found in marked respiratory distress. On physical examination, he has a regular HR with a loud audible click over the precordium. A CXR is performed, as shown in Figure 13.14. What does this patient have?

a. He has a pulmonary embolism and should be treated with thrombolytics.

b. He has a hiatal/diaphragmatic hernia with compression of the heart by the fundus of stomach.

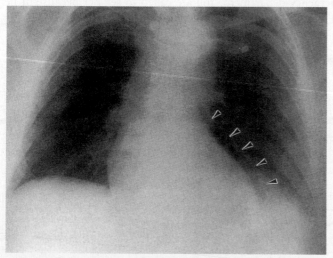

Figure 13.14 • (From Spodick DS. *The Pericardium: A Comprehensive Textbook.* New York: Marcel Dekker; 1997, with permission.)

 c. He has an iatrogenic pneumohydropericardium; immediate drainage and surgical attention are needed.

 d. He has a recurrence of atrial fibrillation.

23. A 59-year-old woman with a history of chronic renal insufficiency presents to the emergency department with anterior left-sided chest pain. She reports that the chest pain started after her last dialysis 7 days ago. She appears lethargic and in mild respiratory distress. The physical examination demonstrates a BP of 160/90 mmHg and an HR of 100 bpm. On cardiac auscultation, a loud friction rub is heard. An ECG is obtained (Fig. 13.15). What is the most important next step in this case?

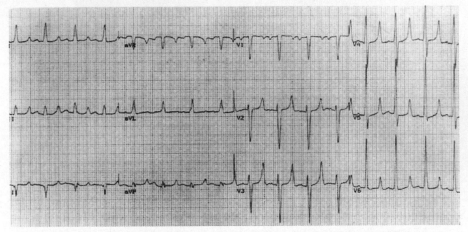

Figure 13.15 • (From Spodick DS. *The Pericardium: A Comprehensive Textbook.* New York: Marcel Dekker; 1997, with permission.)

 a. Perform emergency dialysis.

 b. Obtain an echocardiogram.

 c. Prepare for pericardiocentesis.

 d. Admit the patient to the cardiac care unit to rule out MI.

24. A 29-year-old woman with known insulin-dependent diabetes mellitus was found unconscious 1 hour after an office party. Initial assessment by the emergency medical service team showed a BP of 90/60 mm Hg. Her pulse was 120, and her blood sugar was 870 mg/dL. She was given SC insulin and rushed to the emergency department. You are called to see her because of her abnormal ECG (Fig. 13.16). She is noted to be semiconscious. The emergency physician has

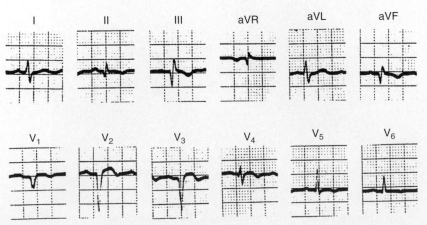

Figure 13.16 • (From Spodick DS. *The Pericardium: A Comprehensive Textbook.* New York: Marcel Dekker; 1997, with permission.)

already started her on IV insulin drip and hydration. What is your recommendation at this juncture?

a. She is having an acute MI, and immediate restoration of coronary flow is essential.

b. She has ECG evidence of hyperkalemia, and she needs IV calcium and, possibly, dialysis.

c. Continue the current management; the ECG will improve with the resolution of ketoacidosis.

d. Her ECG predicts high-degree atrioventricular block; a standby external pacemaker should be available.

25. Which of the following is the most common neoplastic pericardial tumor in adults?

a. Neuroma

b. Hemangioma

c. Mesothelioma

d. Teratoma

ANSWERS

1. **a.** Presence of an ASD. The presence of the iatrogenic ASD after the transseptal puncture for the radiofrequency ablation/pulmonary vein isolation procedure equates right atrial (RA) and left atrial (LA) pressures with inspiration. The predicted decrease in LV filling during inspiration due to interventricular dependence and exaggerated RV filling and septal shift toward the LV is mitigated by the presence of an ASD. With inspiration, the decrease in intrathoracic pressure is transmitted to both atria and thus preload to the LV is maintained and interventricular dependence is not as pronounced. Thus, the variation in systolic blood pressure is not as prominent, resulting in minimal to no pulsus paradoxus. Administration of excess fluid would stave off circulatory collapse in tamponade; however, it would not diminish the pulsus. Answer b is incorrect as with severe LV dysfunction, patients can have a pulsus alternans (variation in peak systolic pressure with every other beat) and Answer c is incorrect as obstructive lung disease can lead to the presence of a pulsus due to exaggerated inspiratory effort and negative intrathoracic pressure.

2. **a.** Ibuprofen 600 TID for 2 weeks followed by taper and colchicine 0.5 mg BID for 3 months. The patient presents with an initial attack of acute pericarditis without any high-risk features (small effusion, negative troponin, no fever/ trauma, or anticoagulant use). The appropriate regimen in this case would be an NSAID (ibuprofen 600 to 800 mg TID or indomethacin 50 mg TID) for a course of 1 to 2 weeks with physician follow-up. In addition, the use of colchicine has been studied in two trials with improvement in symptom resolution and maintenance of remission at a dose of 0.5 mg (daily for <70 kg; BID for >70 kg) for a fixed period of 3 months.

   Aspirin and colchicine can be used together; however, the dosing is incorrect for Answer **b** (650 to 1,000 mg TID) and the colchicine should still be continued for 3 months. Prophylactic Proton-pump inhibitor (PPI) should be utilized during the high-dose NSAID use to prevent gastric ulcer. Answer **c** is incorrect (dosing of ibuprofen is incorrect). Answer **d** is incorrect since steroid therapy is only reserved for patients with NSAID or acetylsalicylic acid (ASA) contraindication or patients having relapsing pericarditis that is refractory to NSAID/ASA therapy.

3. **a.** Aspirin 650 TID for 2 weeks with taper to 81 mg daily + colchicine 0.5 mg BID for 3 months. The patient has postinfarction pericarditis with a typical presentation after reperfusion for late-presenting MI. Although not as frequent, postinfarction pericarditis (Dressler syndrome) is still seen in a small percentage of patients after large MI, and cardiac/pericardial trauma. The regimen used in these patients is modified to include aspirin (instead of NSAIDs) for two reasons: (a) aspirin is required for patients with CAD, with or without recent stenting; and (b) NSAIDs are postulated to impair scar formation and wound healing after an MI. Colchicine is still part of the regimen despite the recent MI and helps with symptom resolution. Correct answer is a—with high-dose aspirin initially with gradual taper once symptoms improve. The clopidogrel is continued despite high doses of aspirin, due to the placement of a recent intracoronary stent.

4. **a.** Initiate steroid therapy (0.25 to 0.5 mg/kg/day) along with colchicine, and initiate PO diuretic. The patient had acute pericarditis, which transformed into a chronic effusive constrictive pericarditis. There is evidence of therapy failure (persistent symptoms and elevated biomarkers) and ongoing inflammation, leading to symptomatic constrictive pericarditis with increasing hemodynamic significance (as demonstrated by symptoms/physical examination and echo findings). The next step would be to escalate anti-inflammatory therapy to include glucocorticoids (prednisone) to help abate the ongoing symptoms and pericardial inflammation. Glucocorticoids are generally not first-line therapy since

patients who receive them early in the course of the disease process are more likely to have relapsing pericarditis and eventually develop constrictive pericarditis. In the case of this patient, he does not have any other treatment options due to his NSAID allergy, so steroids should be initiated at a low dose and maintained with very gradual taper (weeks to months) that involves assessment of his symptoms, biomarker trend (ESR/hsCRP), as well as MRI findings to assess for inflammation/edema within the pericardium to help quell the disease process.

Admission for IV diuresis is not necessary as the patient has not proven resistance to PO diuretics and although a cardiac catheterization may be required alternative noninvasive diagnostic modalities should be performed prior to catheterization to make the diagnosis. Answer c is incorrect since the patient has demonstrated treatment failure with progression of symptoms in the interim. Answer d is incorrect as medical therapy options (steroids, diuresis) are still available. Pericardiectomy is generally reserved in medically refractory cases.

5. **a.** Tuberculous pericarditis. The patient presents with acute tuberculous pericarditis with large exudative effusion. Indolence of the effusion is likely over months; however, the salient findings in the fluid analysis are the elevated interferon gamma, ADA, and normal peripheral white blood cell count with pericardial lymphocyte predominance. The presence of interferon gamma elevation had a 92% sensitivity, 100% specificity, and 100% positive predictive value for tuberculous pericarditis. ADA was also linked to tuberculous pericarditis; however, it was not as sensitive or specific (87%/92%).

Although Answers b and c are epidemiologically possible, the fluid analysis is not suggestive of either. Pericardial biopsy (Answer d) is incorrect as tuberculous pericarditis can be defined by the interferon gamma and ADA elevation. Also Acid-Fast Bacilli (AFB) staining will reveal AFB + organisms confirming diagnosis. Biopsy should be reserved for patients with unrevealing fluid analysis who are still symptomatic and require further diagnostic testing to make a diagnosis.

6. **a.** Annulus reversus refers to reversal of septal and lateral mitral tissue Doppler velocities (E′ septal > E′ lateral) and annulus paradoxus refers to inverse correlation of E/E′ and LV end-diastolic pressure. The annulus reversus phenomenon describes a reversal of mitral lateral and septal tissue Doppler velocity. Normally, E′ lateral > E′ septal; however, in constrictive pericarditis it is postulated that tethering of the free wall prevents longitudinal motion of the annulus at the lateral border, thus decreasing the lateral E′ and the septal E′ concurrently is mildly exaggerated.

The annulus paradoxus phenomenon was initially described after data looking at the correlation between the E/E′ ratio and pulmonary capillary wedge pressure were established. In a small subset of patients with constrictive pericarditis, inversion of the correlation between E/E′ and PCWP was noted, and named annulus paradoxus.

7. **a.** Lack of preload due to overdiuresis. Volume loading is required to elucidate the diagnostic findings described above. Constrictive pericarditis is a preload-dependent condition and with overdiuresis and low central venous pressure, the hemodynamic findings of elevated and equal end-diastolic ventricular pressure waveforms as well as respiratory discordance of the LV/RV waveforms are not seen. Often in these cases, the patient is given a bolus of 1 to 2 L of normal saline to increase the RA pressure >12 to 15 mmHg and the study is performed once they are adequately volume loaded. Of note, in cases of atrial fibrillation, the patient may require a temporary venous pacemaker to regularize the rhythm for analysis purposes.

8. **c.** Reassure the patient and observe him over the next 3 months for worsening of symptoms. The natural history of acute viral or idiopathic pericarditis is usually

short and self-limited. Occasionally, mild forms of constriction may develop weeks after the initial event, but they usually resolve without any specific treatment. No further treatment is indicated unless he becomes more symptomatic or develops signs of cardiac tamponade.

9. **c.** Give a nonsteroidal anti-inflammatory medication. The clinical presentation of a few days of severe chest pain does not favor an acute MI. Furthermore, the ECG tracing supports the diagnosis of pericarditis. Therefore, cardiac catheterization and thrombolytics are not appropriate. The only reasonable answer is to start the patient on anti-inflammatory medications and obtain a TTE to rule out pericardial effusion.

10. **a.** Constrictive pericardial disease. This patient did not have evidence of ischemia on a recent stress test. Furthermore, there is no evidence of obstructive disease in his coronaries or grafts. His tracings mostly support the diagnosis of constriction, given the diastolic equalization of pressures in the cardiac chambers and the typical square root sign. Amyloidosis would typically show signs of restrictive hemodynamics with no respiratory variation. Echocardiography typically shows increased LV wall thickness. Additionally, a diagnosis of tamponade should have been evident by echocardiography, which the patient had before heart catheterization. Otherwise, hemodynamic tracings of cardiac tamponade would look exactly the same as for constriction.

11. **b.** This patient has significant diastolic dysfunction, and his prognosis is guarded. He has evidence of restrictive LV filling (advanced diastolic dysfunction) in the absence of CAD. The differential diagnosis in his age group includes amyloidosis (especially considering concomitant renal dysfunction), hemochromatosis, and other infiltrative processes.

12. **c.** His symptoms are related to impairment of RV filling and pericardial disease. This patient with the main presentation of dyspnea has an increased cardiac silhouette. The nuclear image provided shows a circumferential echolucency surrounding the heart. This is consistent with a large pericardial effusion, and he most likely has RA and RV diastolic compromise. There is no evidence of a perfusion defect to suggest ischemia.

13. **c.** He is showing signs of early postinfarction pericarditis, and a nonsteroidal anti-inflammatory medication should be started. This patient had an MI 72 hours ago that was successfully treated with thrombolytics. The ECG shows diffuse ST elevation with PR depression. These findings support the diagnosis of post-MI pericarditis. The ECG changes are new and nonlocalizing. Most patients improve with nonsteroidal anti-inflammatory medications.

14. **a.** He has a pericardial cyst that is benign; no further treatment should be offered. The TTE and CXR show a pericardial cyst. Pericardial cysts are usually smooth structures containing transudative fluid. They are frequently only 2 or 3 cm in diameter, often located at the right cardiodiaphragmatic angle, and clinically silent. However, cysts can be associated with chest pain, dyspnea, cough, and arrhythmias likely caused by compression of adjacent tissues. They can also become secondarily infected. In this patient, whose nonspecific symptoms appear to be resolving, no further treatment is needed.

15. **a.** The patient should have immediate surgical intervention. This patient has evidence of acute type A aortic dissection with extension to the pericardium, as evidenced by the pericardial effusion on the TEE. He should be immediately referred for surgical repair. If the diagnosis were not certain based on the TEE, then CT, MRI, or aortic angiography would be needed to better define the anatomy. The safest and most efficient management of patients with aortic dissection is to carry out all diagnostic procedures in the operating room. Pericardial drainage often

gives only temporary relief or no relief of the tamponade, and the subsequent increase in BP disrupts sealing clots, accelerating intrapericardial leakage.

16. **a.** Immediate surgical exploration of the pericardium. The TTE and TEE demonstrate a pericardial hematoma compromising RA and RV filling. This is an indication for surgical exploration and evacuation of the hematoma.

17. **b.** IV hydration. This patient has evidence of pericarditis likely related to uremia, as he is close to requiring dialysis. Although his TTE shows signs of tamponade (RA collapse, moderate-sized effusion, and respiratory variation across the mitral inflow), there is no jugular venous distention, and the inferior vena cava is small sized, indicating that this patient has been overdiuresed. His hypotension and tachycardia are related to dehydration. He should, therefore, be treated with IV hydration.

18. **b.** Admit the patient for observation on telemetry with a follow-up TTE. The ECG shows findings consistent with an anterior wall injury, and the TTE shows a small pericardial effusion. Given this patient's history, he most likely has a cardiac contusion. Although the prognosis for recovery is generally excellent, these patients require careful monitoring and follow-up for late complications, which range from ventricular arrhythmias to cardiac rupture. Hence, the most logical answer to this question is to admit the patient to a telemetry bed with follow-up TTE.

19. **d.** Proceeding with chemotherapy without further cardiac evaluation. This patient's MRI shows congenital absence of the pericardium. This is a benign condition usually found incidentally. No specific cardiac treatment is needed unless there is entrapment of one of the cardiac chambers.

20. **d.** A surgical evaluation for pericardiectomy is necessary because the findings on his TTE indicate that he will develop problems in the future if this is not taken care of soon. The patient is currently symptomatic with edema of the lower extremities. Furthermore, he has a pericardial friction rub suggestive of an active pericardial process likely related to his rheumatologic disease process. He is already on methotrexate and prednisone as anti-inflammatory medications. Pericardial effusions related to rheumatoid arthritis often progress to constriction despite anti-inflammatory therapy, and early management consisting of pericardial stripping is recommended.

21. **b.** Immediate pericardiocentesis. The next step is an immediate pericardiocentesis. This patient has signs of early sepsis. Furthermore, the CXR shows pneumopericardium that likely developed secondary to gastric perforation from the esophagogastroduodenoscopy and cauterization of the ulcer. This patient needs immediate referral to surgery for repair.

22. **c.** He has an iatrogenic pneumohydropericardium; immediate drainage and surgical attention are needed. This patient had a TEE that most likely resulted in an esophageal tear with communication to the pericardial sac. On the CXR, there is a lucent triangle outlining the pericardium with pericardial passage over the aortic arch.

23. **a.** Perform emergency dialysis. This patient has missed her dialysis session and is now presenting with hyperkalemia (note peaked T waves on ECG) and uremic pericarditis. The most essential step is to start dialysis to treat the hyperkalemia.

24. **c.** Continue the current management; the ECG will improve with the resolution of ketoacidosis. Patients presenting with diabetic ketoacidosis can have ECG features that are typical of stage I pericarditis and hypokalemia. The treatment is usually that of ketoacidosis. The ECG returns to normal after resolution of the acidosis.

25. **c.** Mesothelioma. Teratoma is the most common pericardial tumor in infancy and childhood. Neuroma and hemangioma are uncommon enough to be considered curiosities.

SUGGESTED READINGS

Buck M, Ingle JN, Giuliani ER, et al. Pericardial effusion in women with breast cancer. *Cancer.* 1987;60(2):263–269.

Ha JW, Oh JK, Ling LH, Nishimura RA, Seward JB, Tajik AJ. Annulus paradoxus: transmitral flow velocity to mitral annular velocity ratio is inversely proportional to pulmonary capillary wedge pressure in patients with constrictive pericarditis. *Circulation.* 2001;105:976–978.

Hoit BD. Management of effusive and constrictive pericardial heart disease. *Circulation.* 2002;105(25):2939–2942.

Imazio M, Brucato A, Cemin R, et al. A randomized trial of colchicine for acute pericarditis. *N Engl J Med.* 2013;369:1522–1528.

Klein AL, Asher CR. Diseases of the pericardium, restrictive cardiomyopathy, and diastolic dysfunction. In: Topol EJ, ed. *Textbook of Cardiovascular Medicine,* 2nd ed. Philadelphia, PA: Lippincott Williams & Wilkins; 2002.

Lange RA, Hillis LD. Clinical practice. Acute pericarditis. *N Engl J Med.* 2004;351:2195.

Reuss CS, Wilansky SM, Lester SJ, et al. Using mitral "annulus reversus" to diagnose constrictive pericarditis. *Eur J Echocardiogr.* 2009;10:372–375.

Reuter H, Burgess L, van Vuuren W, Doubell A. Diagnosing tuberculous pericarditis. *QJM.* 2006;99:827–839.

Spodick DS. *The Pericardium: A Comprehensive Textbook.* New York: Marcel Dekker; 1997.

chapter 14

Cardiac Imaging

Ellen Mayer Sabik • Brian P. Griffin

QUESTIONS

1. The three-dimensional (3D) transesophageal echocardiographic (TEE) image in Figure 14.1 demonstrates a patient with

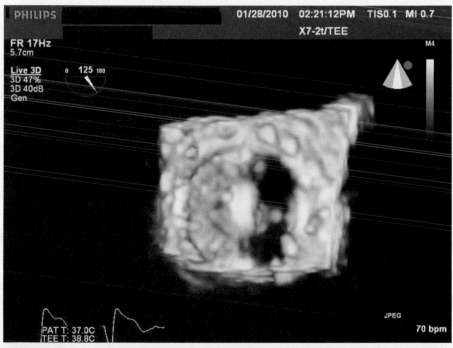

Figure 14.1

   a. normally functioning bioprosthetic mitral valve replacement (MVR).
   b. normally functioning bileaflet mechanical MVR.
   c. mitral valve (MV) endocarditis with a vegetation.
   d. abnormal mechanical MVR.
   e. abnormal bioprosthetic MVR.

2. The images in Figure 14.2A–E come from an 18-year-old young man with marked shortness of breath (SOB). The most appropriate course of action would be

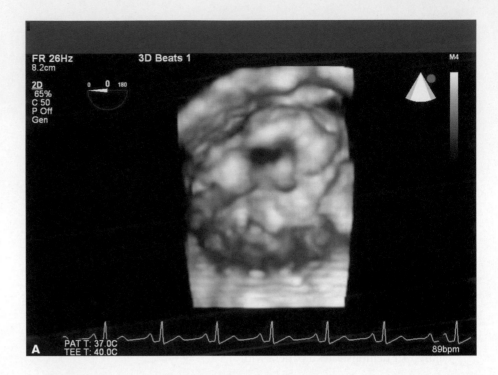

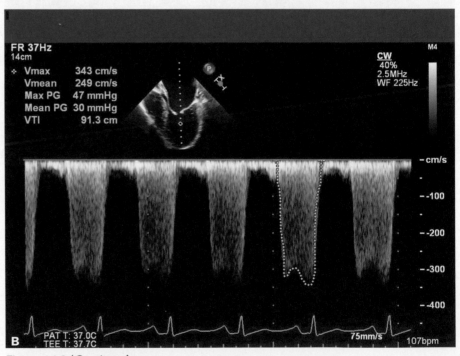

Figure 14.2 (*Continued*)

a. closed mitral commissurotomy because he has a split score of 0 to 4 and minimal mitral regurgitation (MR).

b. percutaneous mitral valvuloplasty (PMV) because he has a split score of 4 to 8 and minimal MR.

c. surgical MVR because he has a split score of 8 to 12 and minimal MR.

d. surgical MVR because he has a split score of 0 to 4 with significant MR.

e. surgical MVR because he has a split score of 4 to 8 and significant MR.

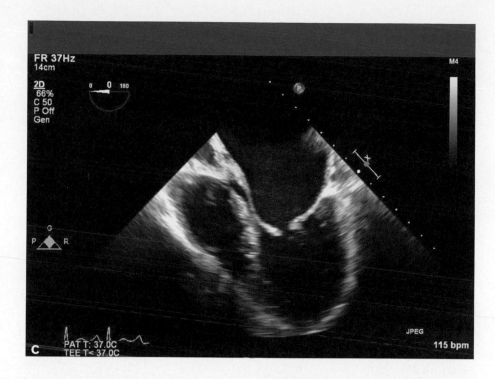

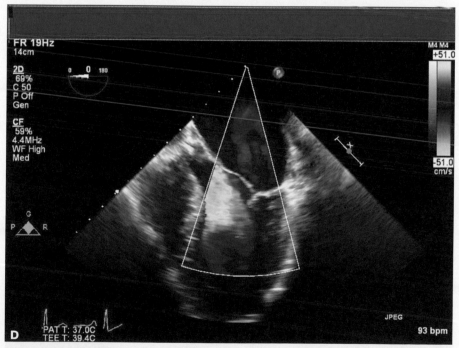

Figure 14.2 (*Continued*)

3. The images in Figure 14.3A–C belong to a 65-year-old woman with lung cancer and a central venous catheter for chemotherapy. The structure seen on these images is most likely to be

   a. prominent Chiari network.

   b. implantable cardioverter-defibrillator (ICD) wire.

   c. right atrial (RA) thrombus or thrombus on central venous catheter.

   d. RA myxoma.

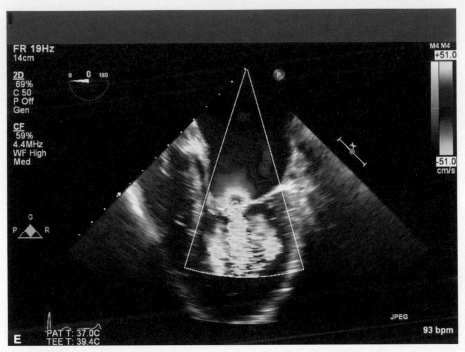

Figure 14.2

4. The images in Figure 14.4A and B are associated with which of the following?

   a. Moderate risk of endocarditis
   b. No risk of heart failure
   c. Large jugular venous v waves
   d. Radiofemoral delay

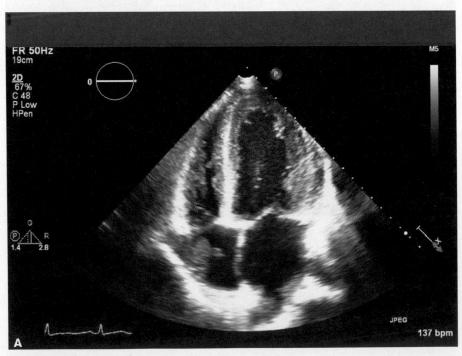

Figure 14.3 (*Continued*)

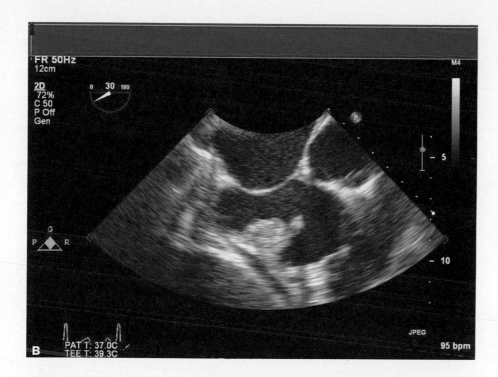

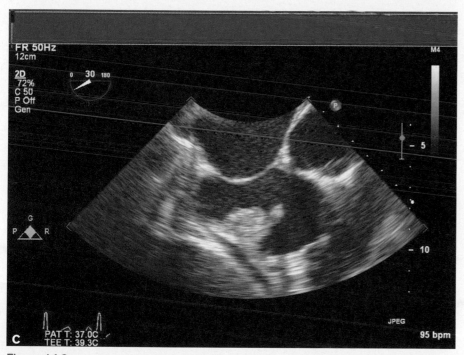

Figure 14.3

5. The images in Figure 14.5A–C are from a 43-year-old s/p carpentier edwards aortic valve replacement (CE AVR) with fevers and night sweats. These images demonstrate all of the following except

   a. paravalvular abscess.

   b. fistula.

   c. aortic stenosis (AS).

   d. aortic insufficiency (AI).

   e. vegetations.

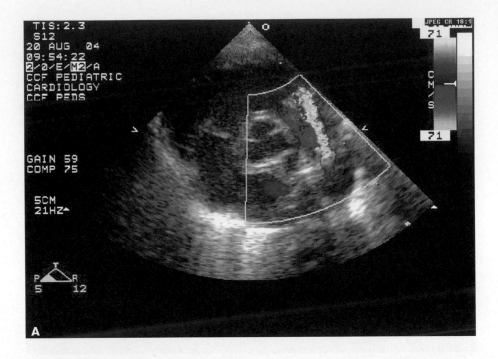

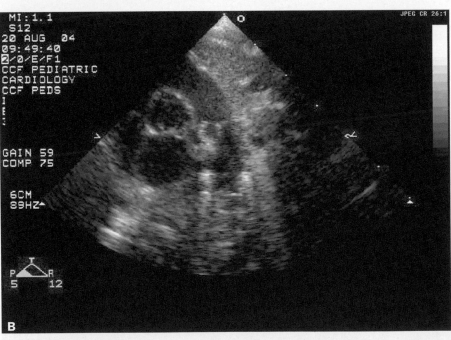

Figure 14.4

6. The images in Figure 14.6A and B are from a transthoracic echocardiogram (TTE) from a patient who is a 57-year-old woman with lung cancer who presents with chest pain (CP) and SOB. The most likely cause of her CP and SOB based on these images is

    a. myocardial infarction (MI).

    b. aortic dissection.

    c. pericardial effusion with pericarditis/tamponade.

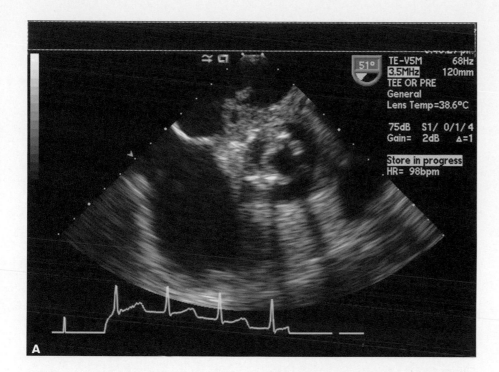

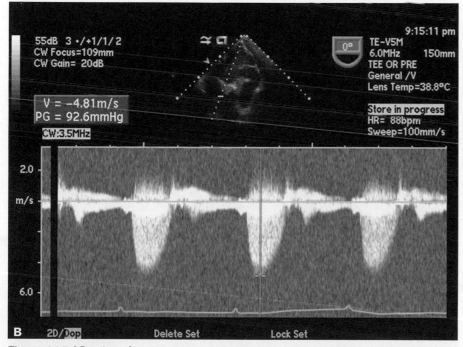

Figure 14.5 (*Continued*)

    d. pulmonary embolus.

    e. pneumonia.

7. The patient is a 70-year-old woman with a history of hypertension, but no prior cardiac history, who comes in with sudden onset of CP, which later migrates to her back. She is diagnosed with a computed tomography (CT) of her chest to have a type I aortic dissection. Her blood pressure is 100/70 mmHg and her heart rate is 115 bpm. Images from her TTE are in Figures 14.7A–C. The next step in her care would be

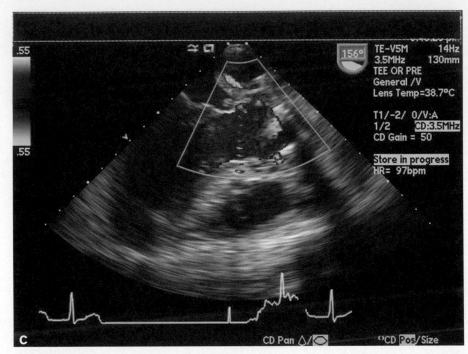

Figure 14.5

a. aortic stent graft.

b. coronary angiography.

c. intraaortic balloon pump placement.

d. pericardiocentesis.

e. emergent cardiac surgery.

8. The finding in the transthoracic images in Figure 14.8A and B is commonly associated with which of the following lesions?

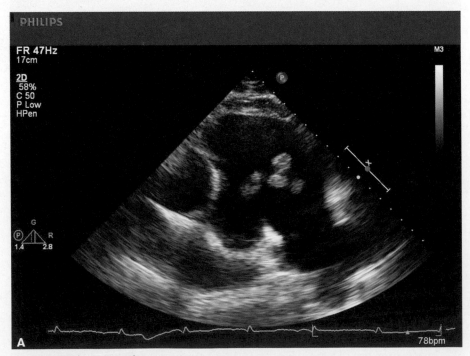

Figure 14.6 (*Continued*)

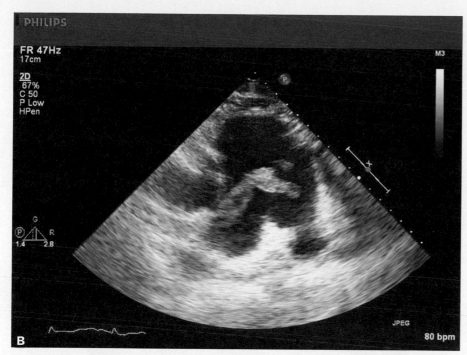

Figure 14.6

    a. Congenitally corrected transposition

    b. Cleft MV

    c. Coarctation of the aorta

    d. Right ventricular (RV) infarction

    e. Bicuspid aortic valve (AV)

9. A 36-year-old man with a history of hypertension on medications for 5 years presents to your office with complaints of dyspnea on exertion and is found by his internist to have a heart murmur. Below are some representative views from his TTE (Fig. 14.9A–E). What is the diagnosis?

    a. Patent ductus arteriosus (PDA)

    b. Rheumatic AV with AI

    c. Rheumatic AS

    d. Coarctation of the aorta with bicuspid AV with AI

    e. Marfan's with aortic dissection

10. A 37-year-old patient presents with fever, weight loss, and blood cultures that are positive for *Pseudomonas* and the transthoracic echo finding in Figure 14.10. The patient's most likely demographic for this clinical scenario is

    a. patient with hypertrophic obstructive cardiomyopathy (HOCM) who had a dental procedure 3 weeks ago.

    b. patient with myxomatous MV disease with mitral valve prolapse (MVP).

    c. patient with subaortic stenosis after dental procedure 3 weeks ago.

    d. patient with a patent ductus.

    e. intravenous (IV) drug abuser.

11. This M-mode tracing (Fig. 14.11) demonstrates a patient with

    a. HOCM with systolic anterior motion (SAM) of the MV leaflets.

    b. MVP.

    c. AS.

    d. rheumatic mitral stenosis (MS).

    e. severe left ventricular (LV) dysfunction.

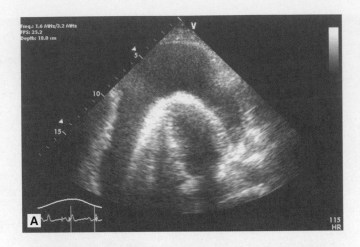

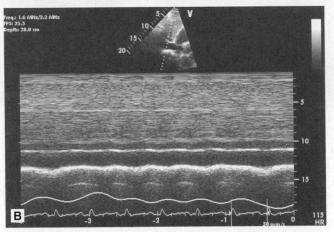

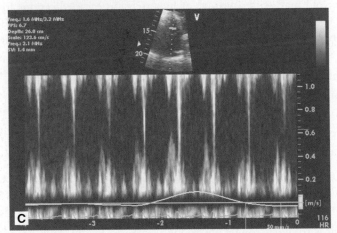

Figure 14.7 • A. Apical four-chamber view (TTE). **B.** M-mode through the IVC in the subcostal view (TTE). **C.** Continuous-wave Doppler through the mitral valve showing mitral valve inflow pattern.

12. The following TEE image (Fig. 14.12) demonstrates a patient with

   a. trileaflet AV.

   b. bicuspid AV with fusion of right coronary cusp (RCC) and noncoronary cusp (NCC).

   c. bicuspid AV with fusion of RCC and LCC.

   d. bicuspid AV with fusion of left coronary cusp (LCC) and NCC.

   e. unicuspid AV.

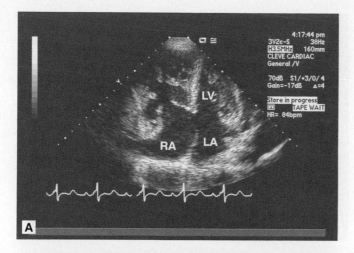

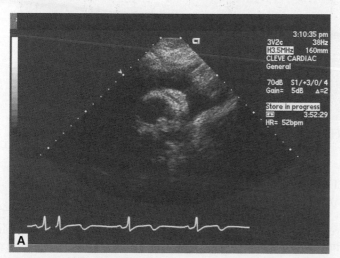

Figure 14.8 • **A.** Apical four-chamber view (TTE). **B.** Apical four-chamber view with color Doppler.

13. The patient is a 22-year-old with a systolic and diastolic murmur with the following echo images (Fig. 14.13A and B). These images demonstrate

   a. membranous ventricular septal defect (VSD).

   b. supracristal VSD.

   c. Ebstein anomaly.

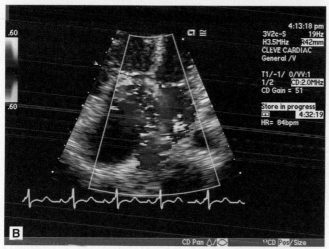

Figure 14.9 (*Continued*)

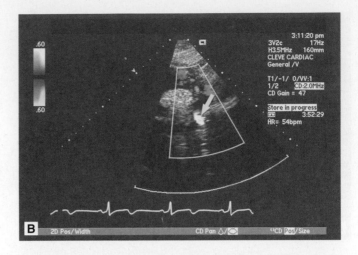

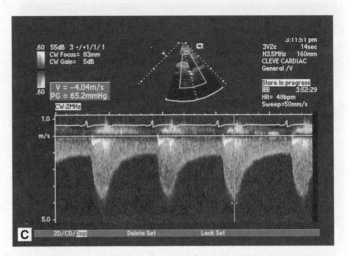

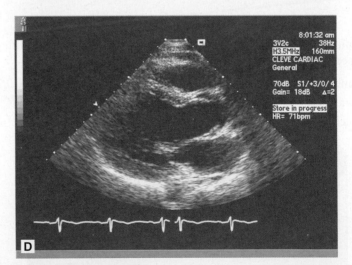

Figure 14.9 (*Continued*)

  d. pulmonic stenosis (PS)/pulmonic insufficiency.

  e. PDA.

14. A 46-year-old woman with dyspnea on exertion with occasional palpitations has the following surface echo images (Fig. 14.14A–D). Her dyspnea on exertion can be explained by

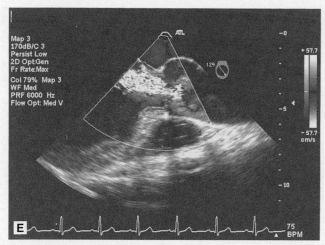

Figure 14.9 • **A.** Suprasternal notch view in 2D (TTE). **B.** Suprasternal notch with color Doppler. **C.** Continuous-wave Doppler in the descending aorta from the suprasternal notch. **D.** Parasternal long-axis view in systole. **E.** Parasternal long-axis view with color Doppler.

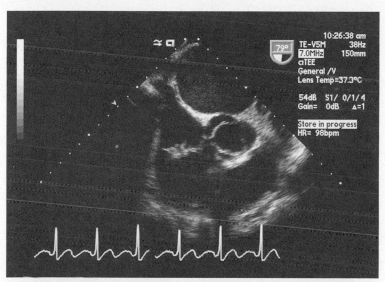

Figure 14.10 • Mid-esophageal short-axis view of the aortic valve (TEE).

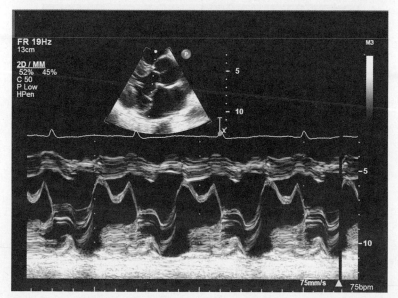

Figure 14.11 • M-mode through the mitral valve.

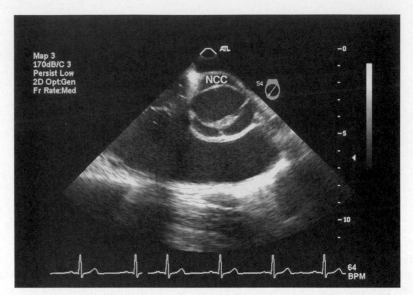

Figure 14.12 • Mid-esophageal short-axis view of the aortic valve (systole).

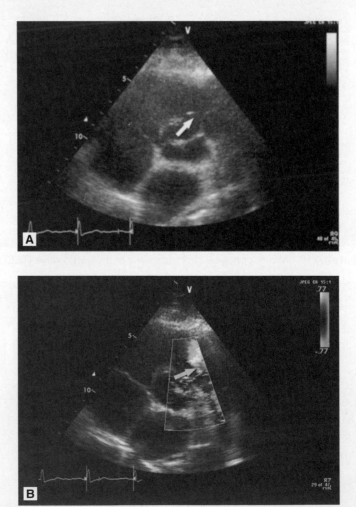

Figure 14.13 • **A.** Parasternal short-axis view. **B.** Parasternal short-axis view with color Doppler.

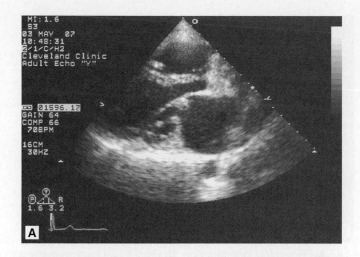

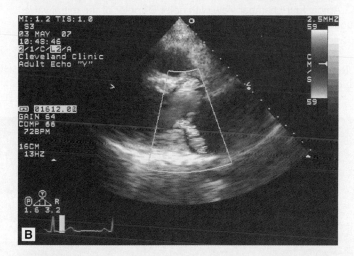

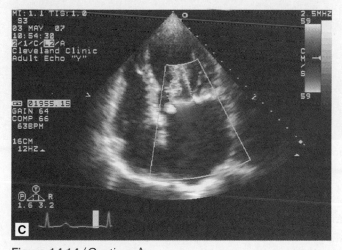

Figure 14.14 (*Continued*)

a. myxomatous MV disease with MR.

b. rheumatic MV disease with MS and MR.

c. endocarditis with vegetation causing MR.

d. severe mitral annular calcification.

e. cleft mitral leaflet.

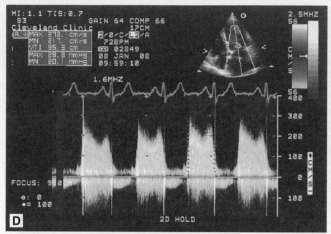

Figure 14.14 • A. Parasternal long-axis view. **B.** Parasternal long-axis view with color Doppler. **C.** Apical four-chamber view with color Doppler of the mitral valve. **D.** Continuous-wave Doppler through the mitral valve.

15. This parasternal short-axis view (Fig. 14.15) would be most consistent with which of the following patients?

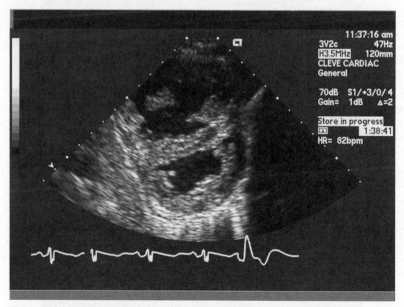

Figure 14.15 • Parasternal short-axis view (diastole).

   a. Patient with severe MR

   b. Patient with severe AI

   c. Patient with severe tricuspid regurgitation (TR)

   d. Patient with severe LV systolic dysfunction

   e. Patient with a subaortic membrane

16. The TEE images below are from a patient who has marked dyspnea on exertion and one episode of presyncope (Fig. 14.16A–C). The patient is now in the operating room for a procedure. The most appropriate operation for this patient would be

   a. MV repair.

   b. septal myectomy.

   c. MVR.

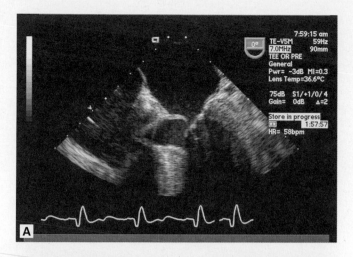

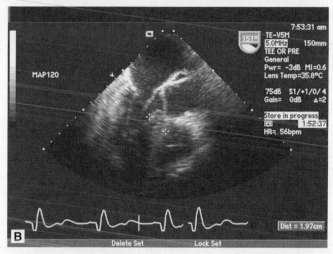

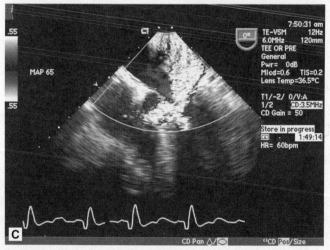

Figure 14.16 • A. Mid-esophageal four-chamber view (TEE). **B.** Mid-esophageal long-axis view (TEE). **C.** Mid-esophageal four-chamber view with color Doppler.

d. coronary artery bypass grafting (CABG).

e. ascending aortic conduit.

17. The following TEE images (Fig. 14.17A and B) demonstrate a large mass noted in the LV apex. This mass is located in a region of myocardial thinning and akinesis in a dilated LV. Although there is some mobility there does not appear to be a stalk. This mass is most likely which of the following possibilities?

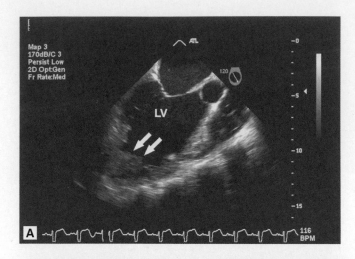

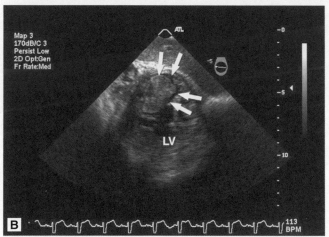

Figure 14.17 • A. Mid-esophageal long-axis view (TEE). **B.** Transgastric short-axis view of the LV (TEE).

a. Teratoma

b. Myosarcoma

c. Fibroelastoma

d. Thrombus

e. Adenocarcinoma

18. The patient is a 56-year-old man with hypertension, diabetes, and obesity who was admitted 6 months ago to an outside hospital with a late presentation of an anterior MI. He presented approximately 3 days post MI and underwent cardiac catheterization at 1 week, which showed a total occlusion in the mid-left anterior descending artery (LAD), severe stenoses of the first and second diagonals, and no significant disease in either the right coronary artery (RCA) or left circumflex artery (LCx). The patient was then referred to your hospital for revascularization. The patient, however, failed to show for his appointment and finally presented 8 months later with CP and SOB. Prior to revascularization you order a positron emission tomography (PET) rubidium (Rb)/fluorodeoxyglucose (FDG) using Rubidium^{82}/F18$_A$ (flourine-18–labeled deoxyglucose) to determine the degree of inducible ischemia and viability. The images obtained are in Figure 14.18. The images from the PET scan demonstrate

a. scar in the LAD territory.

b. inducible ischemia in the LAD territory.

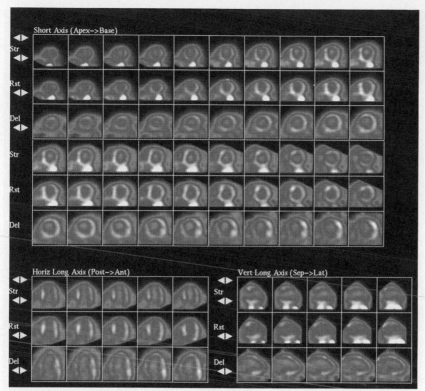

Figure 14.18 • Rubidium/FDG PET scan with the stress images displayed on top, the rest images next, and the delayed metabolic FDG images displayed on the bottom.

   c. hibernating myocardium in the LAD territory.

   d. a combination of inducible ischemia and hibernation in the LAD territory.

   e. scar in the RCA territory.

19. The patient is a 75-year-old man with hypertension, diabetes, hypercholesterolemia, and coronary artery disease (CAD) who is 10 years s/p CABG: left internal mammary artery to LAD, saphenous vein graft (SVG) to RCA, and SVG to first obtuse marginal. He is asymptomatic on a good medical regimen, although he is relatively sedentary. TTE demonstrated normal LV systolic function with left ventricular ejection fraction (LVEF) 60%, moderately severe left ventricular hypertrophy (LVH), and no significant valvular disease. The patient is now sent for cardiac evaluation prior to surgery on his dilated abdominal aorta (7.5 cm in diameter). An adenosine nuclear stress test is ordered for preoperative risk assessment. During the adenosine stress he remained asymptomatic although he developed 2-mm ST depressions in I, L, and V_2–V_6. There were no significant changes in blood pressure. Figure 14.19 shows the scan. The scan demonstrates

   a. marked attenuation.

   b. multivessel ischemia.

   c. infarct but no ischemia.

   d. mixture of infarct and ischemia.

   e. motion artifact.

20. The patient is a 62-year-old man with CAD risk factors including diabetes (16 years), hypertension, family history of CAD, and obesity. The patient had a silent inferior MI 2 years earlier detected by ECG. The patient is now sent for preoperative evaluation for bilateral knee surgery. The patient has no CP with exertion; however, his exercise capacity is limited by knee pain. He does

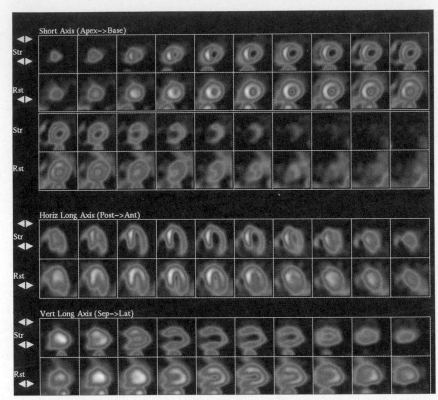

Figure 14.19 • Adenosine technetium-99m nuclear stress test with the stress images on top and the resting images below.

occasionally have mild post-prandial dyspnea. His medications include insulin, a statin, an angiotensin-converting enzyme inhibitor, a β-blocker, and an aspirin. A pharmacologic dual-isotope (Thal/Tc) scan was performed and is shown in Figure 14.20. The gated images showed an LVEF of 42% with a wall motion abnormality in the inferolateral wall. There were no ECG changes or symptoms during the adenosine infusion. The rest and post-stress images demonstrate

a. scarred RCA/LCx territory.

b. scarred LAD territory.

c. normal test with artifacts.

d. scar and ischemia in the LCx/RCA territory.

e. scar and ischemia in the LAD territory.

21. The patient is a 60-year-old man with hypertension, diabetes (newly diagnosed), and CAD (s/p percutaneous coronary intervention with drug-eluting stent in his mid-LAD 5 years ago, and bare metal stent to distal RCA, and a posteroventricular branch 7 years ago). The patient is now sent for symptom evaluation. The patient notes the onset of CPs with exertion while playing squash approximately 2 months ago. The pain occurs only with activity and resolves within a few minutes with rest. He denies other associated symptoms or discomfort at rest. A treadmill nuclear stress test was performed. The patient exercised using a standard Bruce protocol having completed eight metabolic equivalents and reached 98% maximum predicted heart rate (MPHR). There was a normal ST-segment response to stress, and there was no CP with exercise. He did, however, develop new ST depressions in recovery and new atrial fibrillation in recovery, requiring treatment with β-blockers. The scan images are shown in Figure 14.21. The appropriate interpretation of this scan is

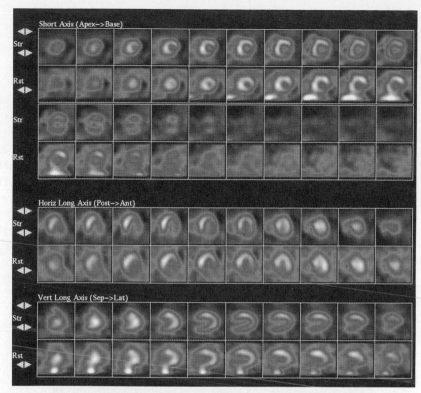

Figure 14.20 • A pharmacologic (adenosine) dual-isotope (Thal/Tc) scan with the stress images displayed on top with the resting images below.

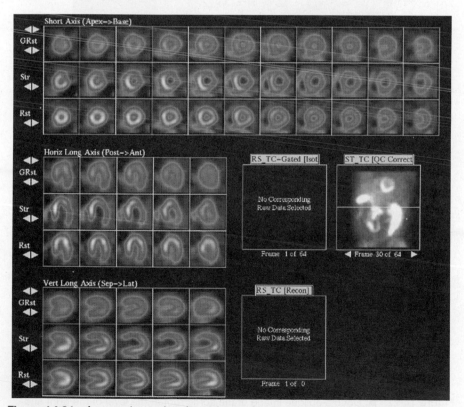

Figure 14.21 • An exercise technetium-99m nuclear stress test with the stress images with the gated images (currently still) on top, the post-stress images next, and the resting images on the bottom.

a. RCA territory infarct.

b. LAD territory infarct.

c. RCA territory ischemia.

d. LAD infarct with peri-infarct ischemia.

e. LAD and LCx versus left main ischemia.

22. A 19-year-old young woman is referred to your office for evaluation of congestive heart failure (CHF) and MR. She has a history of complete heart block and has previously undergone pacemaker implantation. On physical examination, her heart rate is 85 bpm, respiratory rate of 16, and blood pressure 108/65 mmHg. Her jugular venous pulse is visible 6 cm above the sternal angle at 45 degrees. The point of maximum impulse is sustained but normal in location. She has a grade II/VI holosystolic murmur at the apex that radiates to the axilla. There is trivial bilateral pedal edema. A posterior–anterior and lateral chest X-ray demonstrates mild cardiomegaly. A TTE reveals moderately reduced LV systolic function with an EF of 35%. There is 2+ to 3+ posteriorly directed MR. A cardiac CT with contrast is obtained to evaluate the coronary arteries (Fig. 14.22A and B). Which of the following is *true* regarding this patient's condition?

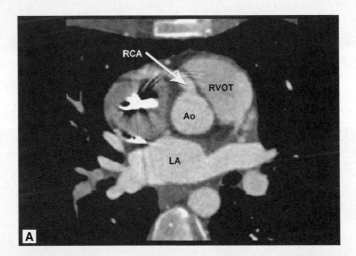

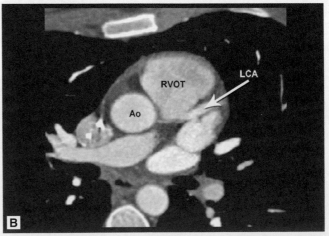

Figure 14.22 • A. Double-oblique image of the aortic root at the level of the right and left sinuses of Valsalva. Ao, aorta; LA, left atrium; RCA, right coronary artery; RVOT, right ventricular outflow tract. **B.** Oblique axial image at the level of the left coronary artery origin. LCA, left coronary artery.

a. This condition is a common cause of sudden cardiac death in athletes.

b. The anomaly shown represents origin of the left coronary artery from the right coronary ostium.

c. Surgical reimplantation of the anomalous coronary artery is indicated.

d. Patients with this condition who survive past childhood often present with varying degrees of heart failure, myocardial ischemia, and MR, depending on the development of collateral circulation.

e. This condition is usually inoperable and best left alone.

ANSWERS

● ● ●

1. **d.** Abnormal mechanical MVR. Figure 14.1 is a 3D echo image showing a malfunctioning bileaflet mechanical MVR. This image demonstrates one leaflet that is open (to the right of the image), while the other remains shut. You can see the sewing ring of the prosthesis well. This is most likely due to thrombus although impingement by a chord or piece of valve could do this as well.

2. **b.** Percutaneous mitral valvuloplasty (PMV) because he has a split score of 4 to 8 and minimal MR. The MV "split score" as it pertains to " splittability" of a rheumatic MV with MS is derived by grading four features of the stenotic valve. The features, which are graded on a scale of 1 to 4, include leaflet thickening, leaflet calcification, leaflet mobility, and involvement of the subvalvular apparatus. Grade 1 denotes the least abnormality while 4 denotes the most severe abnormality. Because each feature is graded on a scale of 1 to 4, the total score can range from 4 (more splittable) to 16 (least splittable). A valve with a score of ≤8 is considered amenable to PMV as long as there is no significant MR. Of note, the degree of MR typically increases by 1 grade when a patient undergoes balloon mitral valvuloplasty. A score of >8 denotes a valve that would not be amenable to PMV and if the patient is symptomatic or has significant pulmonary hypertension or other indication for an intervention (other than maximizing medical therapy), the patient would undergo a surgical valve replacement as long as they were considered a surgical candidate. The images presented for this example show a patient with severe MS due to rheumatic disease with minimal leaflet thickening or calcification, and no subvalvular involvement with preserved mobility. The stenosis is due almost entirely to commissural fusion and as such has a split score of 4. In addition, the color Doppler still frame in systole showed only trivial MR. For these reasons, the patient is an ideal candidate for PMV. The images in Figure 14.23A and B were taken following the balloon inflations during the PMV.

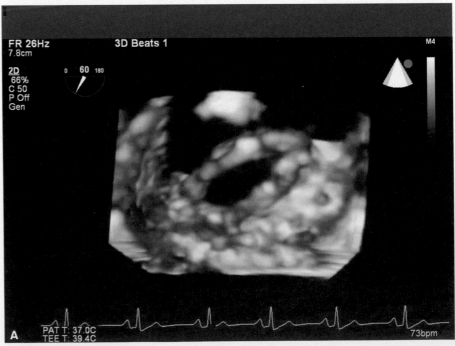

Figure 14.23 (*Continued*)

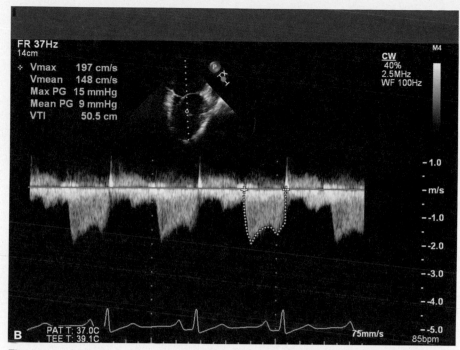

FR 37Hz
14cm

÷ Vmax   197 cm/s
  Vmean   148 cm/s
  Max PG 15 mmHg
  Mean PG 9 mmHg
  VTI   50.5 cm

CW
40%
2.5MHz
WF 100Hz

M4

- 1.0
- m/s
- -1.0
- -2.0
- -3.0
- -4.0
- -5.0

B   PAT T: 37.0C
     TEE T: 39.1C   75mm/s   85bpm

Figure 14.23 • A. Three-dimensional images of the mitral valve showing a larger orifice and the split commissures compared with the pre-PMV image. **B.** The transmitral gradient post balloon inflation. The mean mitral gradient has decreased from 30 to 9 mmHg.

3. **c.** Right atrial (RA) thrombus or thrombus on central venous catheter. The patient discussed in this question has a malignancy and is likely in a hypercoagulable state. The mass noted within the RA appears to be broad based and may be in association with her central venous catheter. In this situation, this is most likely to be an RA thrombus. The prosthetic appearing structure within the RA appears to be the central venous catheter and does not go through the tricuspid valve (TV) into the RV, and therefore is not an ICD. An RA myxoma typically has a thin stalk and is most often associated with the interatrial septum. It can be seen within the RA or left atrium (LA). Figure 14.24A and B demonstrates a classic myxoma, one showing surgical pathology and the other showing an echo image of a myxoma. A Chiari network is a more fenestrated mobile structure seen at the junction of the vena cava and RA.

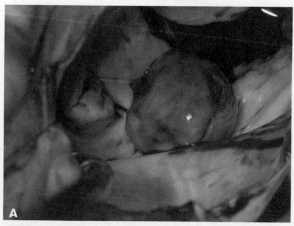

Figure 14.24 (*Continued*)

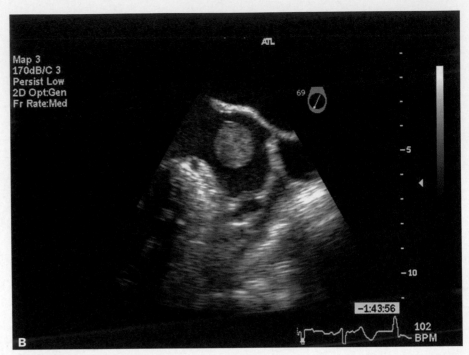

Figure 14.24

4. **a.** Moderate risk of endocarditis. The images in Figure 14.4 demonstrate a PDA. This is seen as the color flow into the pulmonary artery (PA). In this example, the PDA is large and its orifice can be seen in the two-dimensional (2D) images opening into the PA. The complications that can be associated with a PDA include the development of CHF and a moderate risk of endocarditis (although antibiotic prophylaxis is not recommended unless the unrepaired PDA is complicated by pulmonary hypertension/Eisenmenger syndrome causing cyanosis). The clinical manifestations of the PDA depend on the size of the left-to-right shunt. The larger the shunt, the worse the clinical manifestations. The murmur associated with a PDA is a continuous murmur (since the left-sided pressures are higher than the right side throughout the cardiac cycle), not a systolic murmur.

5. **d.** Aortic insufficiency (AI). Although all of the answers are possible complications of infective endocarditis, the images displayed in Figure 14.5 do not show any significant AI. Figure 14.5A shows the short axis of a bioprosthetic AV with a paravalvular abscess with vegetations. It also shows the valve during systole which although it is open, the opening is restricted suggestive of AS which is confirmed by the peak AV gradient of 92.6 mmHg shown in Figure 14.5B. Figure 14.5C shows the long-axis TEE view of the AV with a small fistula into the LA (seen at the top of the image).

6. **d.** Pulmonary embolus. The images in Figure 14.6 show the parasternal short axis showing specifically the main PA/PA bifurcation. Both images show a large multilobulated echodensity or mass within the main PA which represents a clot in transit. The patient is hypercoagulable due to her malignancy and has developed a deep venous thrombosis which has embolized and is on its way to the lungs. The multilobular appearance shows that this mass is a cast from a deep vein in the leg. The remaining answers are causes of CP; however, these answers do not describe the situation found on TTE. Patients with malignancy can present with tamponade from a pericardial effusion but no effusion is seen on these images.

7. e. Emergent cardiac surgery. The images demonstrate a patient with cardiac tamponade. Findings include significant respiratory variation of MV inflows (>25%) and RV diastolic collapse, RA inversion, and inferior vena cava plethora (dilated >2 cm and does not collapse normally with inspiration). A patient with a type I dissection and cardiac tamponade needs to go to emergent cardiac surgery as soon as possible for drainage of the pericardium and repair of the aorta. Pericardiocentesis could potentially cause complete rupture of the flap into the pericardium, causing cardiac arrest and death. An aortic stent graft is currently not the treatment of choice for a type I dissection and could certainly not address the problem of tamponade. Coronary angiography in this patient would only delay the definitive therapy (surgery) as well as possibly further propagate the dissection flap. Recall that delay of surgery in a patient with a type I dissection is associated with a 1% per hour increase in mortality in the first 48 hours of the process. (Note that this patient has not had prior cardiac surgery—if the person had prior cardiac surgery, that would likely change the need for cardiac catheterization prior to surgery, although in this patient emergent surgical drainage of the pericardium would be needed.)

8. b. Cleft MV. The image displays an apical four-chamber view of a patient with a primum ASD. (Note Fig. 14.8B with color Doppler shows left-to-right shunting through the ASD.) This is part of either a partial or complete AV canal defect. A complete AV canal defect includes a primum ASD, a cleft anterior mitral leaflet, and a widened anteroseptal tricuspid commissure. A partial AV canal defect is as above but without the VSD. Note that because of the long-term, significant right-to-left shunt through the ASD in this patient the right side is dilated and there is right ventricular hypertrophy from pulmonary hypertension. The short-axis view of the MV (Fig. 14.25A) demonstrates the cleft anterior mitral leaflet, which "splits" in the center, as opposed to opening like a fish mouth as is seen with normal MVs. Figure 14.25B is a drawing showing normal short axis of MV versus cleft MV.

9. d. Coarctation of the aorta with bicuspid AV with AI. The patient is a young man with hypertension beginning in his late 20s or early 30s. Secondary hypertension must be considered and ruled out in this patient. When he was initially diagnosed he should have had his blood pressure checked in both arms and legs in consideration of a coarctation of the aorta. Note: Someone may also notice rib notching on a chest X-ray. Other etiologies that should have been excluded include renal artery stenosis (more commonly seen in women if caused by fibromuscular dysplasia), pheochromocytoma, Cushing syndrome, or primary aldosteronism. This patient's heart murmur was a diastolic murmur from AI caused by prolapse

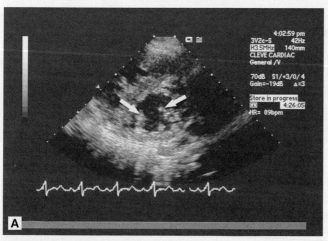

Figure 14.25 (*Continued*)

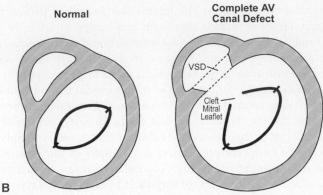

Normal | Complete AV Canal Defect

B

Figure 14.25 • A. Parasternal short-axis view of the mitral valve (TTE). **B.** Drawing comparing the parasternal short-axis view of a normal mitral valve to the opening of a cleft anterior mitral leaflet.

of a bicuspid AV. At least 50% of patients with a coarctation have a bicuspid AV. Fewer patients with bicuspid AV have a coarctation. Note that bicuspid AVs dome (doming aortic leaflets are seen in Fig. 14.9D) and could be mistaken on initial glance in long axis with a rheumatic AV. However, in addition to doming there is prolapse of the conjoined cusp (which would not be seen in a rheumatic valve) and the anatomic situation could be clarified with a good short-axis view.

10. e. Intravenous (IV) drug abuser. Right-sided endocarditis is less common than left-sided endocarditis. The TEE image (Fig. 14.26) shown demonstrates a patient with a vegetation on the tricuspid valve, and the organism identified by culture is *Pseudomonas*. This is associated with IV drug use with contamination at the time of injection. Although the other clinical situations listed are at increased risk for endocarditis (typically left sided), *Pseudomonas* would be a very unusual pathogen in those situations.

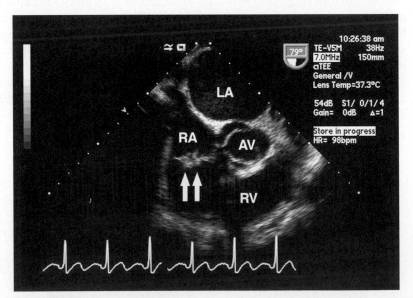

Figure 14.26

11. b. MVP. The M-mode trace is performed through the MV in a patient with myxomatous MV disease with bileaflet prolapse. Note the marked dip backward of the MV leaflets after the closure point (see Fig. 14.11). Note that there is full systolic range of motion creating the "M" trace of the anterior mitral leaflet and the normal "W" trace of the posterior leaflet. This is in contrast with a normal MV M-mode, which would not have the systolic dip (Fig. 14.27A). Thus, there is no rheumatic MS, which would look like Figure 14.27B in which there are still pliable but tethered leaflets causing a loss of the normal "M" and "W" appearance of the mitral leaflets. More advanced MS with thickened and calcified leaflets would have thicker and brighter appearance of the leaflets together with more restriction of the leaflet motion (Fig. 14.27C). M-mode for a patient with HOCM and SAM would appear like the images in Figure 14.27D and E. Note the SAM of the

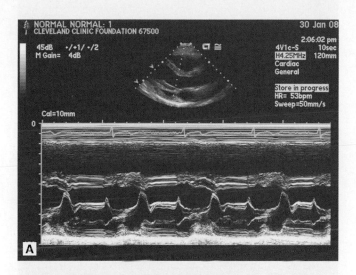

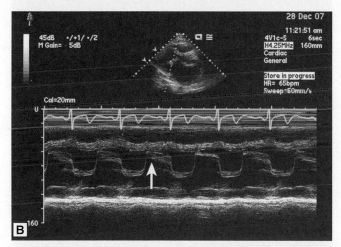

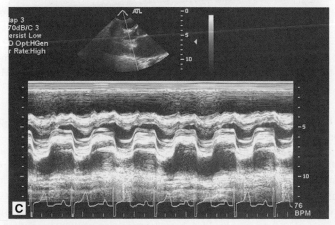

Figure 14.27 (*Continued*)

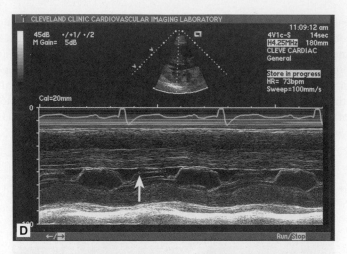

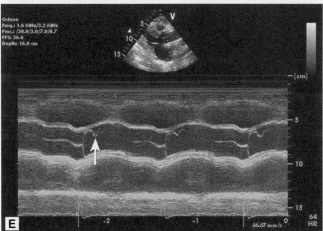

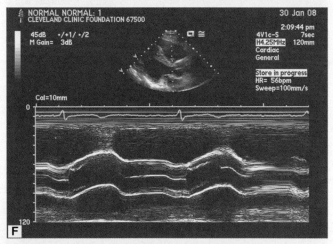

Figure 14.27 • A. M-mode through the mitral valve. **B.** M-mode through the mitral valve. **C.** M-mode through the mitral valve. **D.** M-mode through the mitral valve. **E.** M-mode through the aortic valve. **F.** M-mode through the aortic valve.

mitral leaflets in Figure 14.27D and the early closure of the AV in Figure 14.27E (compared with the M-mode of a normal AV [Fig. 14.27F]).

12. **c.** Bicuspid AV with fusion of the RCC and LCC. The 2D TEE mid-esophageal view (see Fig. 14.12) demonstrates a bicuspid AV in short axis. To determine cusp anatomy one must view the AV in systole. If one looks for a "Mercedes Benz" image of the valve in short axis during diastole (Fig. 14.28A), one may mistake a bicuspid valve for a tricuspid valve, not realizing that one of the arms in the

Mercedes Benz sign is actually a calcified raphe between two fixed cusps. Thus, it is important to look at the valve in systole to determine the true cusp anatomy. The most common form of bicuspid AV is fusion of the RCC and LCC. Bicuspid AVs are also associated with a dilated aorta with an aortopathy involving cystic medial necrosis. Another form of bicuspid AV is fusion of the RCC and NCC (Fig. 14.28B). There are other congenitally abnormal AVs, including unicuspid valves (Fig. 14.28C) and quadricuspid valves (Fig. 14.28D). The unicuspid and quadricuspid valves are much less common than bicuspid valves.

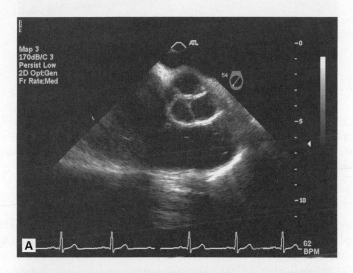

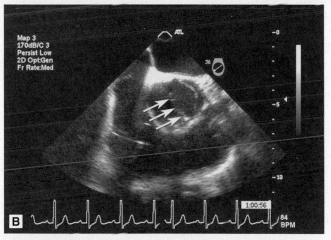

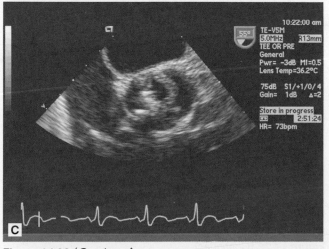

Figure 14.28 (*Continued*)

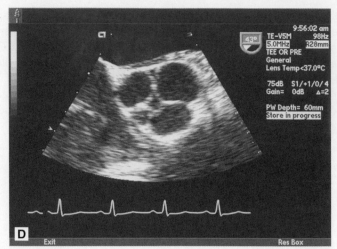

Figure 14.28 • **A.** Mid-esophageal short-axis view of the aortic valve (diastole). **B.** Mid-esophageal short-axis view of a bicuspid aortic valve with fusion of the RCC and NCC. **C.** Mid-esophageal short-axis view of a unicuspid aortic valve. **D.** Mid-esophageal short-axis view of a quadricuspid aortic valve.

13. **b.** Supracristal VSD. This image demonstrates a supracristal VSD. The VSD is located just under the pulmonic valve, best seen in the parasternal short-axis view (seen at 1 o'clock). A membranous VSD would be seen at 10 or 11 o'clock in short-axis view (Fig. 14.29A). Ebstein anomaly involves apical displacement of the tricuspid valve with atrialization of some of the RV (Fig. 14.29B). Patent ductus can also be seen in the parasternal short-axis view seen best by color Doppler showing a flow entering the PA (from the aorta) (Fig. 14.29C). PS is seen on 2D in the parasternal short-axis view with doming pulmonic valve leaflets with color acceleration across the valve. In diastole there may also be some PI as the leaflets may have restricted closing.

14. **b.** Rheumatic MV disease with MS and MR. The images shown demonstrate a doming anterior mitral leaflet and a fixed posterior leaflet. There is color acceleration across the MV, suggestive of MS, which is supported by the high gradients found by continuous-wave Doppler through the MV. There is also significant MR (posteriorly directed) seen in the systolic frame with color Doppler. The mechanism of MR in this case is restricted leaflet motion. Myxomatous MV disease (Fig. 14.30), in contrast, is characterized by markedly redundant, prolapsing

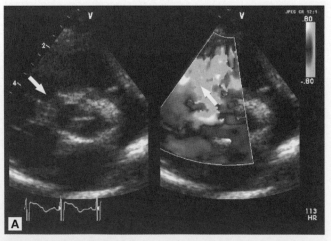

Figure 14.29 (*Continued*)

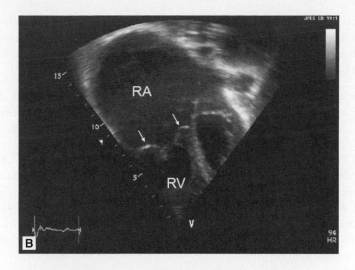

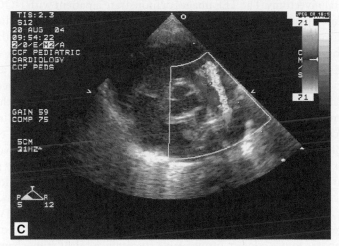

Figure 14.29 • **A.** Parasternal short-axis view (both 2D and with color Doppler). **B.** Apical four-chamber view (pediatric display with atria at the top of the screen). **C.** Parasternal short-axis view.

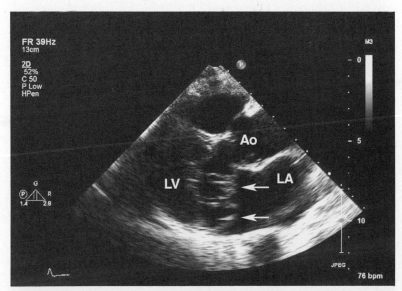

Figure 14.30 • Parasternal long-axis view of a patient with mitral valve prolapse.

leaflets, which prolapse back into the LA, occasionally with a torn chord causing a flail leaflet. Typically, the jet of MR is very eccentric if only one leaflet is involved (the jet is in the opposite direction from the most involved leaflet). If there is balanced bileaflet prolapse, the jet is usually centrally directed.

15. **c.** Patient with severe tricuspid regurgitation (TR). The parasternal short-axis still frame in diastole demonstrates a patient with diastolic septal flattening. This is found in a patient with right-sided *volume* overload. You can also see patients with systolic septal flattening, which is consistent with right-sided pressure overload. The patient with severe TR has right-sided volume overload and would have diastolic septal flattening as shown. Patients often have both diastolic and systolic septal flattening if they have both volume and pressure overload on the right side, for example, in a patient with chronic pulmonary embolisms who has developed pulmonary hypertension and also developed significant TR. The lesions of MR and AI are volume loads for the LV, and the subaortic membrane is a pressure load on the LV.

16. **b.** Septal myectomy. The TEE images demonstrate a patient with HOCM. There is septal hypertrophy and the systolic frame demonstrates SAM, which is SAM of the mitral leaflets (Fig. 14.31). The color Doppler images for this patient demonstrate severe MR that is posteriorly directed, which is classic for MR caused by SAM of the mitral leaflets. SAM can involve either the anterior or posterior leaflet alone, or a patient may have bileaflet SAM. Typically, if the mitral leaflet has not been too damaged by years of contact with the septum, performing a septal myectomy can fix the severe MR by eliminating the left ventricular outflow tract (LVOT) obstruction and eliminating the SAM. This type of MR is often hemodynamically labile depending on the loading conditions of the LV. The SAM can be brought out or accentuated by giving the patient amyl nitrite or isuprel. The SAM is decreased by volume loading the ventricle or increasing the systemic pressure. If the mitral leaflets, however, have been scarred by years of contact with the septum, a simultaneous MV repair or replacement may need to be performed. If the MV has to be replaced, often the surgeon has to use a lower-profile valve (typically a bileaflet mechanical valve) because of the narrowed LVOT. Neither a CABG nor an ascending aortic conduit would help this patient unless he had concomitant CAD or an ascending aortic aneurysm, in which case these procedures would have to be performed in addition to the myectomy.

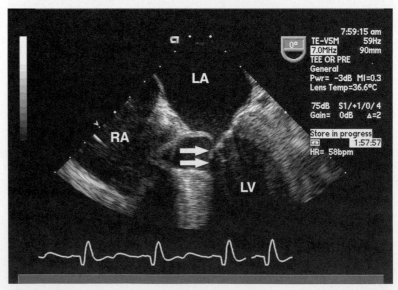

Figure 14.31

17. d. Thrombus. This patient had a very large anterior MI and has significant thinning and akinesis of the anterior wall and LV apex. Because of this significant wall motion abnormality, there is stasis of the blood and the patient is at risk for forming a thrombus, which this patient has done. The homogeneous nature of the mass with an echogenicity similar to that of the myocardium (or slightly less echogenic than the myocardium) suggests that the thrombus is relatively fresh. As this heals or organizes over time, calcium may be deposited, and old, organized thrombi in the heart are often quite echogenic. A sarcoma, on the other hand, would be an invasive mass and would not respect the boundaries of the myocardium, but rather would infiltrate the myocardium. Teratomas if found in the heart arise from the pericardium, not within the LV cavity. These are typically benign although may compress the heart. A teratoma would also have a more heterogeneous appearance on echo. Myxomas are the most common benign tumor of the heart and 80% of those are located in the LA, and most of the remaining ones are found in the RA. Papillary fibroelastomas are the second most common benign cardiac tumors and are typically pedunculated (with a stalk) and mobile. Most (>80%) are located on heart valves.

18. c. Hibernating myocardium in the LAD territory. There is a matched defect in the LAD territory seen on the resting and post-stress images involving the apex and four periapical segments as well as the mid-anterior and anteroapical segments. This is consistent with a large LAD territory infarct without any inducible ischemia. The metabolic FDG images show a perfusion/metabolism mismatch with FDG uptake seen in the previously mentioned LAD segments, suggesting a large region of hibernation in the LAD territory without any significant scar. (Note that there is significant gastrointestinal [GI] uptake near the inferior wall.) The degree of hibernation involved 40% of the myocardium (6% for each involved segment except for the apex, which represents 4% of the myocardium). A study by Hachamovitch et al.[1] in 2003 showed that revascularization was superior to medical therapy if the amount of myocardium at risk (ischemic and hibernating) exceeded 20%. Since the above patient demonstrated a large area of hibernating myocardium in the LAD territory, the patient would benefit from revascularization of the LAD territory as well as the diagonals. This patient underwent surgical revascularization of all three vessels.

19. b. Multivessel ischemia. The resting scan showed GI activity, but overall normal tracer uptake. There was increased septal uptake caused by the moderately severe LVH. Post stress there is severely reduced tracer uptake involving the mid- and apical anterior, entire anteroseptal, and inferolateral walls and inferior wall and apex. There was also cavity dilation post stress. This is known as transient ischemic dilation (TID). The gated images that accompanied this study demonstrated hypokinesis of the above segments. Note that the post-stress gated images are acquired post stress, but at rest. That is to say that there is a delay between stress and imaging, which may allow for some recovery of function. This scan is of high risk in that there is ischemia in all three vascular territories with TID and extensive wall motion abnormalities. Although the patient was asymptomatic under his baseline conditions, it was appropriate to order the adenosine nuclear stress test since the patient is diabetic with prior revascularization and with a questionable functional status who was going to undergo a high-risk surgical procedure (aortic aneurysm repair).

20. d. Scar and ischemia in the LCx/RCA territory. The full interpretation of the study was that there was marked GI activity in the rest images, but there was also a severe resting perfusion defect involving the basal and mid-inferolateral segments. Although GI activity can make the basal and mid-inferior segments difficult to interpret at rest, the post-stress images clearly show that the defect now involves the entire inferolateral and inferior walls, showing infarct with peri-infarct ischemia in the LCx/RCA territory. Cardiac catheterization demonstrated a total obstruction of the proximal LCx (a dominant LCx) with collaterals from the RCA and LAD. There were no obstructions in the RCA and LAD. Important points from this case include that diabetics are at high risk for CAD and clinical parameters do not predict ischemia (from the detection of ischemia in asymptomatic diabetes (DIAD) trial). Myocardial perfusion imaging can be performed safely post MI to assess infarct size and the amount of myocardium at risk. It is also a good test to assess the adequacy of collateral blood flow.

21. **e.** LAD and LCx versus left main ischemia. The resting images demonstrate normal perfusion. Post stress, however, there are significant perfusion defects in the anterior, anterolateral, and inferolateral walls. There is also cavity dilatation, which is consistent with either left main disease or multivessel ischemia. The gated images showed new wall motion abnormalities in the LAD and LCx territories. The presence of stress-induced perfusion defects in multiple vascular territories as well as TID and new wall motion abnormalities on the gated images are all findings associated with high-risk scans. The cardiac catheterization in this patient demonstrated 70% stenosis in the proximal LAD, while the stent in the mid-LAD was patent. There was a large obtuse marginal with a 90% proximal stenosis. There was mild disease in the proximal RCA, and the stents in posterior descending artery and posteroventricular branch were patent.

22. **d.** Patients with this condition who survive past childhood often present with varying degrees of heart failure, myocardial ischemia, and MR, depending on the development of collateral circulation. This CT demonstrates an anomalous origin of the left coronary artery from the pulmonary artery (ALCAPA). Also known as Bland-White-Garland syndrome, ALCAPA is a rare but serious congenital anomaly. It is caused by either (a) abnormal septation of the conotruncus into the aorta and PA or (b) persistence of the pulmonary buds together with involution of the aortic buds that eventually form the coronary arteries. Occurrence is similar between men and women and is not considered an inheritable congenital cardiac defect. Because of the low pulmonary vascular resistance, left coronary artery flow reverses and enters the pulmonic trunk (coronary steal phenomena). As a result, the LV myocardium remains underperfused, leading to infarction of the anterolateral LV wall. This often causes anterolateral papillary muscle dysfunction and variable degrees of mitral insufficiency. Consequently, the combination of LV dysfunction and significant MV insufficiency leads to CHF symptoms (e.g., tachypnea, poor feeding, irritability, and diaphoresis) in the young infant. Collateral circulation between the right and left coronary systems eventually develops. Approximately 85% of patients present with clinical symptoms of CHF within the first 1 to 2 months of life. Left untreated, the mortality rate in the first year of life is 90% secondary to myocardial ischemia or infarction and MV insufficiency leading to CHF. In unusual cases, the clinical presentation with symptoms of myocardial ischemia may be delayed into early childhood. Rarely, a patient may stabilize following infarction and may present with MV regurgitation, periodic dyspnea, angina pectoris, syncope, or sudden death later in childhood or even adulthood, as in this patient. Treatment consists of surgical ligation of the anomalous coronary artery origin and bypass grafting to the left coronary artery. Reimplantation onto the native aortic root is typically not possible because of the friable quality of the anomalous left coronary artery ostium.

REFERENCE

1. Hachamovitch R, Hayes SW, Friedman JD, et al. Comparison of the short-term survival benefit associated with revascularization compared with medical therapy in patients with no prior coronary artery disease undergoing stress myocardial perfusion single photon emission computed tomography. *Circulation*. 2003;107(23):2900–2907.

chapter 15

Electrocardiographic Interpretation

Donald A. Underwood

CODING SHEET ● ● ●

General Features

1. Normal electrocardiogram (ECG)

2. Borderline ECG or normal variant (specify in other section)

3. Incorrect electrode placement

P-Wave Abnormalities

4. Right atrial abnormality

5. Left atrial abnormality

6. Nonspecific atrial abnormality

7. Sinoventricular condition with absent P wave

Supraventricular Rhythms

8. Normal sinus rhythm (without other abnormalities of rhythm or atrioventricular (AV) conduction)

9. Sinus rhythm (in presence of abnormality of rhythm or AV conduction)

10. Sinus arrhythmia

11. Sinus bradycardia

12. Sinus tachycardia

13. Sinus pause or arrest

14. Sinoatrial exit block

15. Ectopic atrial or junctional rhythm

16. Wandering atrial pacemaker

17. Atrial premature beats, normally conducted

18. Atrial premature beats, nonconducted

19. Atrial premature beats with aberrant intraventricular conduction

20. Atrial tachycardia (regular, sustained, 1:1 conduction)

21. Atrial tachycardia, repetitive (short paroxysms)

22. Atrial tachycardia, multifocal (chaotic atrial tachycardia)

23. Atrial tachycardia with AV block

24. Atrial flutter

25. Atrial fibrillation

26. Retrograde atrial activation

27. Supraventricular tachycardia, unspecified

Atrioventricular Junctional Rhythms

28. AV junctional premature beats

29. AV junctional escape beats or escape rhythm

30. AV junctional rhythm, accelerated rhythm (nonparoxysmal junctional tachycardia)

31. AV junctional tachycardia

Ventricular Rhythms

32. Ventricular premature beat(s), uniform, fixed coupled

33. Ventricular premature beats, R on T phenomenon

34. Premature ventricular contractions, in pairs

35. Ventricular parasystole

36. Ventricular tachycardia

37. Accelerated idioventricular rhythm

38. Ventricular escape beats or rhythm

39. Ventricular fibrillation

Atrioventricular Conduction Abnormalities

(Also see items 48 to 53)

40. AV block, primary

41. AV block, secondary—Mobitz type I (Wenkenbach)

42. AV block secondary—Mobitz type II

43. AV block, 2;1, 3:1, 4:1

44. AV block, complete

45. AV block, varying

46. Short PR interval (with sinus rhythm and normal QRS duration)

47. Preexcitation (Wolff-Parkinson-White) syndrome(s)

Atrial Ventricular Interactions in Arrhythmias

(Also see items 40 to 47)

48. Fusion beats

49. Reciprocal (echo) beats

50. Ventricular capture beats

51. AV dissociation (without complete AV block)

52. Isorhythmic AV dissociation

53. Ventriculophasic sinus arrhythmia

Abnormalities of QRS Voltage or Axis

54. Low voltage, limb leads only

55. Low voltage, limb and precordial leads

56. Left axis deviation (>30 degrees)

57. Right axis deviation (>+100 degrees)

58. Electrical alternans

Ventricular Hypertrophy

59. Left ventricular hypertrophy by voltage only

60. Left ventricular hypertrophy by left ventricular hypertrophy by voltage and ST-T segment (secondary repolarization changes)

61. Right ventricular hypertrophy

62. Combined ventricular hypertrophy

Intraventricular Conduction Disturbances

63. Right bundle branch block (RBBB), incomplete

64. RBBB, complete

65. Left anterior fascicular block

66. Left posterior fascicular block

67. Left bundle branch block (LBBB), complete with ST-T waves suggestive of acute myocardial injury or infarction

68. LBBB, complete

69. Intraventricular conduction disturbance, nonspecific type

70. Aberrant intraventricular conduction with supraventricular arrhythmia (specify rhythm)

Transmural Myocardial Infarction

(Also see items 88 and 89)

	Age Recent or Probably Acute	Age Indeterminate or Probably Old
Anterolateral	71	72
Anterior	73	74
Anteroseptal	75	76
Lateral or high lateral	77	78
Inferior (diaphragmatic)	79	80
Posterior	81	82

83. Probable ventricular aneurysm

ST-, T-, and U-Wave Changes

84. Subendocardial or subepicardial nontransmural infarction

85. Normal variant, early repolarization

86. Normal variant, juvenile T wave

87. Nonspecific ST- and/or T-wave changes

88. ST- and/or T-wave changes suggesting myocardial ischemia

89. ST- and/or T-wave changes suggesting myocardial injury

90. ST- and/or T-wave changes suggesting acute pericarditis

91. ST-T segment changes secondary to intraventricular conduction distribution or hypertrophy

92. Post extrasystolic T waves

93. Isolated J-point depression

94. Peaked T waves

95. Prolonged QT interval

96. Prominent U waves

Suggested Probable Clinical Disorder

97. Digitalis effect

98. Digitalis toxicity

99. Hyperkalemia

100. Hypokalemia

101. Hypercalcemia

102. Hypocalcemia

103. Atrial septal defect, secundum

104. Atrial septal defect, primum

105. Dextrocardial, mirror image

106. Mitral valve disease

107. Chronic lung disease

108. Acute cor pulmonale including pulmonary embolus

109. Pericardial effusion

110. Acute pericarditis

111. Hypertrophic obstructive cardiomyopathy (idiopathic hypertrophic subaortic stenosis)

112. Hypertrophic obstructive cardiomyopathy; apical

113. Coronary artery disease

114. Central nervous system (CNS) disorder

115. Myxedema

116. Hypothermia

117. Sick sinus syndrome

118. Cardiac transplant

ECG INTERPRETATION AND CODING

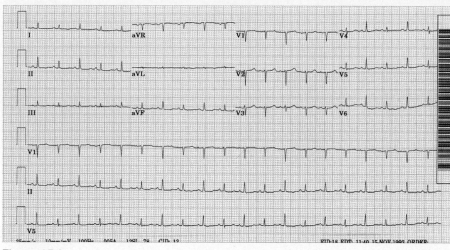

Figure 15.1

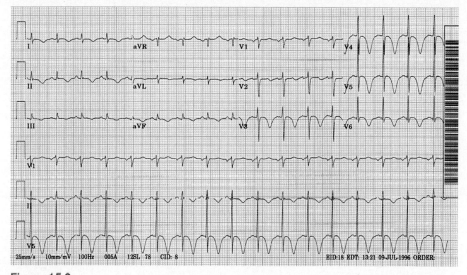

Figure 15.2

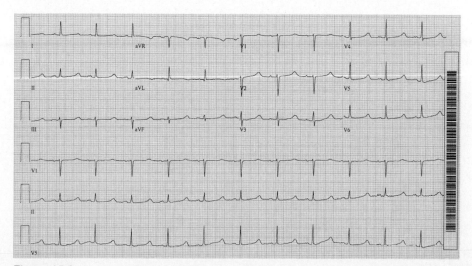

Figure 15.3

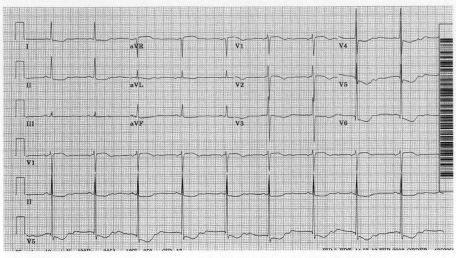

Figure 15.4

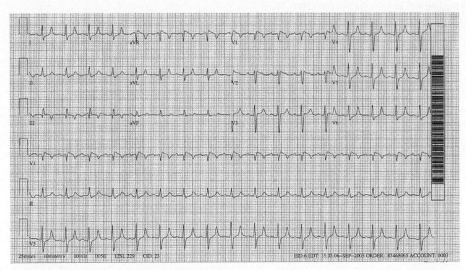

Figure 15.5

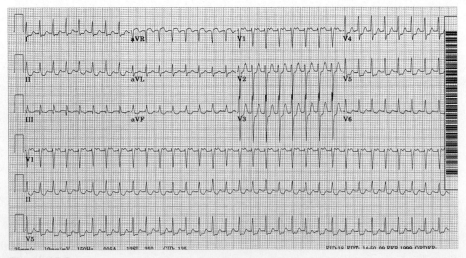

Figure 15.6

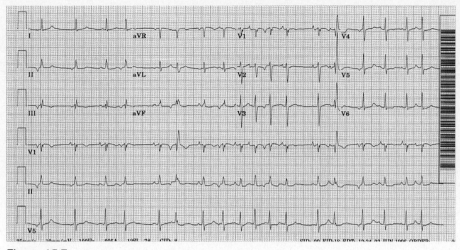

Figure 15.7

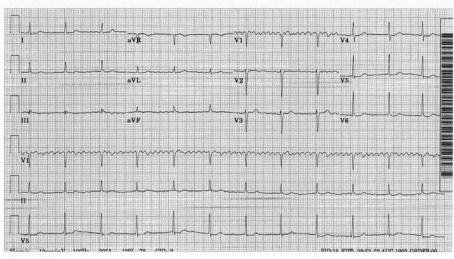

Figure 15.8

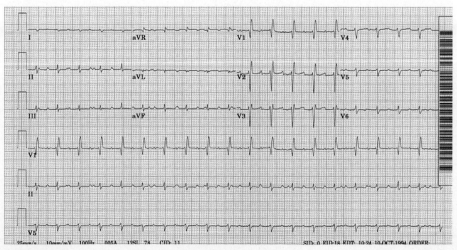

Figure 15.9

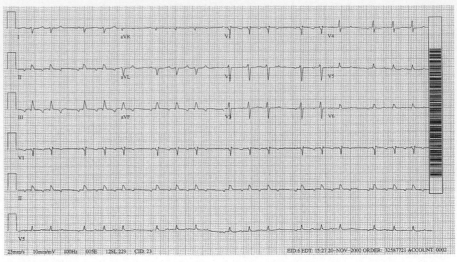

Figure 15.10

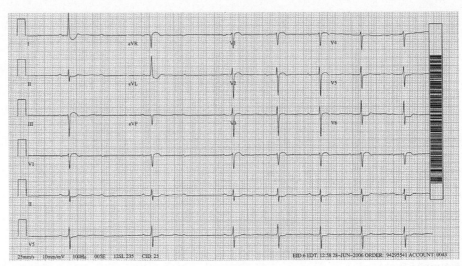

Figure 15.11

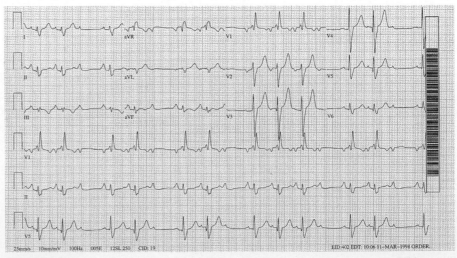

Figure 15.12

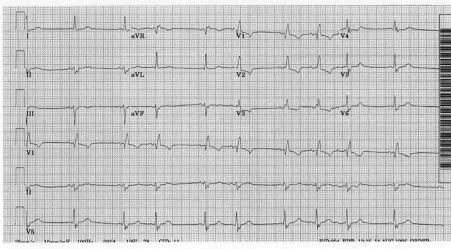

Figure 15.13

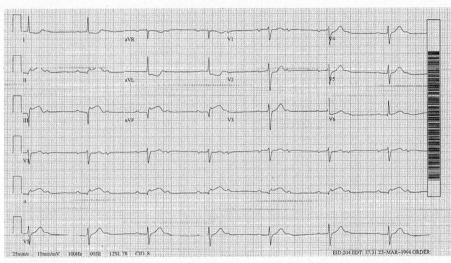

Figure 15.14

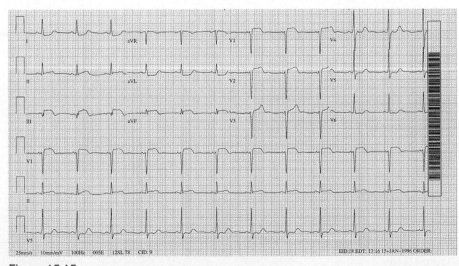

Figure 15.15

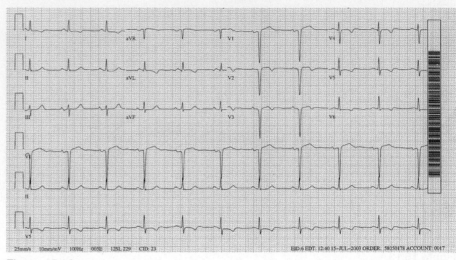

Figure 15.16

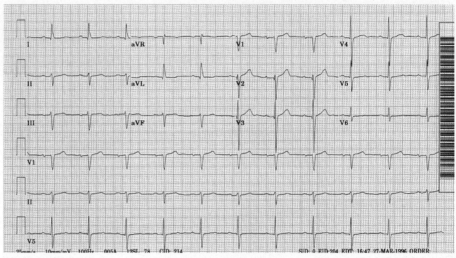

Figure 15.17

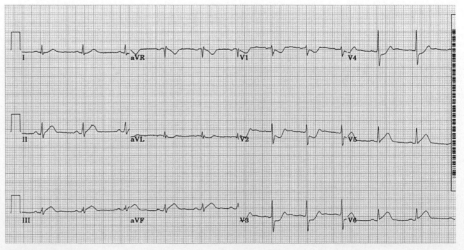

Figure 15.18

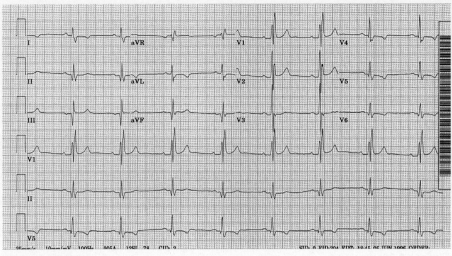

Figure 15.19

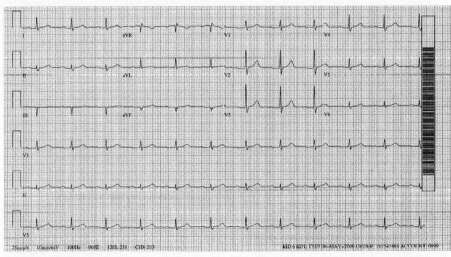

Figure 15.20

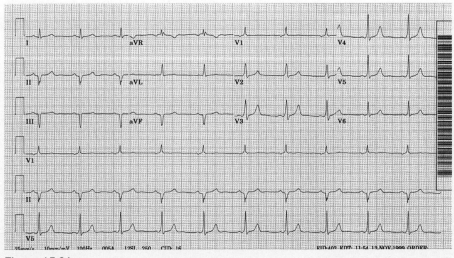

Figure 15.21

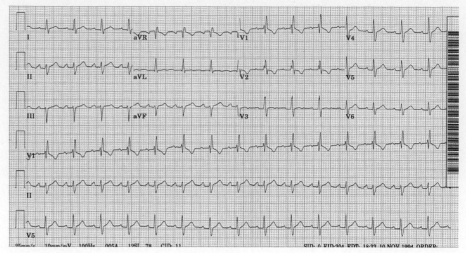

Figure 15.22

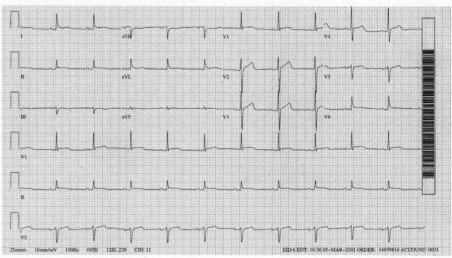

Figure 15.23

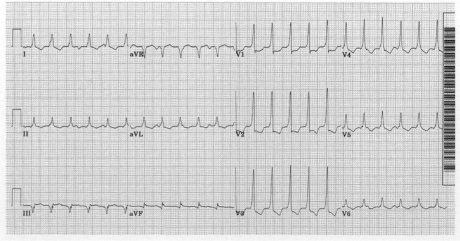

Figure 15.24

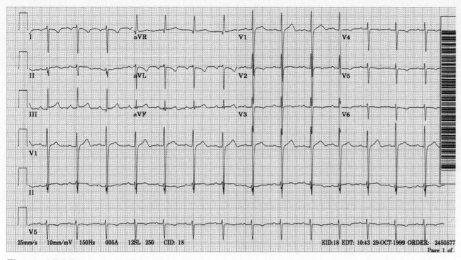

Figure 15.25

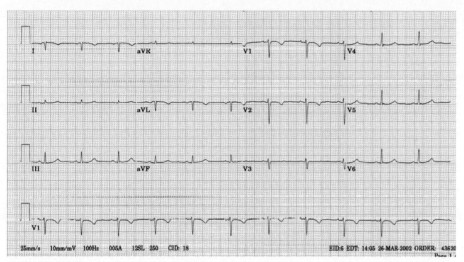

Figure 15.26

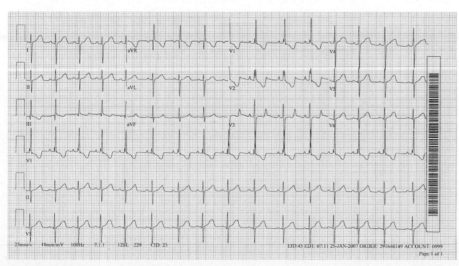

Figure 15.27

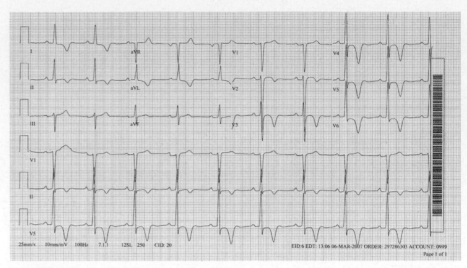

Figure 15.28

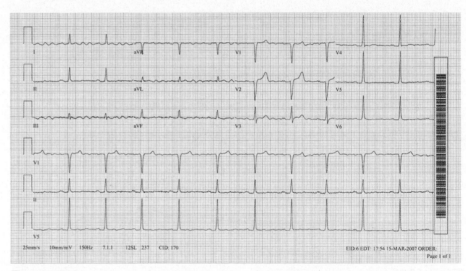

Figure 15.29

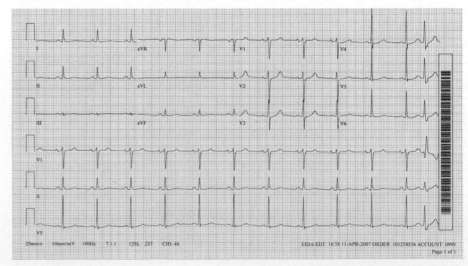

Figure 15.30

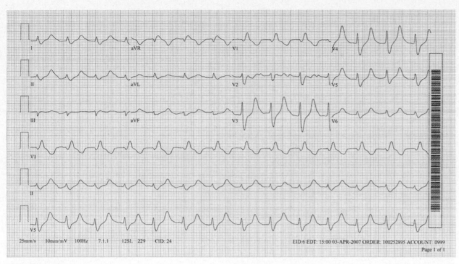

Figure 15.31

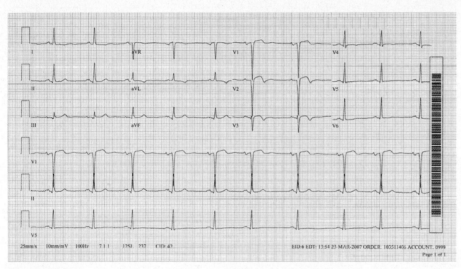

Figure 15.32

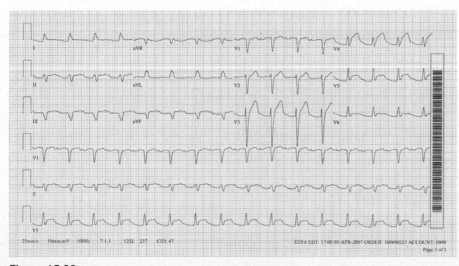

Figure 15.33

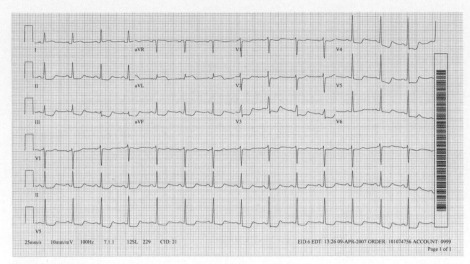

Figure 15.34

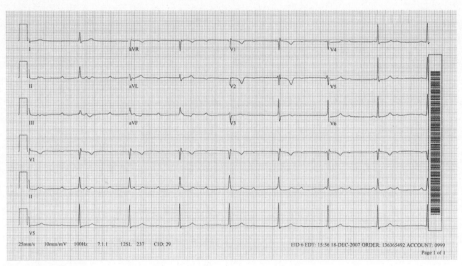

Figure 15.35

1. FIGURE 15.1: On this electrocardiogram, there is a sinus tachycardia. The voltage is low and in the V_1 and II rhythm strips, electrical alternans can be seen. This is an ECG from a patient with cardiac tamponade. Electrocardiographic coding is 12, 58, and 109.

2. FIGURE 15.2: This electrocardiogram shows a sinus tachycardia. There is a generalized T-wave inversion. The T waves are symmetric, deep, and have a long QT interval. This is an electrocardiogram from a patient with a major CNS event such as a subarachnoid or intraventricular hemorrhage. Electrocardiographic coding would be 12, 95, and 114.

3. FIGURE 15.3: This electrocardiogram shows a sinus rhythm. There is prolongation of the QT interval. The T wave has a fairly normal duration and contour, however. This is an example of hypocalcemia. (Type III congenital long QT syndrome also has this appearance.) Electrocardiographic coding would be 8, 95, and 102.

4. FIGURE 15.4: On this electrocardiogram, there is a sinus rhythm. It is sinus bradycardia. There is a prolongation of the QT interval. In this case, there is ST-segment depression, T-wave flattening, and TU fusion with prominent

U waves in the lateral precordial leads. This should suggest hypokalemia. Another possibility is digitalis plus an antiarrhythmic drug's effects (such as quinidine or procainamide). Electrocardiographic coding would be 11, 96, and 100.

5. Figure 15.5: This patient has a sinus tachycardia. There is symmetry of the T waves and there is a degree of QT prolongation. This is an example of a mixed electrolyte abnormality, hyperkalemia, and hypocalcemia. Values at the time were potassium of 7.2 and calcium of 80. This would be coded 12, 94, 95, 99, and 102.

6. FIGURE 15.6: On this electrocardiogram, there is a narrow complex tachycardia. The complexes are regular. In lead V_1, there is an atrial wave that has a short RP, long PR relationship. This is an example of supraventricular tachycardia or AV nodal reentrant tachycardia (AVNRT). If the atrial wave seen in V_1 extends to 70 or 80 milliseconds out into the ST segment, then this type of tracing could be an example of AV reentrant tachycardia (AVRT), which usually involves a larger reentrant loop and a bypass tract. Electrocardiographic coding is 27.

7. FIGURE 15.7: Here there is a narrow complex tachycardia. It is chaotically irregular and there are multiple P-wave vectors. This is not atrial fibrillation, which also is chaotic, but instead is a multifocal atrial tachycardia. This patient also shows aberrancy in the 6th and 14th beats. Electrocardiographic interpretation is 22, 87, 70, and 107.

8. FIGURE 15.8: This patient has a regular rhythm, but the baseline as seen in lead V_1 is chaotic. It is an example of atrial fibrillation with a regular ventricular response. This is actually an accelerated junctional rhythm most likely caused by digitalis excess. In lead V_6 there is ST-segment sagging that is smooth and associated with QT interval shortening. This suggests digitalis "effect." Digitalis effect is seen in the repolarization changes with ST-segment scooping. Digitalis "excess" is usually suggested by arrhythmias and in this case the accelerated junctional rhythm. The coding would be 25, 30, 97, and 98.

9. FIGURE 15.9: This patient shows an rSR' pattern in lead V_1 that might suggest a volume-overload right ventricular hypertrophy (RVH). That is supported in part by the right axis deviation. However, in looking at the rhythm strip in lead II, there is a basic sinus rhythm with a first-degree AV block and in addition there is a second atrial rhythm that is dissociated from the basic PQRS sequence. This is accessory atrial activity related to cardiac transplantation. This would be coded 9, 40, 57, 63, and 118.

10. FIGURE 15.10: On this electrocardiogram, there is a regular atrial activity, but the P waves are inverted in the inferior leads, suggesting an ectopic atrial tachycardia. This conducts with group beating and gradual PR prolongation. This is an example of atrial tachycardia with Mobitz type I AV block. This would be coded 23 and 41.

11. FIGURE 15.11: This electrocardiogram shows a sinus rhythm. There is a first-degree AV block and intermittent 2:1 block. In addition, there is ST-segment depression that is scooping in quality in the lateral leads. This is an example of digitalis excess with intermittent second-degree AV block and digitalis effect. It would be coded 11, 41 or 42, 97, and 98.

12. FIGURE 15.12: This patient has a right bundle branch block and left axis deviation. He also has pauses. In this case, the P waves are regular and the PR intervals do not change. This is an example of a Mobitz type II second-degree AV block.

The P-wave vectors are prominent in both leads II and V$_1$, suggesting left atrial enlargement. This would be coded 8, 42, 5, 56, and 64.

13. FIGURE 15.13: This patient has a right bundle branch block. There is also left axis deviation which probably is enough to qualify as an anterior hemiblock. There are occasional pauses. In this case, the pauses are preceded by P waves, which are within the preceding T waves, and so this is an example of blocked PACs and not an example of more advanced AV block associated with bifascicular block. This would be coded 11, 18, 56, 64, and 65.

14. FIGURE 15.14: This patient shows a sinus rhythm with a 2:1 AV block. This can either be a Mobitz type I or II AV block. It is impossible to tell which. This also shows ST-segment elevation with Q waves in the inferior leads with reciprocal changes in leads I and aVL and is an example of an acute inferior infarction with 2:1 AV block. This would be coded 8, 43, and 79.

15. FIGURE 15.15: This patient shows a sinus rhythm. There is ST elevation in the inferior leads, especially leads III and aVF. There are reciprocal depressions in leads I and aVL. In leads V$_1$ and V$_2$, there is also ST elevation. This is an acute inferior infarction plus acute right ventricular infarct. This would be coded 8 and 79. At least on this code sheet, the ability to call right ventricular infarction would not be available to you.

16. FIGURE 15.16: This electrocardiogram has a sinus rhythm. There are lateral T-wave changes that are not specific, and there are QS waves in leads V$_1$ through V$_3$. This is an anteroseptal infarction of uncertain age. It would be coded 8, 76, and 87.

17. FIGURE 15.17: Here, there is a normal sinus rhythm and marked left axis deviation. There are small Q waves in leads I and aVL with a slight activation delay in aVL. This is anterior hemiblock. Anterior hemiblock produces small Q waves in the right precordial leads. The QRS pattern seen in V$_2$ is often very suggestive of anteroseptal infarction, but the specificity is much less in the presence of anterior fascicular block. This would be coded 8 and 65.

18. FIGURE 15.18: In this patient, there are symmetric, prominent T waves that are upright. These are seen in the inferolateral leads and are associated with ST depression in leads V$_1$, V$_2$, and V$_3$. There are no Q waves so this is not an acute infarct, but it is an acute current of injury. The rhythm is sinus. Electrocardiographic coding would be 8 and 89.

19. FIGURE 15.19: On this electrocardiogram, there is a sinus rhythm. It is slow so sinus bradycardia. There are significant inferior Q waves and also Q waves in leads V$_5$ and V$_6$. There is also a prominent R-wave vector in lead V$_1$, and the T waves are upright despite the presence of a right bundle branch block. Usually with a right bundle branch block, ST-segment and T-wave inversion are expected. In this case, the upright T wave is an example of a "primary" T wave. A prominent initial vector and upright T wave in V$_1$, associated with inferior and lateral Q waves, are interpreted as an inferoposterior and lateral infarct. Electrocardiographic coding is 11, 80, 82, 78, and 64.

20. FIGURE 15.20: This electrocardiogram has a sinus rhythm. There is a prominent initial vector in lead V$_1$ that is greater than the S wave. T wave is upright. This is compatible with posterior infarct. That is supported by the presence of pathologic Q waves in leads III and aVF. Electrocardiographic coding would be 8, 80, and 82.

21. Figure 15.21: This electrocardiogram shows a sinus rhythm. There are inferior Q waves and prominent R vector in leads V_1 and V_2. This might suggest infero-posterior infarction, but in leads V_3 and V_4, especially there is a short PR interval and a delta wave suggesting that this is preexcitation or Wolff-Parkinson-White syndrome. Electrocardiographic coding would be 8 and 47.

22. FIGURE 15.22: This patient has a sinus rhythm. Lead II does suggest left atrial enlargement with a P wave that is broad and notched. There is an rSR′ pattern in lead V_1 with T-wave inversion and R′ greater than S. This type of pattern is commonly seen in volume-overload-type RVH. Volume-overload RVH and left axis should suggest ostium primum ASD. Usually an ASD will not affect P waves greatly, at least in the early phases of the process. Ostium primum ASDs, however, very often have mitral valve and notable mitral insufficiency plus left atrial enlargement. Electrocardiographic coding would be 8, 5, 63, 61, 56, and 104.

23. FIGURE 15.23: This electrocardiogram shows a sinus rhythm. There was a very prominent vector in lead V_1 associated with upright T waves. This drops down to a more typical appearance in lead V_2. This is not an example of posterior infarction but instead is an example of switched leads, V_1 and V_5 having been transposed. There is also ST-segment elevation throughout and perhaps some PR-segment elevation in aVR. This suggests acute pericarditis. Electrocardiographic coding would be 8, 3, and 90.

24. FIGURE 15.24: This patient has a wide complex tachycardia. There is AV dissociation and there is anterior, positive concordance in the chest leads. This is ventricular tachycardia. Electrocardiographic coding would be 9, 51, and 36.

25. FIGURE 15.25: This patient has marked right axis deviation and loss of voltage across the precordium. The P waves are inverted in leads I and aVL. Inverted P waves in leads I and aVL (if it is not an ectopic atrial rhythm) are caused by either dextrocardial or switched arm wires. Loss of voltage across the precordium suggests that this is dextrocardia. Electrocardiographic coding would be 8 and 105.

26. FIGURE 15.26: This patient has a sinus rhythm and right axis deviation. The vectors in leads I and aVL are incompatible with those seen in the other lateral leads, V_5 and V_6. The discrepancies are explained by the inverted P waves in leads I and aVL, which suggest switched arm wires. This is a normal ECG with a technical error. This would be coded 8 and 3.

27. FIGURE 15.27: The patient is a 6-year-old with an outflow tract murmur. Rhythm is sinus with a narrow complex. V_1 shows small rSR′ with a large R′. There is right axis deviation. This is right ventricular hypertrophy. It is a volume-overload-type pattern. Most likely an ostium secundum ASD. Coded 8, 57, 61, and 103.

28. FIGURE 15.28: Here there is sinus bradycardia with left ventricular hypertrophy (voltage) and secondary T-wave changes extending into the right precordium. Most likely this is a hypertrophic cardiomyopathy with apical hypertrophy. This is occasionally called Yamaguchi syndrome after the initial describer of the variant. Coded 11, 60, and 112.

29. FIGURE 15.29: Although leads I, aVL, and III might suggest an atrial tachycardia, other leads clearly show a sinus rhythm. This is a motion artifact due to unilateral tremor and Parkinson disease. Coded 8 and 87.

30. FIGURE 15.30: Here is a sinus rhythm with minor lateral T-wave flattening. The last beat is premature and is an aberrant PAC. Characteristics of aberrancy are preceding atrial activity (seen in the T wave) and initial narrow vector with broadening toward the end of the complex and often a right bundle branch block type of pattern. Coded 8, 19, and 87.

31. FIGURE 15.31: This shows a sinus rhythm with first-degree AV block, generalized broadening of the QRS (with a right bundle branch block-like pattern), and symmetric broadening of the T wave. This is hyperkalemia. Potassium at the time was 6.2 mEq/L. Coded 8, 64, and 99.

32. FIGURE 15.32: Here is a sinus bradycardia with a sinus arrhythmia. There is terminally a symmetric T-wave inversion in leads V_2 and V_3 plus a qrS pattern in V_3. This is an anteroseptal infarct of uncertain age. Also there are lateral T-wave changes that are not specific. Coded 11, 76, 87, and 113.

33. FIGURE 15.33: Rhythm is sinus with a first-degree AV block. There was a wide complex without septal Q waves in leads I and V_6 (a left bundle branch block pattern) and left axis deviation. ST and T waves are "discordant" in the anterolateral leads (and also generally). There is also PR-segment elevation in lead aVR. This could be anterior "injury," but more suggests acute pericarditis. Coded 8, 40, 56, 68, and 90.

34. FIGURE 15.34: There is a sinus rhythm with ST-segment elevation in lead aVL and reciprocal changes in the inferior and lateral leads. This is an acute high lateral infarct. Coded 8, 77, and 113.

35. FIGURE 15.35: A sinus rhythm with AV dissociation (complete heart block) and junctional escape. V_1 shows an incomplete right bundle branch block pattern. T waves are not entirely normal in V_3. Coded 12, 44, 63, and 87.

Index

Page numbers followed by f refer to figures; those followed by t refer to tables

RRS1409